T0248799

Physiology of Hematology

Physiology of Hematology

Edited by **Brian Jenkins**

FOSTER
ACADEMICS

New Jersey

Published by Foster Academics,
61 Van Reypen Street,
Jersey City, NJ 07306, USA
www.fosteracademics.com

Physiology of Hematology
Edited by Brian Jenkins

International Standard Book Number: 978-1-63242-323-8 (Hardback)

This book contains information obtained from authentic and highly regarded sources. Copyright for all individual chapters remain with the respective authors as indicated. A wide variety of references are listed. Permission and sources are indicated; for detailed attributions, please refer to the permissions page. Reasonable efforts have been made to publish reliable data and information, but the authors, editors and publisher cannot assume any responsibility for the validity of all materials or the consequences of their use.

The publisher's policy is to use permanent paper from mills that operate a sustainable forestry policy. Furthermore, the publisher ensures that the text paper and cover boards used have met acceptable environmental accreditation standards.

Trademark Notice: Registered trademark of products or corporate names are used only for explanation and identification without intent to infringe.

Printed in the United States of America.

Contents

Preface

This book gives an extensive analysis of the physiology of hematology. Hematology encircles the physiology and pathology of blood and of the blood-forming organs. In similar areas of medicine, the pace of improvements in hematology has been rapid over the recent years. Now various treatment options are available to the modern hematologist and a great advanced outlook for the broad majority of patients with blood disorders. Developments in the clinic depict, and in various aspects are driven by, improvements in scientific grasping of hematological procedures under normal as well as in disease conditions. This book consists of a selection of research work which focuses on the physiology of hematology by analysing the molecular mechanisms behind the functioning of blood systems. It serves as a reference informing both experts and amateur readers about some of the latest developments in hematology, in both laboratory and clinic.

This book is a result of research of several months to collate the most relevant data in the field.

When I was approached with the idea of this book and the proposal to edit it, I was overwhelmed. It gave me an opportunity to reach out to all those who share a common interest with me in this field. I had 3 main parameters for editing this text:

1. Accuracy – The data and information provided in this book should be up-to-date and valuable to the readers.
2. Structure – The data must be presented in a structured format for easy understanding and better grasping of the readers.
3. Universal Approach – This book not only targets students but also experts and innovators in the field, thus my aim was to present topics which are of use to all.

Thus, it took me a couple of months to finish the editing of this book.

I would like to make a special mention of my publisher who considered me worthy of this opportunity and also supported me throughout the editing process. I would also like to thank the editing team at the back-end who extended their help whenever required.

Editor

Blood Physiology

Mechanisms Controlling Hematopoiesis

Katja Fiedler and Cornelia Brunner
University Ulm
Germany

1. Introduction

Hematopoiesis – the generation of blood cells that proceeds mainly in the bone marrow - is a well-controlled process constantly occurring throughout the live of the mammalian organism. Generally, blood cells are relatively short-lived cells with a life span ranging from few hours to several weeks causing the need for a sustained replenishment of functional erythroid, lymphoid and myeloid cells. The development of mature hematopoietic cells in a hierarchical manner from a pluripotent hematopoietic stem cell over multipotent progenitors that further develop to oligopotent and then to lineage-restricted progenitors requires several control mechanisms at different levels. Transcription factors important for the expression of lineage-specific genes play a major role in the regulation of hematopoietic stem cell maintenance as well as hematopoietic lineage decision. Moreover, the discovery of so-called master transcription factors determining the fate of a terminally differentiated cell population indicates on one side the coordinated processes of hematopoietic cell differentiation but on the other side the complex mechanisms of transcriptional activation and/or repression of specific genes. However, what in turn regulates the expression of transcription factors that finally determine the lineage and differentiation choice of a certain progenitor or immature cell? Is the development into one or another cell type a definitive event or is there some plasticity observed? Which factors are necessary and which sufficient for hematopoietic cell differentiation? These and several other important questions concerning the regulation of development and differentiation of blood cells will be discussed. This chapter summarizes the current knowledge about cell intrinsic, environmental as well as epigenetic mechanisms involved in the control of hematopoiesis under homeostatic as well as infectious conditions.

1.1 Hematopoiesis

The hematopoietic system is traditionally categorized into two separate lineages, the lymphoid lineage responsible for adaptive immunity and the myeloid lineage embracing morphologically, phenotypically and functionally distinct cell types like innate immune cells as well as erythrocytes and platelets. Mature hematopoietic cells, except some rare lymphoid cell types, are relatively short-lived with life spans ranging from few hours for granulocytes to a couple of weeks for erythrocytes demanding a continued replenishment of functional cells. This process is named hematopoiesis and takes place primarily in the bone marrow, where few hematopoietic stem cells give rise to a differentiated progeny following a series of more or less well-defined steps of multipotent progenitors and lineage-restricted precursors leading to a hierarchical structure of the process. During the course of hematopoiesis cells lose their proliferative potential as well as multi-lineage differentiation capacity and progressively acquire characteristics of terminally differentiated mature cells.

1.2 Hematopoietic stem cells

In the hematopoietic differentiation hierarchy, the most primitive cells with highest multipotent activity are long-term repopulating hematopoietic stem cells (LT-HSC). One of the first definitions of true HSC meaning LT-HSC came from bone marrow transplantation experiments in mice determining HSC by their capacity to reconstitute several times the hematopoietic system of lethally irradiated adult organisms. Such experiments have demonstrated that HSC possess multi-potentiality as well as the ability to produce exact replicas upon cell division, named self-renewal capacity. In contrast to real HSC, short-term repopulating HSC (ST-HSC) defined by their ability to contribute transiently to the production of lymphoid and myeloid cells in lethally irradiated recipients, are often described misleadingly as self-renewing cells. The contemporary model of hematopoietic stem cells proposes the affiliation of ST-HSC to the group of multipotent progenitors (MPP), which are characterized by a more limited proliferative potential, but retained ability to differentiate into various hematopoietic lineages (Kondo et al., 2003; Weissman & Shizuru, 2008). Concerning MPP hierarchy, a defined model is not available at the moment, because several studies have demonstrated different types of multipotent progenitors with myelo-lymphoid or myelo-erythroid potential, such as the lymphoid-primed multipotent progenitor (LMPP) (Iwasaki & Akashi, 2007).

Additionally, a lot of research concerning prospective isolation and characterization of HSC and multipotent progenitors has provided insight into the surface marker expression on these types of cells leading to the definition of HSC and multipotent progenitors as cells being mainly negative for lineage markers but positive for the surface markers Sca1 and Kit. This fraction of bone marrow cells is also named LSK-fraction (Lin-Sca1+Kit+) and comprises all stem cell capacity of the hematopoietic system, whereby HSC are defined as Lin-Kit+Sca1+Flt3- and MPP as Lin-Kit+Sca1+Flt3+. Furthermore, the Slam (signaling lymphocyte activation molecule) family receptors CD150 and CD48 are useful surface markers allowing to distinguish inside the LSK-fraction between HSC (CD150+CD48-) and multipotent progenitors (CD150-CD48-) as well as the most restricted progenitors (CD48+) (Kiel et al., 2005).

Under homeostatic conditions, the number of HSC remains relatively constant and the majority of HSC stays in a quiescent state that contributes not only to their long-term maintenance, but also allows a rapid cell cycle entry upon a variety of differentiation cues. The minority of HSC is in an active and dividing state and gives rise to all hematopoietic cells meaning that these few active HSC not only have to self-renew, but also have to produce all differentiated progeny. These different cell fates can only be achieved by an asymmetric division of the HSC, which allows the generation of two non-identical daughter cells, one maintaining stem cell identity and the other becoming a differentiated cell. Two different mechanisms are proposed by which asymmetry could be achieved: first by divisional asymmetry that is introduced by unequally redistributed cell-fate determinants in the cytoplasm (Florian & Geiger, 2010). An alternative possibility would be the environmental asymmetry, which is caused by different extrinsic signals provided by distinct local microenvironments and provokes different cell fate decisions of two identical daughter cells (Wilson, A. & Trumpp, 2006).

1.3 Lineage-committed progenitors

Downstream of the HSC and MPP populations with high proliferative and self-renewal capacity starts the differentiation process in hematopoiesis leading to oligopotent and later on to lineage-committed progenitors with a diminished proliferation but increased differentiation. The contemporary model of hematopoiesis (Figure 1) assumes that the decision for differentiation into the lymphoid/myeloid or megakaryocyte/erythrocyte lineages probably occurs very early in hematopoiesis. Several studies have demonstrated that multipotent progenitors like the lymphoid-primed multipotent progenitor (LMPP, Lin⁻Kit⁺Sca1⁺CD150⁻CD34⁺Flt3^hi) retain only minor megakaryocyte/erythrocyte lineage potential, whereas the vast majority of progenitors appears to be committed to the granulocyte/monocyte as well as the lymphoid lineage (Iwasaki & Akashi, 2007).

In the next step of ongoing differentiation oligopotent progenitors with differentiation capacity for several hematopoietic lineages develop from an ancestor, the common lymphoid progenitor (CLP) (Kondo et al., 1997) and the common myeloid progenitor (CMP) (Akashi et al., 2000). The CLP is the earliest population in the lineage-negative fraction that upregulates the receptor for interleukin 7 (IL-7), an essential cytokine for T and B cell development. Furthermore, the CLP carries differentiation potential for all types of lymphoid cells including B cells, T cells and NK cells. The surface marker profile of CLP is defined as Lin⁻Sca1^loKit^loIL7Rα⁺ (Kondo et al., 1997). In contrast to CLP, the CMP resides in the Lin⁻Sca1⁻Kit⁺ population in bone marrow that can be further fractioned by expression of the Fcγ receptor II/III (FcγRII/III) and CD34 leading to three distinct progenitor populations.

The CMP is defined as FcγRII/III^loCD34⁺ and can give rise to all types of myeloid colonies in clonogenic assays, while the FcγRII/III^hiCD34⁺ granulocyte-monocyte progenitor (GMP) is restricted to granulocytes and macrophages. The FcγRII/III^loCD34⁻ megakaryocyte-erythrocyte progenitor (MEP) is delimitated to megakaryocytes and erythrocytes (Akashi et al., 2000).

Still a matter of dispute is the dendritic cell (DC) development, because DC mainly are the progeny of GMP, but can also be generated from lymphoid progenitors such as CLP and pro T cells under certain conditions (Manz et al., 2001). However, the majority of plasmacytoid DC (pDC) and conventional or myeloid DC (mDC) develop successively by several commitment steps downstream of the GMP in the bone marrow. The first step is the development of the monocyte/macrophage and DC precursor (MDP) (Fogg et al., 2006) (MDP) out of the GMP that has lost differentiation potential for granulocytes and expresses the FcγRII/III and CD34 at a comparable level to the GMP, but is also Kit^loCX₃CR1⁺. Further differentiation of MDP, which is accompanied by the loss of monocyte potential, leads to the common DC precursor (CDP) defined as Lin⁻Kit^intFlt3⁺M-CSFR⁺ population that can only give rise to pDC and mDC (Geissmann et al., 2010; Naik et al., 2007; Onai et al., 2007).

Besides the characterization of MDP and CDP by several studies, further progenitor populations for eosinophils, basophils and mast cells have been isolated downstream of the GMP and their position in the hematopoietic hierarchy is depicted in Figure 1. Moreover,

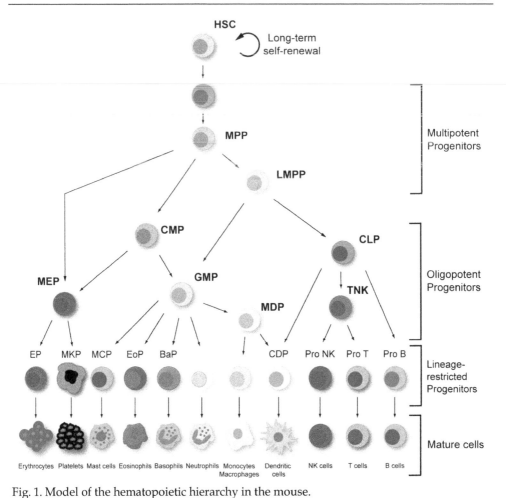

Fig. 1. Model of the hematopoietic hierarchy in the mouse.
The developmental course shown in the scheme is proposed using results generated by prospective isolation and characterization of different progenitors. HSC, hematopoietic stem cell; MPP, multipotent progenitor; LMPP, lymphoid-primed multipotent progenitor; CLP, common lymphoid progenitor; CMP, common myeloid progenitor; MEP, megakaryocyte-erythrocyte progenitor; GMP, granulocyte-macrophage progenitor; MDP, monocyte-dendritic cell progenitor; TNK, T cell NK cell progenitor; EP, erythroid progenitor; MKP, megakaryocyte progenitor; MCP, mast cell progenitor; EoP, eosinophil progenitor; BaP, basophil progenitor; CDP, common dendritic cell progenitor.

the monopotent megakaryocyte lineage-committed progenitor (MKP) (Pronk et al., 2007) and erythroid progenitor (EP) (Terszowski et al., 2005) have been described downstream of the MEP. Only for the monocyte/macrophage lineage and the neutrophil granulocytes, a putative committed precursor downstream of the GMP has not been identified to date (Iwasaki & Akashi, 2007). With regard to lymphoid development one committed precursor downstream of the CLP is the bipotent T/NK cell progenitor that resides in the bone marrow and is able to generate thymic- and bone marrow-dependent NK cells as well as T cells (Nozad Charoudeh et al., 2010).

1.4 Factors involved in the regulation of hematopoiesis

The highly regulated differentiation process of quiescent HSC towards different progeny of mature hematopoietic cells is associated with a variety of cell fate choices at every single step of hematopoiesis. These different choices comprise quiescence, self-renewal or differentiation at HSC level as well as proliferation, lineage commitment and terminal differentiation at the progenitor or precursor level. Of course, different cell fate choices require at each step in the hematopoietic hierarchy a process of decision-making that is presumed to be dependent on and regulated by a combination of intrinsic factors that embrace lineage-determining transcription factors and their epigenetic regulation as well as extrinsic regulators such as cytokines.

1.4.1 Maintenance of HSC characteristics

For the maintenance of HSC with respect to quiescence, self-renewal and suppression of differentiation, the major intrinsic factors belong to the Bmi1-p53 axis of cell cycle regulators and the PI3K signaling pathway. Bmi1 is a member of the Polycomb group gene family that controls cell proliferation via repression of the *Ink4/Arf* locus. Therefore, Bmi1 supports self-renewal by suppressing transcription of the cell cycle inhibitors p16^{Ink4a} and p19^{ARF}, which are encoded in the *Ink4/Arf* locus, whereas the tumor suppressor p53 contributes to the regulation of HSC quiescence via inhibition of cell cycle (Warr et al., 2011). In contrast, the PI3K signaling pathway controls cell proliferation, growth and survival via integration of numerous upstream signals, including growth factors, nutrients and oxygen status.

Additionally, several extrinsic factors have been identified that are necessary for preservation of HSC stemness. The extrinsic regulators embrace soluble membrane-bound extrinsic factors including cytokines (fms-related tyrosine kinase 3-ligand, stem cell factor), chemokines (CXCL12) and growth factors (Angiopoietin-1, granulocyte-CSF, granulocyte-macrophage-CSF), as well as Wnt (wingless type), Notch, Hedgehog and the TGFβ (transforming growth factor β) family of cytokines. These extrinsic factors are provided by a specialized microenvironment in the bone marrow, the so-called stem cell niche that resides in the endosteal and vascular compartments of the bone. In these areas, the bone marrow cells of hematopoietic and non-hematopoietic origin like megakaryocytes, osteoblasts, endothelial cells and CXCL12-abundant reticular (CAR) cells create a supportive microenvironment via physical interaction with HSC and production of soluble factors (Warr et al., 2011).

1.4.2 Transcription factors involved in lineage commitment

At the cellular level the differentiation process from HSC into lineage-committed hematopoietic cells involves the selective activation of lineage-specific genes as well as the silencing of lineage-foreign genes and developmental regulators in a defined order. The orchestration of such complex lineage-determining programs is dependent on several factors, but extensive research has emphasized the essential role of gene regulatory networks in directing cell fate choice and lineage restriction. These gene regulatory networks are composed of several master transcription factors that join special features, such as mutual regulation of transcriptional activity by antagonism as well as lineage-determining functions via activation of lineage-specific genes and repression of lineage-foreign genes. The first example pointing out the importance of such transcription factors is the transition from self-renewing HSC towards more committed MPP that is dependent on the transcription factor CCAAT-enhancer binding protein α (C/EBPα). The prototype of the C/EBP family displays all characteristic features of the transcription factor family, such as the N-terminal transactivation domain as well as the C-terminal DNA-binding domain consisting of a highly conserved basic region and a leucine zipper dimerization domain. Prerequisite for binding of C/EBPα to the cognate DNA-site is the homo- or heterodimerization with another transcription factor via the leucine zipper domain that in turn allows the basic region to bind to the CCAAT motif (Johnson, 2005; Lekstrom-Himes, J. & Xanthopoulos, 1998). Evidences for the function of C/EBPα in hematopoietic differentiation revealed from studies on conditional C/EBPα-deficient mice, which demonstrated a competitive advantage of C/EBPα-deficient HSC over wild type HSC in reconstitution experiments. Further analyses of the transcriptome of C/EBPα-deficient HSC have confirmed that the expression of the self-renewal factor Bmi1 is increased in these cells, suggesting C/EBPα as a pro-differentiation factor in HSC fate decision (Zhang et al., 2004).

1.4.2.1 Erythroid-megakaryocyte lineage commitment

Probably, the next step in decision-making during differentiation is the choice for erythroid versus myeloid-lymphoid lineage restriction at the transition from MPP to LMPP or MEP that is regulated by the E-twenty six (Ets) family transcription factor PU.1 and the transcription factor GATA-binding protein 1 (GATA-1). GATA-1 is expressed in erythroid, megakaryocyte and mast cell as well as eosinophil lineages and contains zinc fingers, which mediate DNA binding to the WGATAR DNA sequence as well as protein-protein interaction (Bresnick et al., 2010; Morceau et al., 2004). In contrast to GATA-1, PU.1 is restricted to monocyte as well as B lymphoid lineages and consists of a N-terminal transactivation domain, a PEST-domain (proline, glutamic acid, serine and threonine rich sequence) and the eponymous Ets-domain at the C-terminus, which mediate DNA binding to an 11 bp sequence with a central GGAA motif (Gangenahalli et al., 2005; Sharrocks, 2001). Additionally, both transcription factors are detectable in MPP and gene disruption studies have demonstrated the indispensable functions of GATA-1 and PU.1 for megakaryocyte/erythrocyte and myeloid/lymphoid development, respectively. Analyses of systemic PU.1-deficient mice revealed a complete loss of CMP, GMP and CLP populations but normal numbers of MEP causing impaired lymphoid and myeloid cell development as well as retained megakaryocyte/erythrocyte development (Scott et al., 1994). In contrast, GATA-1-deficient mice die between embryonic day 10.5 and 11.5 due to severe anemia resulting from a maturation arrest of erythroid cells (Fujiwara et al., 1996). Further support for the lineage instructive role of GATA-1 originated from the forced expression of GATA-1 in lineage-committed progenitors like GMP and CLP that exclusively leads to megakaryocyte/erythrocyte development (Iwasaki et al., 2003). Several other studies dealing with certain aspects of the molecular interaction of PU.1 and GATA-1 as well as their gene regulatory capacity revealed the cross-antagonism between these proteins involving direct physical interaction of both factors that results in an inhibition of the transactivation potential of the counterpart (Laslo et al., 2008). Based on these findings,

GATA-1 is prospected as the erythrocyte/megakaryocyte lineage determinant, whereas PU.1 is regarded as the myeloid/lymphoid lineage determinant. Regarding the regulation of erythrocyte versus megakaryocyte development, the detailed molecular mechanisms are not fully understood, but several transcription factors involved in this process are described such as Friend of GATA-1 (FOG-1), Fli-1 or Krueppel-like factor 1 (KLF1) (Kerenyi & Orkin, 2010; Szalai et al., 2006).

1.4.2.2 Myeloid lineage commitment

Downstream of LMPP, lineage choice embraces myeloid, as well as B or T lymphoid lineage and mainly depends on the transcription factors PU.1, early B cell factor 1 (EBF1) and Notch. For myeloid lineage restriction, a high expression level of PU.1 is necessary, whereas low levels of PU.1 plus EBF1 expression establish the B lymphoid lineage restriction and Notch instructs the T lymphoid lineage choice. Regarding granulocyte and monocyte development, besides PU.1, the transcription factor C/EBPα has to be enumerated. Studies have demonstrated that conditional deletion of C/EBPα in bone marrow cells of mice using the Mx1-Cre system leads to a total lack of mature granulocytes and a partial lack of monocytes due to a differentiation block at the transition from CMP to GMP (Zhang et al., 2004). Moreover, lineage choice between monocytes and granulocytes depends on the expression level of PU.1 and C/EBPα, which has been shown by studies using different mouse as well as *in vitro* models for diminished PU.1 expression in the hematopoietic system. In all experimental setups, reduced expression of PU.1 is followed by an augmented granulopoiesis to the disadvantage of monopoiesis. Additionally, gene expression analyses of PU.1-deficient progenitors have demonstrated a decreased or even absent expression of several monocyte-specific genes, like the macrophage scavenger receptor or the M-CSF receptor. Furthermore, the need for C/EBPα during the transition from CMP to GMP is possibly due to the transcriptional upregulation of PU.1, since forced C/EBPα expression in hematopoietic progenitors favors monopoiesis and not granulopoiesis, whereas exogenous C/EBPα in myeloid cell lines directs granulopoiesis (Friedman, 2007). Nevertheless, C/EBPα is probably indispensable for granulocyte development due to the transcriptional upregulation of several granulocyte-specific factors. One of these factors is the transcriptional repressor growth factor independent 1 (Gfi1), which is necessary for the repression of proliferation and of monocyte lineage-promoting factors such as M-CSF (Borregaard, 2010). Another important target of C/EBPα is the transcription factor C/EBPε that is important for terminal granulocyte differentiation, because of the transcriptional control of granule-specific genes (lactoferrin and gelatinase) as well as genes necessary for cell cycle regulation (Borregaard, 2010).

Besides the upregulation of other transcription factors, C/EBPα forces granulocyte development additionally by transactivation of various genes, such as G-CSF receptor (Hohaus et al., 1995; Smith, L. T. et al., 1996) or myeloperoxidase (MPO) (Wang, W. et al., 2001), and downregulation of proliferation by direct interaction with the cell cycle regulator E2F (D'Alo et al., 2003; Theilgaard-Monch et al., 2005). In line with these experimental results is the association of inactivating C/EBPα mutations with hematopoietic malignancies like acute myeloid leukemia and high-risk myelodysplastic syndrome proposing that C/EBPα possesses the ability to arrest cell proliferation and to drive terminal differentiation (Koschmieder et al., 2009). Taken together, the plethora of studies implicates the following model for monocyte versus granulocyte lineage choice: First

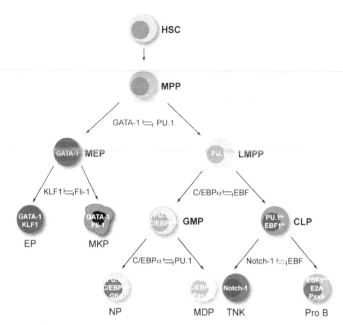

Fig. 2. Transcription factor network regulating lineage commitment.
The scheme displays a simplified overview of gene regulatory networks, which have a major influence on hematopoietic lineage choice during hematopoiesis. Supposed (dashed lines) and proved (continuous lines) cross-antagonisms between key transcription factors which function to regulate binary cell fate choices are noted in the scheme. Additionally, transcription factors that are important for the generation of particular intermediates are noted in white. HSC, hematopoietic stem cell; MPP, multipotent progenitor; LMPP, lymphoid-primed multipotent progenitor; CLP, common lymphoid progenitor; CMP, common myeloid progenitor; MEP, megakaryocyte-erythrocyte progenitor; GMP, granulocyte-macrophage progenitor; NP, neutrophil progenitor; MDP, monocyte-dendritic cell progenitor; TNK, T cell NK cell progenitor; EP, erythroid progenitor; MKP, megakaryocyte progenitor.

of all, C/EBPα is needed for the transition from CMP to GMP by induction of PU.1 expression. High protein levels of PU.1 induce monopoiesis via interaction with other transcription factors like interferon regulatory factor 8 (IRF8) or activating protein-1 family transcription factors (AP-1/Jun proteins) and the transcriptional activation of monocyte-specific genes (Friedman, 2007). However, AP-1 family transcription factors are also able to heterodimerize with C/EBPα (Cai et al., 2008) implicating an inhibition mechanism of PU.1 for granulocyte development by sequestering the binding partners of C/EBPα. In contrast to the high protein levels of PU.1 that favor monopoiesis, insufficient activation of PU.1 transcription allows C/EBPα to induce the granulopoiesis program accompanied by suppression of monopoiesis (Figure 2).

Terminal granulopoiesis starts with the myeloblast and promyelocyte state, where the switch from proliferation to differentiation takes place, displayed by the loss of ability for cell division after the promyelocyte state. Moreover, the formation of the first granules starts, which are named primary or azurophilic granules. The most important transcription factors at myeloblast/promyelocyte stage are C/EBPα and Gfi1, which are necessary for the suppression of monocyte development and proliferation as well as for the transcriptional activation of granulocyte-specific genes like *MPO*, *ELANE* or *CEBPE* (Borregaard, 2010; Koschmieder et al., 2009; Theilgaard-Monch et al., 2005). The importance of Gfi1 and ELANE has been demonstrated by studies analyzing the genetic background of severe congenital neutropenia (SCN) and other forms of neutropenia. These studies revealed that one of the major causes for loss of neutrophil differentiation beyond promyelocyte state are mutations in the *ELANE* gene (Dale et al., 2000; Horwitz et al., 1999), but in rare cases of SCN also mutations of the *GFI1* gene have been described (Person et al., 2003). Detailed analyses of Gfi1 in mice further supported the function of Gfi1 as molecular switch towards granulocyte development by suppression of monocyte-specific genes, like *Csf1* (M-CSF) and *Csf1r* (M-CSFR) (Zarebski et al., 2008).

Ongoing differentiation beyond promyelocytes leads to the development of myelocytes and metamyelocytes, which are defined by the beginning of nuclear segmentation and the appearance of secondary (also called specific) granules as well as the exit from cell cycle. The regulation of secondary granule protein expression and the exit from cell cycle mainly depends on the transcription factor C/EBPε, whose expression peaks in myelocytes and metamyelocytes (Bjerregaard et al., 2003; Theilgaard-Monch et al., 2005). Based on studies using C/EBPε-deficient mice, which displayed neutrophil-specific defects including bilobed nuclei, abnormal respiratory burst and compromised bactericidal activity as well as impaired chemotaxis (Lekstrom-Himes, J. & Xanthopoulos, 1999; Yamanaka et al., 1997), the genetic cause of a very rare congenital disorder named neutrophil specific granule deficiency (SGD) has been delineated to the *CEBPE* locus (Lekstrom-Himes, J. A. et al., 1999). Additional studies have revealed the essential functions of C/EBPε for the expression of secondary and tertiary granule proteins (Verbeek et al., 1999; Yamanaka et al., 1997) and demonstrated the direct interaction of C/EBPε with E2F1 and Rb protein, finally leading to cell cycle exit (Gery et al., 2004).

The last step of terminal granulopoiesis, the differentiation into band and segmented neutrophils leads to mature neutrophils with finally segmented nuclei and tertiary as well as secretory granules. In the course of neutrophil terminal differentiation, C/EBPα expression gradually diminishes during the myeloblast stage. C/EBPε peaks at the myelocyte/metamyelocyte stage, whereas the expression level of the transcription factors PU.1, C/EBPβ, C/EBPδ and C/EBPγ increases subsequently to the metamyelocyte stage (Bjerregaard et al., 2003). However, gene deletion studies using C/EBPβ- or C/EBPδ-deficient mice revealed no hematopoietic abnormalities with regard to terminal granulopoiesis. Still, Hirai and colleagues have demonstrated the indispensable role of C/EBPβ during emergency granulopoiesis in response to cytokine treatment or fungal infection in contrast to C/EBPα and C/EBPε, which were not upregulated under these conditions (Hirai et al., 2006). In the case of the transcription factor PU.1, a conditional gene deletion model has evidenced a PU.1-dependent transcriptional activation of *gp91phox*, a component of the NADPH oxidase, as well as of *Mac-1/CD11b* (Dakic et al., 2005) (Figure 3).

Terminal differentiation during monopoiesis leads to monocytes, macrophages as well as dendritic cells and involves again the selection of specific gene expression programs to

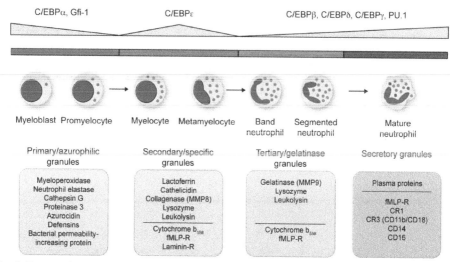

Fig. 3. Terminal granulopoiesis in the bone marrow.
The terminal granulopoiesis that is characterized by sequential formation of different granule types and segmentation of the nucleus starts at the myeloblast/promyelocyte stage and ends with mature neutrophils. Granule types not only differ in the time point at which they are formed, but also in their specific content, which is described at the bottom of the figure. Above the line in the boxes matrix content is depicted and beneath the proteins that are located to the vesicle membrane. At different stages of terminal granulopoiesis several transcription factors, which are indicated on top of the figure, are important for the regulation of maturation and timed expression of granule proteins.

determine cell fates. Additionally, several subtypes of macrophages or DC have been described in recent years bringing more complexity into monopoietic differentiation. Nevertheless, some key transcription factors with indispensable functions for monopoiesis are known already. For example, PU.1 is not only required for myeloid lineage commitment, but also for macrophage versus DC lineage choice during late myelopoiesis. Intermediate PU.1 expression at GMP stage results in the activation of the macrophage-specific transcription factors Egr-1 and Egr-2 (Laslo et al., 2006), whereas high expression of PU.1 promotes the induction of DC fate via repression of the macrophage-inducing transcription factors c-Maf and MafB (Bakri et al., 2005). In addition, gain-of-function experiments have demonstrated that ectopic expression of MafB, c-Maf, Egr-1 or IRF8 in early progenitors can drive monocyte or macrophage lineage commitment. In contrast, RelB induces DC differentiation and SpiB pDC differentiation in monocytic intermediates (Auffray et al., 2009; Geissmann et al., 2010). However, the detailed molecular mechanisms driving terminal monopoiesis remains to be elucidated.

1.4.2.3 B cell lineage commitment

B cells develop from CLP in the bone marrow, where several stages of B cell development have been defined. The earliest B lineage precursors are the pre/pro B cells, which begin to express the B lineage specific marker B220 at their surfaces. The transition of pre/pro B cells to the pre B cell stage is characterized by the upregulation of the surface marker CD19 as well as by the rearrangement of the immunoglobulin (Ig) heavy chain gene locus. Successful rearrangement of the Ig light chain locus is the prerequisite for the development to immature IgM expressing B cells. At this stage the antigen-independent phase of B cell development is almost complete. IgM⁺ cells are ready to leave the bone marrow to enter peripheral secondary lymphoid organs where they first develop via the IgM⁺IgD⁺ stage to mature IgD⁺ B cells. These cells undergo final maturation during the antigen-dependent phase of B cell development.

In addition to cytokines and cytokine receptors, several key transcription factors have been identified necessary for the B lineage commitment as well as for the maintenance of the B cell fate, like Ikaros, Gfi1, PU.1, E2A, EBF1 and Pax5. Prior to the differentiation of CLP, PU.1 is involved in the expression of components of the IL-7 signaling pathways (DeKoter et al., 2007) essential for EBF1-dependent lineage restriction in early lymphoid progenitors (Tsapogas et al., 2011). Additionally, the level of PU.1 expression predicts the decision between the myeloid and the B cell lineage. Low levels of PU.1 favors B cell development whereas high levels promote myeloid cell differentiation (DeKoter & Singh, 2000). The upregulation of the transcriptional repressor Gfi1 was suggested to be responsible for the down-modulation of PU.1 expression in early progenitors by displacing PU.1 from its upstream autoregulatory element and therefore for the promotion of B lineage decision (Spooner et al., 2009). In MPP, Gfi1 is upregulated by Ikaros to antagonize PU.1 expression, thus favoring B cell development (Spooner et al., 2009). CLP begin to express genes associated with committed B cells including E2A as well as EBF1 at the onset of B lymphopoiesis (Roessler et al., 2007; Seet et al., 2004; Smith, E. M. et al., 2002). The deficiency of these factors leads to a block of B cell development at a very early stage, even before D$_H$-J$_H$ rearrangement of the IgH gene (Bain et al., 1994; Lin, H. & Grosschedl, 1995; Zhuang et al., 1994). In contrast, forced expression of E2A and EBF1 revealed that both factors cooperate in the upregulation of several B cell-specific genes, like Pax5, the surrogate light chain *λ5* gene, the *VpreB*, *Igα* and *Igβ* genes, plus the genes coding for *Rag1* and *Rag2* (Kee & Murre, 1998; O'Riordan & Grosschedl, 1999; Sigvardsson et al., 1997). In addition, the transcriptional co-activator *Pou2af1 (BOB.1/OBF.1; OCA-B)* and the transcription factor *FoxO1* were identified as direct targets of EBF1 (Zandi et al., 2008). In CLP the expression of Pax5 is still low. Consistent with the observation that Pax5 is essential for B lineage commitment, CLP still retain T cell developmental potential. The expression of Pax5 is detectable at the pro B cell where Pax5 antagonizes T cell development by blocking Notch1 (Souabni et al., 2002). Additionally, Pax5 interferes with the developmental potential to differentiate into several other hematopoietic lineages, since in the absence of Pax5 but in the presence of appropriate cytokines pro B cells are able to differentiate *in vitro* into NK cells, dendritic cells, macrophages, granulocytes and osteoclasts (Nutt, S. L. et al., 1999) indicating that the expression E2A and EBF1 is not sufficient to commit B cell progenitors to the B cell lineage in the absence of Pax5. Therefore, Pax5 plays an essential and dual role in B lineage development, it represses non-B cell-specific genes, like the genes coding for the M-CSFR or for MPO (Nutt, S. L. et al., 1999), whereas in the same time it activates the B lineage-specific gene program (Nutt, S. L. et al., 1998; Schebesta et al., 2002). Thus, Pax5 controls the pre-BCR signaling by promoting the V to DJ recombination at the *IgH* locus (Nutt, S. L. et al., 1997) and also by regulating directly the expression of the signaling molecule BLNK (Schebesta et al., 2002). Additionally, Pax5 is essential for the upregulation of *CD19* and *Igα* gene expression (Kozmik et al., 1992; Nutt, S. L. et al., 1997). Pax5-deficient

B cells are arrested at the pro B cell stage while expressing normal levels of E2A and EBF1 as well as of their target genes (Nutt, S. L. et al., 1998; Nutt, S.L. et al., 1997), indicating that E2A and EBF1 are upstream of Pax5 in the hierarchical order of lineage-determining transcription factor expression.

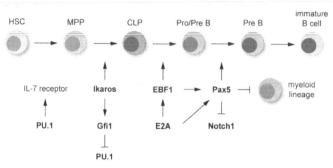

Fig. 4. Key transcription factors involved in B lymphopoiesis.
B cell development is driven by the consecutive activation of lineage-determining transcription factors like E2A, EBF1 and Pax5 and the repression of lineage-foreign genes. Transcription factors are highlighted in bold. HSC, hematopoietic stem cell; MPP, multipotent progenitor; CLP, common lymphoid progenitor.

However, sustained expression of EBF1 in Pax5-deficient hematopoietic precursor cells efficiently blocks myeloid and T lineage potential *in vivo*. Moreover, overexpression of EBF1 in Pax5-deficient pro B cells represses alternative lineage potential indicating that EBF1 promotes the commitment of the B cell lineage independently of Pax5 (Pongubala et al., 2008) (Figure 4). E2A in turn is required for the initiation but also for the maintenance of the expression of EBF1, Pax5 and the B cell-specific gene program at the pro B cell stage (Kwon et al., 2008). E2A exerts its instructive role not only in the bone marrow at the pro and pre B cell stage as well as at the immature B cell stage, but also in peripheral lymphatic organs during the formation of germinal center B cells (Kwon et al., 2008). In contrast, E2A is dispensable for Ig class switch recombination as well as for the generation of mature splenic subpopulations, like marginal zone B cells, follicular B cells and B1 cells. Also, the memory B cell subpopulation and the plasma cell generation is unaffected by the loss of E2A (Kwon et al., 2008).

Conditional inactivation of Pax5 revealed its requirement for the maintenance of B cell identity also during late B cell development in peripheral lymphatic organs (Horcher et al., 2001). Upon exposure to an antigen B lymphocytes can either maintain their B cell identity and differentiate into memory B cells or rapidly change their gene expression program and develop into germinal center (GC) and plasma cells (PC). During GC formation pre GC B cells upregulate the expression of the transcriptional repressor Bcl6 that controls the GC B cell differentiation. Bcl6-deficiency results in a complete block of GC B cell reaction, necessary for the generation of high-affinity antibodies by somatic hypermutation and class-switch recombination. In contrast, plasma cell generation occurs normally in Bcl6-deficient mice (Dent et al., 1997; Fukuda et al., 1997). The transcription factor IRF8 directly regulates, possibly in concert with other transcription factors, Bcl6 upregulation in GC B cells (Lee, C. H. et al., 2006). Bcl6 is able to repress several targets including the transcriptional repressor Blimp1 (B lymphocyte induced maturation protein 1) (Shaffer et al., 2000; Tunyaplin et al.,

2004). Therefore, during the GC reaction, Bcl6 represses the gene program for plasma cell generation in GC B cells (Shaffer et al., 2000).

Blimp1 is a key transcription factor for plasma cell (PC) differentiation, where it initiates a gene program, which leads to the inhibition of cell division, to the repression of genes defining the identity of GC B cells, and to the induction of genes necessary for Ig secretion (Kallies et al., 2007; Shaffer et al., 2002). Besides Blimp1, the transcription factors XBP-1 and IRF4 play an essential role for PC differentiation (Sciammas et al., 2006; Shaffer et al., 2004). During PC generation the GC gene program should be downregulated, which is achieved by Blimp1 that represses the expression of Bcl6 and also Pax5 (Diehl et al., 2008; Lin, K. I. et al., 2002) (Figure 5).

In general, the hierarchical expression and the cooperative action of transcription factors as well as epigenetic modulators cause the initiation of a gene program characteristic and irreversible for a certain committed lineage. However, under certain conditions, committed lineages exhibit a high degree of plasticity. For example, TLR engagement drives lymphoid progenitor cells to differentiate into dendritic cells (Nagai et al., 2006), a mechanism that possibly ensures the generation of sufficient numbers of myeloid cells during an acute infection. Today we know that the overexpression of few transcription factors Oct3/4, Sox2, c-Myc and Klf4 in adult murine or human fibroblasts can re-differentiate these cells into multipotent embryonic stem cell-like cells with pluripotent potential *in vitro* as well as *in vivo* (Takahashi et al., 2007; Takahashi & Yamanaka, 2006; Wernig et al., 2007). Therefore, it is not longer surprising that in the hematopoietic system the overexpression of lineage-determining transcription factors in committed cells leads to re-differentiation and lineage conversion. Thus, T cell progenitors could be converted into dendritic cells and mast cells by ectopic expression of PU.1 or GATA-3, respectively (Laiosa et al., 2006; Taghon et al., 2007). Also B cells could be re-differentiated into macrophages upon overexpression of C/EBPα (Xie et al., 2004). Nevertheless, these studies revealed the high instructive capacity of lineage-determining transcription factors.

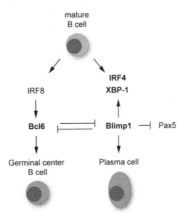

Fig. 5. Cross-regulatory control of germinal center B cell versus plasma cell fate.
Cell fate decision of mature B cells upon antigen exposure is regulated by key transcription factors (bold) that activate cell-specific genes and mutually repress transcription factors necessary for alternative cell differentiation.

In B cells, the lineage commitment and the maintenance of the B cell fate throughout B cell development is achieved by a single transcription factor – Pax5 (Cobaleda et al., 2007; Nutt, S. L. et al., 1999). As already mentioned, deletion of Pax5 leads to a block of B cell development at the pro B cell stage and Pax5-/- pro B cells can be re-differentiate in the presence of appropriate cytokines into osteoclasts, NK cells, dendritic cells, macrophages and granulocytes (Nutt, S. L. et al., 1999). More recently it was shown, that the conditional deletion of Pax5 in mature B cells from peripheral lymphoid organs, despite their advanced differentiation state, leads to a de-differentiation back to early uncommitted progenitors in the bone marrow, which even rescued T cell development in T cell-deficient mice (Cobaleda et al., 2007). However, the molecular mechanisms for these reprogramming processes are not finally clear. Since the complete loss of Pax5 in mature B cells also caused the development of aggressive lymphomas, Pax5 was identified as a tumor suppressor for the B cell lineage (Cobaleda et al., 2007).

1.4.2.4 T cell lineage commitment

Multiple bone marrow-derived hematopoietic precursor populations that belong mainly to the MPP or the CLP subsets are able to enter the thymus (Saran et al., 2010; Serwold et al., 2009), where they represent the population of early thymic progenitors (ETP), the initial source for the development of T cells. At this developmental stage the ETP still retain beside the T cell developmental potential also the capability to develop into B cells, macrophages, granulocytes, dendritic cells, and NK cells. Thymic environmental factors, like IL-7, Kit-ligand as well as ligands activating Notch signaling, operate in an inductive manner to force T cell development (Petrie & Zuniga-Pflucker, 2007) and at the same time to down-modulate the capacity to develop into the NK, B or myeloid lineage. Notch signaling blocks these alternative developmental processes and, in addition, is necessary to maintain T cell specification and differentiation (Feyerabend et al., 2009; Franco et al., 2006; Laiosa et al., 2006; Schmitt et al., 2004; Taghon et al., 2007). Very recently it became evident, that besides blocking alternative lineage development Notch signaling drives T cell lineage commitment by upregulating the expression of T lineage-specific transcription factors like TCF-1 necessary for the induction of several T cell-specific genes, like *GATA-3*, *Bcl11b*, and genes coding for components of the T cell receptor (Weber et al., 2011). The Krueppel-like C2H2 type zinc finger transcription factor Bcl11b in turn is required for the repression of NK cell associated genes as well as for the downregulation of stem cell or progenitor cell genes not longer required for committed T cells (Li, L. et al., 2010) (Figure 6).

After initial T lineage commitment a subsequent lineage decision is made – the choice to develop into either αβ or γδ T cell sub-lineages. At the double negative stage (DN; CD4-CD8) thymocytes begin to rearrange their TCRβ, γ and δ genes. These cells that productively rearranged their TCRγ and δ genes develop to γδ T cells, which remain largely CD4-CD8-. Thymocytes that rearranged efficiently their TCRβ locus are committed to the αβ lineage and express a pre-TCR complex composed of functional TCRβ chains paired with the invariant pre-TCRα (pTα) chain. Committed αβ T cells undergo a strong proliferative burst and develop further to CD4+CD8+ double positive (DP) thymocytes that start to rearrange their TCRα locus. The precise mechanisms by which DN thymocytes develop into αβ or γδ T cells are not well understood. Currently mainly two models are discussed: the stochastic and the TCR signal strength model, where strong TCR signals favor γδ and weak signals αβ lineage choice (reviewed in (Kreslavsky et al., 2010)). Beside TCR signaling also the

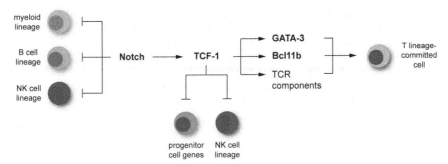

Fig. 6. T lineage-determining transcription factors.
The key transcription factor for T lineage commitment is Notch that suppresses lineage-foreign gene programs and upregulates the lineage-determining transcription factor TCF-1. Finally, lineage commitment is achieved by upregulation of the transcription factors GATA-3 and Bcl11b. Transcription factors are highlighted in bold.

Lymphotoxin-mediated as well as Notch signaling are important for the αβ versus γδ lineage commitment (Ciofani et al., 2004; Garbe et al., 2006; Garcia-Peydro et al., 2003; Hayes et al., 2005; Kang et al., 2001; Silva-Santos et al., 2005; Van de Walle et al., 2009). Additionally, several transcription factors were identified as important regulators of αβ versus γδ lineage decision. The high-mobility group transcription factor Sox13, for example, promotes γδ T cell development while opposing αβ T cell differentiation by antagonizing TCF-1 (Melichar et al., 2007), which is required, similar to RORγt (Guo, J. et al., 2002), for the survival of CD4+CD8+ αβ thymocytes (Ioannidis et al., 2001). Also, the TCR-signal strength dependent upregulation of the Zn-finger transcription factor ThPOK (T-helper inducing POZ-Krueppel factor) was shown to be an important regulator of γδ T cell development and maturation (Park, K. et al., 2010). Additionally, by integrating TCR and Notch signals as well as by interacting with and thereby suppressing E protein targets, also the helix-loop-helix transcription factor Id3 promotes γδ T cell fate (Lauritsen et al., 2009). The AP-1 family member c-Jun in turn controls directly the expression of the *IL-7Rα* gene important for thymocyte development. Deletion of c-Jun results in an enhanced γδ T cell generation indicating the importance of IL-7 receptor signaling for the regulation of αβ/γδ T cell fate decision (Riera-Sans & Behrens, 2007).

CD4+CD8+ DP cells expressing a mature αβTCR further undergo positive and negative selection processes based on their ability to recognize self-peptide:self-MHC-complexes as well as their affinity to such complexes. During these selection processes DP cells develop to functionally competent single positive CD4+CD8- or CD4-CD8+ T cells equipped with a specific gene expression program characteristic for CD4+ T helper or CD8+ cytotoxic T lymphocytes. Mainly two transcription factors – ThPOK and Runx3 – are important for directing the development of DP thymocytes either into the CD4+ T helper or CD8+ cytotoxic T cell population (Egawa & Littman, 2008; He et al., 2008; Taniuchi et al., 2002; Wang, L. et al., 2008). Therefore, ThPOK is required for the commitment to CD4+ T helper cells by repressing the characteristic genes for CD8+ cells including Runx3, whereas Runx3 mediates the silencing of the *CD4* locus in CD8+ cells. These dual regulative processes, leading to the exclusion of Runx3 expression in CD4+ cells by ThPOK as well as the exclusion of the expression of ThPOK in CD8+ cells by Runx3, result finally in CD4-CD8 lineage commitment. Transcription factors involved in ThPOK upregulation in MHCII-restricted T lymphocytes are GATA-3 (Wang, L. et al., 2008) together with the HMG protein Tox (Aliahmad & Kaye, 2008). In contrast, IL-7-mediated activation of the STAT5 transcription factor promotes the upregulation of Runx3 in CD8+ cells (Park, J. H. et al., 2010) indicating a differential requirement of cytokine signaling for CD4 and CD8 lineage development. After CD4+ or CD8+ single positive αβ T cells are generated they are ready to leave the thymus and enter via the blood stream peripheral lymphatic organs, where their terminal differentiation occurs.

From the CD4+CD8+ DP pool of thymocytes not only conventional αβ T cells arise, but also natural killer (NK) T cells. In contrast to conventional αβ T cells that are restricted by MHCI or MHCII molecules, invariant NK T cells undergo positive and negative selection processes during their thymic maturation, which are mediated by the recognition of glycolipids presented by the MHCI-like molecule CD1d. Additionally, they also require signals from the Slam family of receptors. Different types of NK T cells are described. However, the most common and best-studied NK T cells are the invariant NK (iNK) T cells expressing an invariant TCR that is composed of a common α-chain in combination with a certain number of β-chains. After antigen recognition iNK T cells secrete high amounts of a large variety of cytokines and chemokines within minutes. Therefore, these cells exhibit rather an innate than an adaptive immune function. Several transcription factors were identified to be important for iNK T cell lineage choice. Among them, the transcription factor PLZF (promyelocytic leukemia zinc finger) is a key regulator for the development of this particular cell type (Kovalovsky et al., 2008; Savage et al., 2008), since in the thymus it is exclusively expressed by iNK T cells. In addition, several other transcription factors like NF-κB (Sivakumar et al., 2003; Stanic et al., 2004), Ets-1 (Lacorazza et al., 2002; Walunas et al., 2000), GATA-3 (Kim, P. J. et al., 2006), T-bet (Matsuda et al., 2006) and Runx proteins (Egawa et al., 2007) contribute to the development, differentiation and survival of iNK T cells. Because these transcription factors are also expressed in other thymic subpopulations they are not exclusively important for the iNK T cell lineage. However, PLZF-deficiency did not prevent iNK T cell development in general but severely interfered with iNK T cell effector differentiation and therefore with their functionality (Kovalovsky et al., 2008; Savage et al., 2008).

In the thymus, a subpopulation of MHC-II-restricted CD4+ T cells further differentiates into CD25+ naturally occurring regulatory T cells (nTregs) characterized by the expression of the transcription factor FoxP3 (Fontenot et al., 2003; Hori et al., 2003). They comprise about 5 to 10% of peripheral CD4+ T cell and play a crucial role for maintaining peripheral tolerance. nTregs are able to suppress the proliferation, cytokine secretion as well as activation of autoreactive effector T cells thereby preventing autoimmunity. FoxP3 plays an essential function for the regulation of nTregs suppressive activity, since the deficiency of a functional FoxP3 leads to a severe autoimmune pathology in mouse (Godfrey et al., 1991; Lyon et al., 1990) and man (Bennett et al., 2001; Wildin et al., 2001). Several transcription factors are implicated in the *FoxP3* gene regulation and therefore for the development and function of nTregs. After activation of PKCθ and/or CD28 engagement, Notch3 together with NF-κB heterodimers composed of p50/p65 are able to bind and to trans-activate the FoxP3 promoter *in vivo* (Barbarulo et al., 2011; Soligo et al., 2011). Also NF-κB c-Rel was identified as a factor able to initiate FoxP3 transcription in thymic Treg precursors (Deenick et al., 2010; Isomura et al., 2009; Long et al., 2009; Ruan et al., 2009). Additionally, the FoxP3 promoter contains several functional NFAT/AP-1 binding sites, which are occupied *in vivo* (Mantel et al., 2006). Moreover, the transcription factor Bcl11b is also able to promote directly FoxP3 as well as IL-10 expression. Deletion of Bcl11b at the DP stage of thymic T cell development or solely in Tregs causes inflammatory bowel disease – a severe autoimmune disorder - due to reduced Treg suppressor activity accompanied with reduced FoxP3 and IL-10 expression (Vanvalkenburgh et al., 2011).

Conventional $\alpha\beta$ T cells leave the thymus and settle peripheral lymphatic organs as naïve T cells. After activation by exposure to their cognate antigens naïve CD4+ cells differentiate into an appropriate T helper cell (TH) lineage that plays an essential role in acquired immunity. Depending on the cytokine milieu produced by antigen presenting cells naïve CD4+ cells undergo differentiation processes resulting in the expression of master transcription factors defining the ability to secrete a certain set of cytokines. Initially, two main TH subpopulations were described (Mosmann et al., 1986). The generation of TH1 cells depends on the presence of IFNγ and/or IL-12 inducing the expression of the master transcription factor T-bet essential for the TH1 phenotype characterized by the production of large amounts of IFNγ, IL-2 and TNFα. TH1 cells mediate the defense against infections by intracellular microbes and the isotype switching to IgG2a and IgG2b. In contrast, TH2 cells are generated in the presence of IL-4 and also secrete, depending on the upregulation of the transcription factor GATA-3, IL-4 together with IL-5 and IL-13. Thereby, humoral responses against parasites and extracellular pathogens are supported and also the class switching to IgG1 and IgE (Mosmann et al., 1986; Mowen & Glimcher, 2004; Szabo et al., 2003). A third TH subpopulation was described, the TH17 cells that is characterized by the secretion mainly of IL-17A and IL17F, but also IL-21 and IL-22, protecting the host against bacterial and fungal infections. Their differentiation is induced by TGFβ together with IL-6 or IL-21, which prompts the expression of the master transcription factor essential for TH17-development – RORγt (Ivanov et al., 2006). More recently, two additional TH subsets were described – TH9 and TH22 expressing predominantly the cytokines IL-9 or IL-22, respectively. The development of TH9 cells is initiated upon antigen receptor stimulation in the presence of IL-4 and TGFβ (Dardalhon et al., 2008; Veldhoen et al., 2008) and requires the upregulation of the transcription factor PU.1 (Chang et al., 2010). TH22, identified in the human skin, are characterized by the expression of the chemokine receptors CCR6, CCR4 and CCR10 as well as by the transcription factor aryl hydrocarbon receptor (AHR) that might be involved in the regulation of *IL-22* gene expression (Duhen et al., 2009; Trifari et al., 2009).

Another T helper subtype that differentiates in the periphery from naïve CD4+ cells is the follicular T helper (TFH) cell subpopulation, characterized by the expression of CXCR5, ICOS and PD-1 as surface markers. They synthesize large quantities of IL-21 and require the upregulation of the transcriptional repressor Bcl6 for their development and also for their function to promote germinal center B cell maturation (Johnston et al., 2009; Nurieva et al., 2009; Yu et al., 2009). Bcl6 expression is regulated by IL-6 and IL-21 (Nurieva et al., 2009) and drives not only the TFH differentiation but also inhibits the development of other CD4+ differentiation pathways by blocking Blimp1 (Johnston et al., 2009).

In the periphery, CD4+ effector T cells can be converted by exposure to TGFβ and IL-2 to inducible regulatory T cells (iTregs) expressing CD25 at the surface and, like nTregs, FoxP3 as a master transcription factor necessary for Treg function (Davidson et al., 2007; Zheng et al., 2007) (Figure 7).

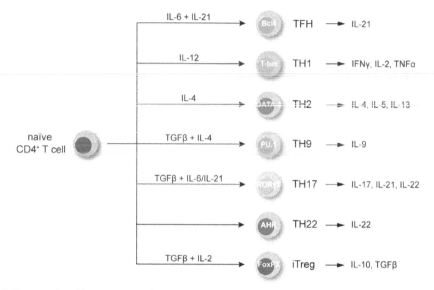

Fig. 7. Terminal Differentiation of CD4⁺ T cells.

Differentiation of CD4⁺ T cells into different T helper cell subpopulations after antigen exposure is driven by the specific cytokine milieu and results in the expression of specific transcription factors (noted in white). Every T helper cell subset releases distinct cytokines, which modulate the immune response of the host.

CD4⁺ T cell master transcription factors as well as lineage-specific cytokines characteristic for the appropriate TH subpopulations are able to block the differentiation of other TH subsets. For example, T-bet in cooperation with Runx3 suppresses the generation of TH2 cells by physical interaction with GATA-3 thereby inhibiting GATA-3 activity (Djuretic et al., 2007; Hwang et al., 2005). Additionally, T-bet also actively represses TH17 differentiation by preventing Runx1-mediated upregulation of RORγt expression (Lazarevic et al., 2011). Also, as already noted, Bcl6 expressed by TFH antagonizes Blimp1 and thereby it inhibits the developmental program necessary for alternative TH cell differentiation (Johnston et al., 2009). However, several studies suggest certain plasticity in the expression of master transcription factors as well in the set of cytokines that differentiated T helper cells secrete. The conversion of peripheral effector CD4⁺ cells to iTregs expressing FoxP3 like nTregs that developed in the thymus was a first hint indicating plasticity of CD4⁺ TH cells (Jonuleit et al., 2001). Moreover, in the presence of TGFβ TH2 cells can acquire IL-9 producing capacity (Veldhoen et al., 2008). Additionally, several studies described the acquisition of IFNγ-producing potential by TH17 cells *in vivo* in mouse and man (Kurschus et al., 2010; Wilson, N. J. et al., 2007) and even a complete conversion of TH17 cells into IFNγ-producers (Bending et al., 2009; Lee, Y. K. et al., 2009; Shi et al., 2008). When stimulated with IL-4, TH17 cells can change into IL4-secreting TH2 cells (Yi et al., 2009). Also, Tregs stimulated with IL-6 can express IL-17 and downregulate FoxP3 expression (Xu et al., 2007). Together, these data indicate the high flexibility of peripheral CD4+ cells in their potential to secrete a certain set of cytokines and therefore to modulate and/or influence the outcome of an ongoing immune response. However, the mechanism(s) underlying the plasticity of "committed" TH cells remain largely unclear.

1.4.3 Epigenetic mechanisms controlling hematopoiesis

The highly coordinated program needed to pass through the diverse developmental stages that comprise hematopoiesis can only be achieved by tight regulation. In fact, every cellular transition and differentiation step is characterized by the activation of a new, lineage-specific, genetic program and the extinction of the previous one. This is achieved by the action of well-defined networks of transcription factors at each developmental step as already described. However, transcription factors are not the only players in the complex differentiation process of hematopoiesis, since there is an increasing body of evidence demonstrating that the regulation of hematopoietic stemness and lineage commitment is dependent on epigenetic mechanisms. Chromatin, the higher order structure of DNA and nucleosomes, can adopt different structural conformations depending on epigenetic modifications, which influence the accessibility of DNA for the gene transcription machinery. Four types of epigenetic regulation can take place: DNA methylation, histone modification, chromatin remodeling and gene silencing via microRNAs.

1.4.3.1 DNA methylation

DNA methylation of cytosines at CpG dinucleotides, except for CpG islands, is established during early embryogenesis by DNA methyltransferases (Dnmt) and is maintained in somatic cells to repress transcription. The DNA methyltransferases Dnmt3a and Dnmt3b are supposed to convey *de novo* methylation, whereas Dnmt1 conserves previously installed methylation states during replication. First hints depicting the importance of DNA methylation for hematopoietic development arose from gene deletion studies in mice revealing the indispensable functions of Dnmt1 for HSC self-renewal and lineage-commitment. The ablation or reduced expression of Dnmt1 in murine HSC led to diminished repopulating capacity of HSC and decreased production of lymphoid progenitors accompanied with retained myelo-erythroid progenitor development (Broske et al., 2009; Trowbridge et al., 2009). Additionally, the examination of genome-wide methylation profiles of the mouse hematopoietic system demonstrated methylation pattern changes during differentiation resulting in the activation of silent genes and the silencing of active genes. Moreover, the study could show that myeloid commitment involved less global DNA methylation than lymphoid commitment (Ji et al., 2010) in line with the findings from the Dnmt1 deletion studies. In contrast to Dnmt1, Dnmt3a/3b deficiency affected only the long-term reconstitution ability of HSC, but not their differentiation into committed progenitors (Tadokoro et al., 2007). Nevertheless, the molecular mechanisms mediating DNA methylation and demethylation during hematopoietic development have not been deciphered, although chromatin-remodeling factors as well as Polycomb group/Dnmt3a/3b complexes recruited by transcription factors were supposed to be involved (Gao et al., 2009; Kirillov et al., 1996; Vire et al., 2006).

1.4.3.2 Histone modification

Another crucial epigenetic mechanism is the posttranslational modification of histones, which embraces acetylation, methylation, phosphorylation and sumoylation among others. These modifications occur at the tails of histones and change the direct interactions between nucleosomes and DNA, thereby affecting gene expression (Campos & Reinberg, 2009). In terms of hematopoietic regulation the methylation of lysine 4 (K4) and 27 (K27) of histone 3 (H3) particularly have to be stressed, since they can serve as repressing, activating and poising marks dependent on the methylation pattern. The concomitant trimethylation of H3K27 (repressing mark) and H3K4 (activating mark) as well as the mono- and dimethylation of H3K4 introduce a bivalent epigenetic modification leading to poised chromatin that is primed for activation of gene transcription (Bernstein, B. E. et al., 2006; Heintzman et al., 2009; Orford et al., 2008). Several studies have demonstrated that a plethora of lineage-specific genes are poised at the beginning of hematopoiesis or achieve poising marks during hematopoietic differentiation. After commitment of the cell to a specific lineage, lineage-foreign genes lose their poising marks and repression of gene transcription occurs (Orford et al., 2008; Weishaupt et al., 2010). Moreover, genome-wide analysis of poised chromatin sites revealed a tight correlation of bivalent histone methylation sites with binding sites of lineage-determining transcription factors such as EBF1, E2A, GATA-1 or PU.1. These sites are independent of the transcription start site and are probably enhancer sites that are involved in the priming for transcriptional activation in later stages of hematopoietic development (Heintzman et al., 2009; Heinz et al., 2010; Lin, Y. C. et al., 2010; Treiber et al., 2010). Similar to DNA methylation, the molecular mechanisms underlying histone modifications have not yet been identified.

1.4.3.3 Chromatin remodeling

Additional epigenetic modifiers of DNA accessibility that were recruited through lineage-specific transcription factors are chromatin-remodeling complexes. Such chromatin remodelers are multi-protein complexes that are able to change nucleosome location or conformation in an ATP-dependent manner, but they additionally contain interchangeable histone modifying enzymes such as deacetylase or acetylase to produce functionally distinct complexes (Bowen et al., 2004). For example, Ikaros, a lymphoid-specific transcription factor crucial for the commitment of LMPP into CLP can recruit Mi2/NuRD complexes in order to repress genes (Kim, J. et al., 1999; Koipally et al., 1999; Sridharan & Smale, 2007). Whereas, EBF1 and E2A are involved in the recruitment of the SWI/SNF complex to the upstream enhancer of the CD19 locus as well as to the CD79a promoter region facilitating the transcriptional activation of these B cell-specific genes (Gao et al., 2009; Walter et al., 2008).

1.4.3.4 MicroRNAs

Besides the already mentioned epigenetic mechanisms established at the level of DNA, the recent discovery of microRNAs (miRNAs) added a further layer of epigenetic regulation that guides the hematopoietic differentiation process. These mRNAs are small, single-stranded, non-coding RNAs, which are able to repress mRNA transcription by the promotion of mRNA degradation due to direct binding to the 3' untranslated regions (UTR) of specific target mRNAs. The first evidences for the importance of miRNAs during hematopoietic development revealed from the deletion of Dicer, an RNase-III-like enzyme that is indispensable for miRNA biogenesis, in mice. These gene ablation leads to embryonal lethality at day 7.5 due to a lack of detectable multipotent stem cells, whereas the conditional deletion in murine embryonic stem cells blocks the ability to differentiate (Bernstein, E. et al., 2003; Kanellopoulou et al., 2005) and the lineage-specific ablation of Dicer in lymphoid progenitors results in severe defects in the B as well as T cell development (Cobb et al., 2005; Koralov et al., 2008; Muljo et al., 2005). Moreover, analyses of miRNA expression in several subsets of human CD34+ HSC and progenitors cells as well as murine hematopoietic tissues have demonstrated the modulated transcription of different miRNA during hematopoiesis (Chen et al., 2004; Georgantas et al., 2007; Liao et al., 2008). With regard to the relative young field of miRNA research, only limited data about the detailed role of single miRNAs in the different steps of HSC maintenance or hematopoietic differentiation are available, but some regulatory mechanisms are already described. At the level of HSC, where decision-making comprises self-renewal and differentiation into committed progenitors, miRNAs of the miR-196 and miR-10 family are highly expressed, which are able to modulate HSC homeostasis and lineage commitment through the regulation of certain *HOX* genes (Mansfield et al., 2004; Yekta et al., 2004), whereas miR-125a has been shown to mediate self-renewal of LT-HSC by targeting the pro-apoptotic protein *Bak-1* (Guo, S. et al., 2010). In contrast, miR-126 conferring lineage commitment and progenitor production via down-modulation of *HOXA9* and the tumor suppressor polo-like kinase 2 that has to be downregulated during differentiation towards multipotent progenitors (Shen et al., 2008).

Downstream of HSC, the introduction of lineage commitment is the most important task of a regulatory mechanism and several miRNAs are involved in these processes in the different progenitor populations. For example, during erythroid lineage differentiation starting from the MEP a progressive downregulation of miR-24, miR-221, miR-222 and miR-223 as well as a upregulation of miR-451 and miR-16 has been reported in differentiating human erythroid progenitors (Bruchova et al., 2007). The down-modulation of miR-221 and miR-222 is necessary for the expression of Kit that in turn allows the expansion of erythroblasts (Felli et al., 2005), whereas the repression of miR-24 permit the expression of activin type I receptor, which promotes erythropoiesis in cooperation with erythropoietin (Wang, Q. et al., 2008). A further activator of erythroid differentiation is the transcription factor and miR-223-target LIM-only protein 2 that along with GATA-1 and others constitutes a multi-protein complex (Felli et al., 2009). In contrast to these down-modulated miRNAs, miR-451 upregulation is indispensable for erythroid maturation and effective erythropoiesis in response to oxidative stress. Several studies have demonstrated that miR-451 targets 14-3-3ζ, a chaperone protein modulating intracellular growth factor signals, and therefore regulating the expression of several genes associated with late erythropoiesis (Patrick et al., 2010; Rasmussen et al., 2010; Zhan et al., 2007). But also megakaryocyte differentiation occurs downstream of the MEP and several studies revealed the importance of miR-150 for lineage commitment during megakaryocyte-erythroid differentiation, since the ectopic expression of miR-150 in MEP drives the differentiation towards megakaryocytes at the expense of erythroid cells by targeting the transcription factor *c-Myb* (Lu et al., 2008). Further support for the lineage-determining function of miR-150 has arose from a study demonstrating the regulation of miR-150 and c-Myb through the megakaryocyte-specific cytokine TPO (Barroga et al., 2008). Other miRNAs downregulated during megakaryopoiesis are miR-130 targeting *MafB* that in turn together with GATA-1 is needed for the induction of the *GbIIb* gene (Garzon et al., 2006) as well as miR-155 that targets the transcription factors *Ets-1* and *Meis-1* (Romania et al., 2008).

With respect to the role of miRNAs in myelopoiesis miR-223 has to be enumerated, which also functions as lineage-determining factor that is upregulated during granulopoiesis and downregulated during monopoiesis (Fazi et al., 2005; Johnnidis et al., 2008). Targets of miR-223 are the cell cycle regulator *E2F1* and the monocyte lineage-promoting gene *Mef2c* leading to suppression of proliferation and induction of granulocyte differentiation (Johnnidis et al., 2008). Moreover, the transcription of miR-223 is activated by the master transcription factor for granulopoiesis C/EBPα that replaces the transcriptional repressor NFI-A upon activation of granulocytic differentiation (Fazi et al., 2005). A similar mechanism has been recently described for miR-34a that is also increased expressed during granulopoiesis by C/EBPα-mediated transcription and targets the cell cycle regulator *E2F3* (Pulikkan et al., 2010). Another lineage-determining mechanism displays the repression of miR-21 and miR-196b by the transcriptional repressor Gfi1 during granulopoiesis, since ectopic expression of both miRNAs in myeloid progenitors results in a complete block of G-CSF induced granulopoiesis (Velu et al., 2009). In favor of monocytic development acts the activation of miR-424 transcription via PU.1 that in turn targets the negative regulator of monopoiesis *NFI-A* (Forrest et al., 2010). Whereas the miR-17/miR-20/miR-106 cluster is repressed during monopoiesis in humans, probably to allow expression of the target AML-1 that consecutively promotes monocyte-macrophage differentiation and maturation (Fontana et al., 2007).

Concerning the function of single miRNAs during lymphopoiesis only few data are available, despite the astonishing effects of Dicer deletion on lymphoid development. However, one study partially explains the phenotype of Dicer deletion by the defective expression of the miR17-92 cluster. This miRNA cluster that is highly expressed in progenitor cells targets the pro-apoptotic factors *Bim* and *Pten*. In line with these findings,

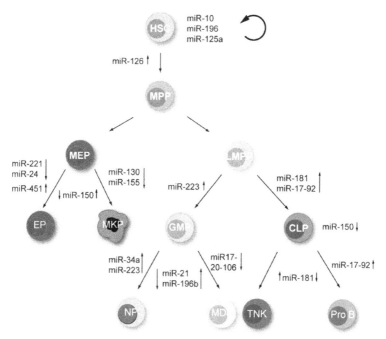

Fig. 8. The regulatory network of miRNAs during hematopoiesis.
Several miRNAs are involved in maintenance of HSC self-renewal, whereas other miRNAs are associated with lineage commitment and development towards differentiated progeny. HSC, hematopoietic stem cell; MPP, multipotent progenitor; LMPP, lymphoid-primed multipotent progenitor; CLP, common lymphoid progenitor; CMP, common myeloid progenitor; MEP, megakaryocyte-erythrocyte progenitor; GMP, granulocyte-macrophage progenitor; NP, neutrophil progenitor; MDP, monocyte-dendritic cell progenitor; TNK, T cell NK cell progenitor; EP, erythroid progenitor; MKP, megakaryocyte progenitor.

ablation of the miR17-92 cluster in mice results in a severe block of B cell development at the pro B to pre B transition due to increased apoptosis of pro B cells (Ventura et al., 2008). A similar block in B cell development at the pro B to pre B transition is caused by the ectopic expression of miR-150 in lymphoid progenitors due to the repression of the transcriptional repressor *c-Myb* (Xiao et al., 2007). The best-described miRNA involved in T lymphocyte development is miR-181, which promotes T cell differentiation through increasing signaling strength of the TCR signaling. In detail, miR-181 targets multiple phosphatases such as *PTPN22* or *DUSP5* and *DUSP6*, which are negative regulators of distinct steps of the TCR signaling pathway leading to an upregulation of ERK1/2 phosphorylation upon TCR engagement. This increased sensitivity of TCR signaling is needed during the positive selection of double-positive T cells in the thymus (Li, Q. J. et al., 2007) (Figure 8).

1.4.4 Role of cytokines in guiding hematopoiesis

Cytokines are a large family of extracellular ligands that stimulate several responses after binding to structurally and functionally conserved cytokine receptors. Biological responses provoked by cytokines cover a broad spectrum of different biological activities, for example survival, proliferation, differentiation, or maturation. In the case of the hematopoietic system, the most important cytokines are interleukins and colony-stimulating factors with supportive functions for several lineages as well as erythropoietin (EPO) and thrombopoietin (TPO) that act on single lineages (Metcalf, 2008). Besides the requirement of cytokines for regulation of basal hematopoiesis, they are also essential for controlling emergency hematopoiesis in response to infections or blood loss. This is reflected by the different origins of cytokines, secreted for example by activated immune cells or by stroma cells as well as by organs, like liver and kidney.

In steady-state conditions, serum concentrations of cytokines are low, but they can be elevated up to 1000-fold by challenging the immune system and possess high picomolar affinities for their corresponding receptors (Metcalf, 2008). On the binding of cytokine molecules follows the activation of the receptor via homodimerization (G-CSFR), oligomerization with a common signaling subunit (GM-CSFR, IL-6R) or conformational changes in preformed receptor dimers (EPOR), which finally leads to activation of Janus kinases (JAK). Upon activation of the tyrosine kinases of JAK family, the cytokine receptors as well as the kinases themselves are phosphorylated to generate docking sites for SH2 domain containing proteins. One example is the STAT protein family that promotes transcriptional activation of target genes after phosphorylation by JAK (Robb, 2007; Smithgall et al., 2000). Additionally, other signaling molecules can be recruited to the cytokine receptors, such as Src kinases, protein phosphatases or PI3K, which mediate the activation of numerous signaling pathways like MAPK-ERK, Ras or PI3K (Baker et al., 2007).

To date, basically two hypotheses exist concerning the role of cytokines in hematopoiesis. The instructive model proposes that cytokines transmit specific signals to multipotent progenitors to direct their lineage commitment. In contrast, the permissive or stochastic model suggests that cytokines only provide permissive growth and survival signals to intrinsically determined and lineage-committed progenitors. Supportive data for the permissive as well as the instructive model of cytokine function originated from different studies, where cytokine receptors were ectopically expressed in lineage-committed progenitors. Studies in favor of the permissive model have demonstrated that viral transduction of fetal liver cells with the M-CSF receptor results in the generation of erythroid colonies upon M-CSF administration (McArthur et al., 1994). Similar results have been obtained by the restoration of definitive erythropoiesis in EPOR-deficient fetal liver cells via the expression of the human GM-CSFR plus GM-CSF treatment (Hisakawa et al., 2001). Furthermore, replacement of the intracellular domain of the G-CSFR with the intracellular domain of EPOR induces no alterations in lineage commitment (Semerad et al., 1999). Oppositional results emanated from the ectopic expression of IL-2Rβ in CLP, which results in rapid generation of granulocytes and macrophages in the presence of IL-2 (Kondo et al., 2000).

Additionally, ectopic expression of the human GM-CSFR in IL-7-deficient CLP was not able to restore lymphopoiesis upon GM-CSF administration (Iwasaki-Arai et al., 2003). Experiments with single GMP cultured in the presence of M-CSF or G-CSF have further supported the hypothesis of lineage instruction by cytokines due to the almost solely development of either macrophages or granulocytes, respectively (Rieger et al., 2009). Nevertheless, gene deletion studies for several cytokine receptors have shown the indispensable function of the most cytokines for hematopoiesis. For example, the knockout of EPO and EPOR in mice leads to embryonic death at E13.5 due to severe anemia, even if erythroid progenitor cells were present (Lin, C. S. et al., 1996; Wu, H. et al., 1995). Analysis of IL-7Rα-deficient mice revealed a lethal phenotype as a result of a severe hypoplasia of all lymphoid lineages, but retained development of the earliest unipotent T and B cell precursors (Peschon et al., 1994). In contrast, mice bearing deletions of colony-stimulating factor receptors demonstrated no lethal phenotypes. Disruption of the G-CSFR in mice results in ineffective granulopoiesis, with chronic neutropenia due to a decrease of mature myeloid cells in the bone marrow and a modest reduction of progenitor cells (Liu et al., 1996), whereas deletion of the common β-chain of IL-3, IL-5 and GM-CSF receptor in mice only lead to reduced numbers of eosinophils (Nishinakamura et al., 1996; Nishinakamura et al., 1996).

Taken together, the present available data do not resolve the question if cytokines only have permissive functions in the guidance of hematopoiesis, especially with regard to differentiation from HSC to restricted progenitors or not. But the plasticity of the transition from multipotent progenitor cells to restricted progenitor cells, especially regarding adaption of hematopoiesis in emergency situations suggests that cytokines have to some extend instructive functions. Furthermore, almost nothing is known about potential functions of cytokines and cytokine signaling regarding gene expression or posttranslational regulation of lineage-determining transcription factors, which would provide a possible link between intrinsic and extrinsic regulation of hematopoiesis (Figure 9).

1.5 Perspectives

The unique property of the hematopoietic system to replenish permanently all hematopoietic cells together with the ongoing progress in the understanding of hematopoietic differentiation processes allows the development of new therapy approaches to treat hemic diseases such as hematologic malignancies, immunodeficiencies or autoimmune diseases. These new therapies are mainly based on the transplantation of hematopoietic stem cells (HSC). Two basic findings promoted the clinical use of HSC transplantation (HSCT) in the last twenty years. First, the definition of human HSC as

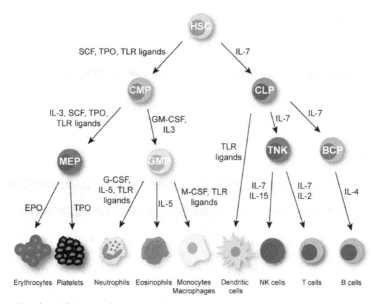

Fig. 9. The role of cytokines in hematopoiesis.
Cytokines act on both multipotent progenitors as well as committed progenitors and provide survival and proliferation signals. HSC, hematopoietic stem cell; CLP, common lymphoid progenitor; CMP, common myeloid progenitor; MEP, megakaryocyte-erythrocyte progenitor; GMP, granulocyte-macrophage progenitor; TNK, T cell NK cell progenitor; BCP, B cell progenitor.

CD34+/CD38- cells that can be found in the bone marrow as well as in the umbilical cord blood (Weissman & Shizuru, 2008), and second, the discovery of the potent function of the cytokine G-CSF in mobilization of stem cells from the bone marrow into peripheral blood (Weaver et al., 1993). In most cases, this method provides several advantages in comparison to bone marrow transplantation, since the isolation of stem cells from peripheral blood via leukapheresis is less invasive for the donor and the recovery of the hematopoietic system occurs faster (Gertz, 2010).

Currently, only two possibilities of HSCT for the treatment of life-threatening hemic diseases or immunodeficiencies are available: the autologous transplantation or the allogeneic transplantation of HSC from a healthy donor. Autologous transplantation of HSC is often used during the cure of hematologic malignancies like myeloma or some types of lymphoma to restore the hematopoietic system after aggressive chemotherapy (Gertz et al., 2000; Linch et al., 1993; Moreau et al., 2011; Philip et al., 1995). In contrast, allogeneic HSC transplantation (HSCT) is the treatment of choice for many otherwise fatal hematologic malignancies (chronic myeloid leukemia, acute leukemia) and genetic disorders such as aplastic anemia, β-thalassemia as well as primary immunodeficiencies (severe combined immunodeficiency, Wiskott-Aldrich syndrome) and requires an almost perfect human leukocyte antigen (HLA) match of donor and recipient (Roncarolo et al., 2011). Additionally, recent trails of allogeneic HSCT provided good results in the cure of autoimmune diseases like multiple sclerosis and rheumatoid arthritis (Sullivan et al., 2010). Nevertheless, the need for an almost perfect HLA match to avoid graft-versus-host reactions, the restricted availability of donors as well as pre-transplant conditioning limits the application of allogeneic HSCT today (Roncarolo et al., 2011).

One possible approach to circumvent the potential risks of allogeneic HSCT is the gene therapy, where defective genes are restored by the introduction of functional counterparts in autologous HSC. The first trails of gene therapy for primary immunodeficiencies employed the retroviral transduction of isolated HSC for gene delivery and afterwards the re-transplantation into patients. But in some of this trails, a certain amount of patients developed hematologic malignancies due to random integration of the transgene into the genome that can lead to the trans-activation of proto-oncogenes when the virus sequence is integrated in their vicinity. Recent efforts for the improvement of viral vectors by the use of retro- and lentiviral vectors with cell-specific promoter sequences may provide gene therapy with a decreased incidence for undesired trans-activation of oncogenes. Another approach could be the development of robust methods for homologous recombination in HSC, which would not only avoid the cancer risk, but also allow the endogenous regulation of the corrected gene (Kohn, 2010). Additionally, new perspectives offered the groundbreaking findings of Takahashi and Yamanaka demonstrating the induction of pluripotent stem cells from mouse fibroblasts by the viral transduction of Oct3/4, Sox2, c-Myc and Klf4 (Takahashi & Yamanaka, 2006). Moreover, several recent improvements in induction of pluripotency in several cell types like dermal fibroblasts, keratinocytes and blood cells by the use of virus-free and/or vector-free techniques render reprogrammed somatic cells to a possible future technology for stem cell plus gene therapy (Wu, S. M. & Hochedlinger, 2011). Some of the advantages of iPS (inducible pluripotent stem) cells are the independency of the cell source, the possibility of prolonged culturing *ex vivo* allowing genetic manipulation, and the differentiation into all cell types. A first proof of principle for use of iPS cells in gene therapy supplied the successful treatment of sickle cell anemia in a mouse model. In this study, autologous skin fibroblasts from humanized sickle cell anemia mice were reprogrammed into iPS cells and the genetic defect was repaired via homologous recombination, afterwards the iPS cells were differentiated into hematopoietic progenitors in vitro and finally transplanted into irradiated recipient mice (Hanna et al., 2007). Nevertheless, these types of therapies need a lot of extensive research before they can be applied in the clinic in future, but our increasing knowledge of the regulation of hematopoietic processes provides the basis for the individual treatment of patients with life-threatening hematologic disorders with autologous cells to abolish side effects associated with allogeneic HSCT, or to cure diseases currently not treatable with peripheral stem cell transplantation.

2. Conclusion

The process of differentiation and lineage commitment during hematopoietic development depends strongly on the defined activation of lineage-determining gene programs as well as the repression of lineage-foreign gene programs. This concerted regulation of genetic programs can only be achieved by the integration of several mechanisms such as activation of lineage-specific transcription factors, modulation of epigenetic marks and extrinsic signals that provide a supportive environment. Moreover, the described mechanisms of hematopoiesis illustrate the complex network involving the synergistic effects of a certain number of key transcription factors that not only induce transcription but also guide epigenetic changes to allow or deny the access of the transcriptional machinery to the DNA or the repression of important genes via gene silencing. Additionally, some of these transcription factors are often involved in several lineage decisions were they induce quite different cell fates depending on the presence of other transcription factors co-expressed in the cell or on the level of protein expression. Therefore, the hematopoietic differentiation process clearly demonstrates the importance of regulatory networks that integrate several intrinsic and extrinsic signals for the outcome of differentiation and cell fate decisions.

3. References

Akashi, K., Traver, D., Miyamoto, T. & Weissman, I.L. (2000). A clonogenic common myeloid progenitor that gives rise to all myeloid lineages. *Nature*, 404, 6774, pp. 193-197.

Aliahmad, P. & Kaye, J. (2008). Development of all CD4 T lineages requires nuclear factor TOX. *J Exp Med*, 205, 1, pp. 245-256.

Auffray, C., Sieweke, M.H. & Geissmann, F. (2009). Blood monocytes: development, heterogeneity, and relationship with dendritic cells. *Annu Rev Immunol*, 27, pp. 669-692.

Bain, G., Maandag, E.C., Izon, D.J., Amsen, D., Kruisbeek, A.M., Weintraub, B.C., Krop, I., Schlissel, M.S., Feeney, A.J., van Roon, M. & et al. (1994). E2A proteins are required for proper B cell development and initiation of immunoglobulin gene rearrangements. *Cell*, 79, 5, pp. 885-892.

Baker, S.J., Rane, S.G. & Reddy, E.P. (2007). Hematopoietic cytokine receptor signaling. *Oncogene*, 26, 47, pp. 6724-6737.

Bakri, Y., Sarrazin, S., Mayer, U.P., Tillmanns, S., Nerlov, C., Boned, A. & Sieweke, M.H. (2005). Balance of MafB and PU.1 specifies alternative macrophage or dendritic cell fate. *Blood*, 105, 7, pp. 2707-2716.

Barbarulo, A., Grazioli, P., Campese, A.F., Bellavia, D., Di Mario, G., Pelullo, M., Ciuffetta, A., Colantoni, S., Vacca, A., Frati, L., Gulino, A., Felli, M.P. & Screpanti, I. (2011). Notch3 and canonical NF-kappaB signaling pathways cooperatively regulate Foxp3 transcription. *J Immunol*, 186, 11, pp. 6199-6206.

Barroga, C.F., Pham, H. & Kaushansky, K. (2008). Thrombopoietin regulates c-Myb expression by modulating micro RNA 150 expression. *Exp Hematol*, 36, 12, pp. 1585-1592.

Bending, D., De la Pena, H., Veldhoen, M., Phillips, J.M., Uyttenhove, C., Stockinger, B. & Cooke, A. (2009). Highly purified Th17 cells from BDC2.5NOD mice convert into Th1-like cells in NOD/SCID recipient mice. *J Clin Invest*, 119, 3, pp. 565-572.

Bennett, C.L., Christie, J., Ramsdell, F., Brunkow, M.E., Ferguson, P.J., Whitesell, L., Kelly, T.E., Saulsbury, F.T., Chance, P.F. & Ochs, H.D. (2001). The immune dysregulation, polyendocrinopathy, enteropathy, X-linked syndrome (IPEX) is caused by mutations of FOXP3. *Nat Genet*, 27, 1, pp. 20-21.

Bernstein, B.E., Mikkelsen, T.S., Xie, X., Kamal, M., Huebert, D.J., Cuff, J., Fry, B., Meissner, A., Wernig, M., Plath, K., Jaenisch, R., Wagschal, A., Feil, R., Schreiber, S.L. & Lander, E.S. (2006). A bivalent chromatin structure marks key developmental genes in embryonic stem cells. *Cell*, 125, 2, pp. 315-326.

Bernstein, E., Kim, S.Y., Carmell, M.A., Murchison, E.P., Alcorn, H., Li, M.Z., Mills, A.A., Elledge, S.J., Anderson, K.V. & Hannon, G.J. (2003). Dicer is essential for mouse development. *Nat Genet*, 35, 3, pp. 215-217.

Bjerregaard, M.D., Jurlander, J., Klausen, P., Borregaard, N. & Cowland, J.B. (2003). The in vivo profile of transcription factors during neutrophil differentiation in human bone marrow. *Blood*, 101, 11, pp. 4322-4332.

Borregaard, N. (2010). Neutrophils, from marrow to microbes. *Immunity*, 33, 5, pp. 657-670.

Bowen, N.J., Fujita, N., Kajita, M. & Wade, P.A. (2004). Mi-2/NuRD: multiple complexes for many purposes. *Biochim Biophys Acta*, 1677, 1-3, pp. 52-57.

Bresnick, E.H., Lee, H.Y., Fujiwara, T., Johnson, K.D. & Keles, S. (2010). GATA switches as developmental drivers. *J Biol Chem*, 285, 41, pp. 31087-31093.

Broske, A.M., Vockentanz, L., Kharazi, S., Huska, M.R., Mancini, E., Scheller, M., Kuhl, C., Enns, A., Prinz, M., Jaenisch, R., Nerlov, C., Leutz, A., Andrade-Navarro, M.A., Jacobsen, S.E. & Rosenbauer, F. (2009). DNA methylation protects hematopoietic stem cell multipotency from myeloerythroid restriction. *Nat Genet*, 41, 11, pp. 1207-1215.

Bruchova, H., Yoon, D., Agarwal, A.M., Mendell, J. & Prchal, J.T. (2007). Regulated expression of microRNAs in normal and polycythemia vera erythropoiesis. *Exp Hematol*, 35, 11, pp. 1657-1667.

Cai, D.H., Wang, D., Keefer, J., Yeamans, C., Hensley, K. & Friedman, A.D. (2008). C/EBP alpha:AP-1 leucine zipper heterodimers bind novel DNA elements, activate the PU.1 promoter and direct monocyte lineage commitment more potently than C/EBP alpha homodimers or AP-1. *Oncogene*, 27, 19, pp. 2772-2779.

Campos, E.I. & Reinberg, D. (2009). Histones: annotating chromatin. *Annu Rev Genet*, 43, pp. 559-599.

Chang, H.C., Sehra, S., Goswami, R., Yao, W., Yu, Q., Stritesky, G.L., Jabeen, R., McKinley, C., Ahyi, A.N., Han, L., Nguyen, E.T., Robertson, M.J., Perumal, N.B., Tepper, R.S., Nutt, S.L. & Kaplan, M.H. (2010). The transcription factor PU.1 is required for the development of IL-9-producing T cells and allergic inflammation. *Nat Immunol*, 11, 6, pp. 527-534.

Chen, C.Z., Li, L., Lodish, H.F. & Bartel, D.P. (2004). MicroRNAs modulate hematopoietic lineage differentiation. *Science*, 303, 5654, pp. 83-86.

Ciofani, M., Schmitt, T.M., Ciofani, A., Michie, A.M., Cuburu, N., Aublin, A., Maryanski, J.L. & Zuniga-Pflucker, J.C. (2004). Obligatory role for cooperative signaling by pre-TCR and Notch during thymocyte differentiation. *J Immunol*, 172, 9, pp. 5230-5239.

Cobaleda, C., Jochum, W. & Busslinger, M. (2007). Conversion of mature B cells into T cells by dedifferentiation to uncommitted progenitors. *Nature*, 449, 7161, pp. 473-477.

Cobb, B.S., Nesterova, T.B., Thompson, E., Hertweck, A., O'Connor, E., Godwin, J., Wilson, C.B., Brockdorff, N., Fisher, A.G., Smale, S.T. & Merkenschlager, M. (2005). T cell lineage choice and differentiation in the absence of the RNase III enzyme Dicer. *J Exp Med*, 201, 9, pp. 1367-1373.

D'Alo, F., Johansen, L.M., Nelson, E.A., Radomska, H.S., Evans, E.K., Zhang, P., Nerlov, C. & Tenen, D.G. (2003). The amino terminal and E2F interaction domains are critical for C/EBP alpha-mediated induction of granulopoietic development of hematopoietic cells. *Blood*, 102, 9, pp. 3163-3171.

Dakic, A., Metcalf, D., Di Rago, L., Mifsud, S., Wu, L. & Nutt, S.L. (2005). PU.1 regulates the commitment of adult hematopoietic progenitors and restricts granulopoiesis. *J Exp Med,* 201, 9, pp. 1487-1502.

Dale, D.C., Person, R.E., Bolyard, A.A., Aprikyan, A.G., Bos, C., Bonilla, M.A., Boxer, L.A., Kannourakis, G., Zeidler, C., Welte, K., Benson, K.F. & Horwitz, M. (2000). Mutations in the gene encoding neutrophil elastase in congenital and cyclic neutropenia. *Blood,* 96, 7, pp. 2317-2322.

Dardalhon, V., Awasthi, A., Kwon, H., Galileos, G., Gao, W., Sobel, R.A., Mitsdoerffer, M., Strom, T.B., Elyaman, W., Ho, I.C., Khoury, S., Oukka, M. & Kuchroo, V.K. (2008). IL-4 inhibits TGF-beta-induced Foxp3+ T cells and, together with TGF-beta, generates IL-9+ IL-10+ Foxp3(-) effector T cells. *Nat Immunol,* 9, 12, pp. 1347-1355.

Davidson, T.S., DiPaolo, R.J., Andersson, J. & Shevach, E.M. (2007). Cutting Edge: IL-2 is essential for TGF-beta-mediated induction of Foxp3+ T regulatory cells. *J Immunol,* 178, 7, pp. 4022-4026.

Deenick, E.K., Elford, A.R., Pellegrini, M., Hall, H., Mak, T.W. & Ohashi, P.S. (2010). c-Rel but not NF-kappaB1 is important for T regulatory cell development. *Eur J Immunol,* 40, 3, pp. 677-681.

DeKoter, R.P., Schweitzer, B.L., Kamath, M.B., Jones, D., Tagoh, H., Bonifer, C., Hildeman, D.A. & Huang, K.J. (2007). Regulation of the interleukin-7 receptor alpha promoter by the Ets transcription factors PU.1 and GA-binding protein in developing B cells. *J Biol Chem,* 282, 19, pp. 14194-14204.

DeKoter, R.P. & Singh, H. (2000). Regulation of B lymphocyte and macrophage development by graded expression of PU.1. *Science,* 288, 5470, pp. 1439-1441.

Dent, A.L., Shaffer, A.L., Yu, X., Allman, D. & Staudt, L.M. (1997). Control of inflammation, cytokine expression, and germinal center formation by BCL-6. *Science,* 276, 5312, pp. 589-592.

Diehl, S.A., Schmidlin, H., Nagasawa, M., van Haren, S.D., Kwakkenbos, M.J., Yasuda, E., Beaumont, T., Scheeren, F.A. & Spits, H. (2008). STAT3-mediated up-regulation of BLIMP1 Is coordinated with BCL6 down-regulation to control human plasma cell differentiation. *J Immunol,* 180, 7, pp. 4805-4815.

Djuretic, I.M., Levanon, D., Negreanu, V., Groner, Y., Rao, A. & Ansel, K.M. (2007). Transcription factors T-bet and Runx3 cooperate to activate Ifng and silence Il4 in T helper type 1 cells. *Nat Immunol,* 8, 2, pp. 145-153.

Duhen, T., Geiger, R., Jarrossay, D., Lanzavecchia, A. & Sallusto, F. (2009). Production of interleukin 22 but not interleukin 17 by a subset of human skin-homing memory T cells. *Nat Immunol,* 10, 8, pp. 857-863.

Egawa, T. & Littman, D.R. (2008). ThPOK acts late in specification of the helper T cell lineage and suppresses Runx-mediated commitment to the cytotoxic T cell lineage. *Nat Immunol,* 9, 10, pp. 1131-1139.

Egawa, T., Tillman, R.E., Naoe, Y., Taniuchi, I. & Littman, D.R. (2007). The role of the Runx transcription factors in thymocyte differentiation and in homeostasis of naive T cells. *J Exp Med,* 204, 8, pp. 1945-1957.

Fazi, F., Rosa, A., Fatica, A., Gelmetti, V., De Marchis, M.L., Nervi, C. & Bozzoni, I. (2005). A minicircuitry comprised of microRNA-223 and transcription factors NFI-A and C/EBPalpha regulates human granulopoiesis. *Cell,* 123, 5, pp. 819-831.

Felli, N., Fontana, L., Pelosi, E., Botta, R., Bonci, D., Facchiano, F., Liuzzi, F., Lulli, V., Morsilli, O., Santoro, S., Valtieri, M., Calin, G.A., Liu, C.G., Sorrentino, A., Croce, C.M. & Peschle, C. (2005). MicroRNAs 221 and 222 inhibit normal erythropoiesis and erythroleukemic cell growth via kit receptor down-modulation. *Proc Natl Acad Sci U S A*, 102, 50, pp. 18081-18086.

Felli, N., Pedini, F., Romania, P., Biffoni, M., Morsilli, O., Castelli, G., Santoro, S., Chicarella, S., Sorrentino, A., Peschle, C. & Marziali, G. (2009). MicroRNA 223-dependent expression of LMO2 regulates normal erythropoiesis. *Haematologica*, 94, 4, pp. 479-486.

Feyerabend, T.B., Terszowski, G., Tietz, A., Blum, C., Luche, H., Gossler, A., Gale, N.W., Radtke, F., Fehling, H.J. & Rodewald, H.R. (2009). Deletion of Notch1 converts pro-T cells to dendritic cells and promotes thymic B cells by cell-extrinsic and cell-intrinsic mechanisms. *Immunity*, 30, 1, pp. 67-79.

Florian, M.C. & Geiger, H. (2010). Concise review: polarity in stem cells, disease, and aging. *Stem Cells*, 28, 9, pp. 1623-1629.

Fogg, D.K., Sibon, C., Miled, C., Jung, S., Aucouturier, P., Littman, D.R., Cumano, A. & Geissmann, F. (2006). A clonogenic bone marrow progenitor specific for macrophages and dendritic cells. *Science*, 311, 5757, pp. 83-87.

Fontana, L., Pelosi, E., Greco, P., Racanicchi, S., Testa, U., Liuzzi, F., Croce, C.M., Brunetti, E., Grignani, F. & Peschle, C. (2007). MicroRNAs 17-5p-20a-106a control monocytopoiesis through AML1 targeting and M-CSF receptor upregulation. *Nat Cell Biol*, 9, 7, pp. 775-787.

Fontenot, J.D., Gavin, M.A. & Rudensky, A.Y. (2003). Foxp3 programs the development and function of CD4+CD25+ regulatory T cells. *Nat Immunol*, 4, 4, pp. 330-336.

Forrest, A.R., Kanamori-Katayama, M., Tomaru, Y., Lassmann, T., Ninomiya, N., Takahashi, Y., de Hoon, M.J., Kubosaki, A., Kaiho, A., Suzuki, M., Yasuda, J., Kawai, J., Hayashizaki, Y., Hume, D.A. & Suzuki, H. (2010). Induction of microRNAs, mir-155, mir-222, mir-424 and mir-503, promotes monocytic differentiation through combinatorial regulation. *Leukemia*, 24, 2, pp. 460-466.

Franco, C.B., Scripture-Adams, D.D., Proekt, I., Taghon, T., Weiss, A.H., Yui, M.A., Adams, S.L., Diamond, R.A. & Rothenberg, E.V. (2006). Notch/Delta signaling constrains reengineering of pro-T cells by PU.1. *Proc Natl Acad Sci U S A*, 103, 32, pp. 11993-11998.

Friedman, A.D. (2007). Transcriptional control of granulocyte and monocyte development. *Oncogene*, 26, 47, pp. 6816-6828.

Fujiwara, Y., Browne, C.P., Cunniff, K., Goff, S.C. & Orkin, S.H. (1996). Arrested development of embryonic red cell precursors in mouse embryos lacking transcription factor GATA-1. *Proc Natl Acad Sci U S A*, 93, 22, pp. 12355-12358.

Fukuda, T., Yoshida, T., Okada, S., Hatano, M., Miki, T., Ishibashi, K., Okabe, S., Koseki, H., Hirosawa, S., Taniguchi, M., Miyasaka, N. & Tokuhisa, T. (1997). Disruption of the Bcl6 gene results in an impaired germinal center formation. *J Exp Med*, 186, 3, pp. 439-448.

Gangenahalli, G.U., Gupta, P., Saluja, D., Verma, Y.K., Kishore, V., Chandra, R., Sharma, R.K. & Ravindranath, T. (2005). Stem cell fate specification: role of master regulatory switch transcription factor PU.1 in differential hematopoiesis. *Stem Cells Dev*, 14, 2, pp. 140-152.

Gao, H., Lukin, K., Ramirez, J., Fields, S., Lopez, D. & Hagman, J. (2009). Opposing effects of SWI/SNF and Mi-2/NuRD chromatin remodeling complexes on epigenetic reprogramming by EBF and Pax5. *Proc Natl Acad Sci U S A*, 106, 27, pp. 11258-11263.

Garbe, A.I., Krueger, A., Gounari, F., Zuniga-Pflucker, J.C. & von Boehmer, H. (2006). Differential synergy of Notch and T cell receptor signaling determines alphabeta versus gammadelta lineage fate. *J Exp Med*, 203, 6, pp. 1579-1590.

Garcia-Peydro, M., de Yebenes, V.G. & Toribio, M.L. (2003). Sustained Notch1 signaling instructs the earliest human intrathymic precursors to adopt a gammadelta T-cell fate in fetal thymus organ culture. *Blood*, 102, 7, pp. 2444-2451.

Garzon, R., Pichiorri, F., Palumbo, T., Iuliano, R., Cimmino, A., Aqeilan, R., Volinia, S., Bhatt, D., Alder, H., Marcucci, G., Calin, G.A., Liu, C.G., Bloomfield, C.D., Andreeff, M. & Croce, C.M. (2006). MicroRNA fingerprints during human megakaryocytopoiesis. *Proc Natl Acad Sci U S A*, 103, 13, pp. 5078-5083.

Geissmann, F., Manz, M.G., Jung, S., Sieweke, M.H., Merad, M. & Ley, K. (2010). Development of monocytes, macrophages, and dendritic cells. *Science*, 327, 5966, pp. 656-661.

Georgantas, R.W., 3rd, Hildreth, R., Morisot, S., Alder, J., Liu, C.G., Heimfeld, S., Calin, G.A., Croce, C.M. & Civin, C.I. (2007). CD34+ hematopoietic stem-progenitor cell microRNA expression and function: a circuit diagram of differentiation control. *Proc Natl Acad Sci U S A*, 104, 8, pp. 2750-2755.

Gertz, M.A. (2010). Current status of stem cell mobilization. *Br J Haematol*, 150, 6, pp. 647-662.

Gertz, M.A., Lacy, M.Q., Inwards, D.J., Gastineau, D.A., Tefferi, A., Chen, M.G., Witzig, T.E., Greipp, P.R. & Litzow, M.R. (2000). Delayed stem cell transplantation for the management of relapsed or refractory multiple myeloma. *Bone Marrow Transplant*, 26, 1, pp. 45-50.

Gery, S., Gombart, A.F., Fung, Y.K. & Koeffler, H.P. (2004). C/EBPepsilon interacts with retinoblastoma and E2F1 during granulopoiesis. *Blood*, 103, 3, pp. 828-835.

Godfrey, V.L., Wilkinson, J.E., Rinchik, E.M. & Russell, L.B. (1991). Fatal lymphoreticular disease in the scurfy (sf) mouse requires T cells that mature in a sf thymic environment: potential model for thymic education. *Proc Natl Acad Sci U S A*, 88, 13, pp. 5528-5532.

Guo, J., Hawwari, A., Li, H., Sun, Z., Mahanta, S.K., Littman, D.R., Krangel, M.S. & He, Y.W. (2002). Regulation of the TCRalpha repertoire by the survival window of CD4(+)CD8(+) thymocytes. *Nat Immunol*, 3, 5, pp. 469-476.

Guo, S., Lu, J., Schlanger, R., Zhang, H., Wang, J.Y., Fox, M.C., Purton, L.E., Fleming, H.H., Cobb, B., Merkenschlager, M., Golub, T.R. & Scadden, D.T. (2010). MicroRNA miR-125a controls hematopoietic stem cell number. *Proc Natl Acad Sci U S A*, 107, 32, pp. 14229-14234.

Hanna, J., Wernig, M., Markoulaki, S., Sun, C.W., Meissner, A., Cassady, J.P., Beard, C., Brambrink, T., Wu, L.C., Townes, T.M. & Jaenisch, R. (2007). Treatment of sickle cell anemia mouse model with iPS cells generated from autologous skin. *Science*, 318, 5858, pp. 1920-1923.

Hayes, S.M., Li, L. & Love, P.E. (2005). TCR signal strength influences alphabeta/gammadelta lineage fate. *Immunity*, 22, 5, pp. 583-593.

He, X., Park, K., Wang, H., Zhang, Y., Hua, X., Li, Y. & Kappes, D.J. (2008). CD4-CD8 lineage commitment is regulated by a silencer element at the ThPOK transcription-factor locus. *Immunity*, 28, 3, pp. 346-358.

Heintzman, N.D., Hon, G.C., Hawkins, R.D., Kheradpour, P., Stark, A., Harp, L.F., Ye, Z., Lee, L.K., Stuart, R.K., Ching, C.W., Ching, K.A., Antosiewicz-Bourget, J.E., Liu, H., Zhang, X., Green, R.D., Lobanenkov, V.V., Stewart, R., Thomson, J.A., Crawford, G.E., Kellis, M. & Ren, B. (2009). Histone modifications at human enhancers reflect global cell-type-specific gene expression. *Nature*, 459, 7243, pp. 108-112.

Heinz, S., Benner, C., Spann, N., Bertolino, E., Lin, Y.C., Laslo, P., Cheng, J.X., Murre, C., Singh, H. & Glass, C.K. (2010). Simple combinations of lineage-determining transcription factors prime cis-regulatory elements required for macrophage and B cell identities. *Mol Cell*, 38, 4, pp. 576-589.

Hirai, H., Zhang, P., Dayaram, T., Hetherington, C.J., Mizuno, S., Imanishi, J., Akashi, K. & Tenen, D.G. (2006). C/EBPbeta is required for 'emergency' granulopoiesis. *Nat Immunol*, 7, 7, pp. 732-739.

Hisakawa, H., Sugiyama, D., Nishijima, I., Xu, M.J., Wu, H., Nakao, K., Watanabe, S., Katsuki, M., Asano, S., Arai, K., Nakahata, T. & Tsuji, K. (2001). Human granulocyte-macrophage colony-stimulating factor (hGM-CSF) stimulates primitive and definitive erythropoiesis in mouse embryos expressing hGM-CSF receptors but not erythropoietin receptors. *Blood*, 98, 13, pp. 3618-3625.

Hohaus, S., Petrovick, M.S., Voso, M.T., Sun, Z., Zhang, D.E. & Tenen, D.G. (1995). PU.1 (Spi-1) and C/EBP alpha regulate expression of the granulocyte-macrophage colony-stimulating factor receptor alpha gene. *Mol Cell Biol*, 15, 10, pp. 5830-5845.

Horcher, M., Souabni, A. & Busslinger, M. (2001). Pax5/BSAP maintains the identity of B cells in late B lymphopoiesis. *Immunity*, 14, 6, pp. 779-790.

Hori, S., Nomura, T. & Sakaguchi, S. (2003). Control of regulatory T cell development by the transcription factor Foxp3. *Science*, 299, 5609, pp. 1057-1061.

Horwitz, M., Benson, K.F., Person, R.E., Aprikyan, A.G. & Dale, D.C. (1999). Mutations in ELA2, encoding neutrophil elastase, define a 21-day biological clock in cyclic haematopoiesis. *Nat Genet*, 23, 4, pp. 433-436.

Hwang, E.S., Szabo, S.J., Schwartzberg, P.L. & Glimcher, L.H. (2005). T helper cell fate specified by kinase-mediated interaction of T-bet with GATA-3. *Science*, 307, 5708, pp. 430-433.

Ioannidis, V., Beermann, F., Clevers, H. & Held, W. (2001). The beta-catenin--TCF-1 pathway ensures CD4(+)CD8(+) thymocyte survival. *Nat Immunol*, 2, 8, pp. 691-697.

Isomura, I., Palmer, S., Grumont, R.J., Bunting, K., Hoyne, G., Wilkinson, N., Banerjee, A., Proietto, A., Gugasyan, R., Wu, L., McNally, A., Steptoe, R.J., Thomas, R., Shannon, M.F. & Gerondakis, S. (2009). c-Rel is required for the development of thymic Foxp3+ CD4 regulatory T cells. *J Exp Med*, 206, 13, pp. 3001-3014.

Ivanov, II, McKenzie, B.S., Zhou, L., Tadokoro, C.E., Lepelley, A., Lafaille, J.J., Cua, D.J. & Littman, D.R. (2006). The orphan nuclear receptor RORgammat directs the differentiation program of proinflammatory IL-17+ T helper cells. *Cell*, 126, 6, pp. 1121-1133.

Iwasaki, H. & Akashi, K. (2007). Hematopoietic developmental pathways: on cellular basis. *Oncogene*, 26, 47, pp. 6687-6696.

Iwasaki, H. & Akashi, K. (2007). Myeloid lineage commitment from the hematopoietic stem cell. *Immunity*, 26, 6, pp. 726-740.

Iwasaki, H., Mizuno, S., Wells, R.A., Cantor, A.B., Watanabe, S. & Akashi, K. (2003). GATA-1 converts lymphoid and myelomonocytic progenitors into the megakaryocyte/erythrocyte lineages. *Immunity*, 19, 3, pp. 451-462.

Iwasaki-Arai, J., Iwasaki, H., Miyamoto, T., Watanabe, S. & Akashi, K. (2003). Enforced granulocyte/macrophage colony-stimulating factor signals do not support lymphopoiesis, but instruct lymphoid to myelomonocytic lineage conversion. *J Exp Med*, 197, 10, pp. 1311-1322.

Ji, H., Ehrlich, L.I., Seita, J., Murakami, P., Doi, A., Lindau, P., Lee, H., Aryee, M.J., Irizarry, R.A., Kim, K., Rossi, D.J., Inlay, M.A., Serwold, T., Karsunky, H., Ho, L., Daley, G.Q., Weissman, I.L. & Feinberg, A.P. (2010). Comprehensive methylome map of lineage commitment from haematopoietic progenitors. *Nature*, 467, 7313, pp. 338-342.

Johnnidis, J.B., Harris, M.H., Wheeler, R.T., Stehling-Sun, S., Lam, M.H., Kirak, O., Brummelkamp, T.R., Fleming, M.D. & Camargo, F.D. (2008). Regulation of progenitor cell proliferation and granulocyte function by microRNA-223. *Nature*, 451, 7182, pp. 1125-1129.

Johnson, P.F. (2005). Molecular stop signs: regulation of cell-cycle arrest by C/EBP transcription factors. *J Cell Sci*, 118, Pt 12, pp. 2545-2555.

Johnston, R.J., Poholek, A.C., DiToro, D., Yusuf, I., Eto, D., Barnett, B., Dent, A.L., Craft, J. & Crotty, S. (2009). Bcl6 and Blimp-1 are reciprocal and antagonistic regulators of T follicular helper cell differentiation. *Science*, 325, 5943, pp. 1006-1010.

Jonuleit, H., Schmitt, E., Steinbrink, K. & Enk, A.H. (2001). Dendritic cells as a tool to induce anergic and regulatory T cells. *Trends Immunol*, 22, 7, pp. 394-400.

Kallies, A., Hasbold, J., Fairfax, K., Pridans, C., Emslie, D., McKenzie, B.S., Lew, A.M., Corcoran, L.M., Hodgkin, P.D., Tarlinton, D.M. & Nutt, S.L. (2007). Initiation of plasma-cell differentiation is independent of the transcription factor Blimp-1. *Immunity*, 26, 5, pp. 555-566.

Kanellopoulou, C., Muljo, S.A., Kung, A.L., Ganesan, S., Drapkin, R., Jenuwein, T., Livingston, D.M. & Rajewsky, K. (2005). Dicer-deficient mouse embryonic stem cells are defective in differentiation and centromeric silencing. *Genes Dev*, 19, 4, pp. 489-501.

Kang, J., Volkmann, A. & Raulet, D.H. (2001). Evidence that gammadelta versus alphabeta T cell fate determination is initiated independently of T cell receptor signaling. *J Exp Med*, 193, 6, pp. 689-698.

Kee, B.L. & Murre, C. (1998). Induction of early B cell factor (EBF) and multiple B lineage genes by the basic helix-loop-helix transcription factor E12. *J Exp Med*, 188, 4, pp. 699-713.

Kerenyi, M.A. & Orkin, S.H. (2010). Networking erythropoiesis. *J Exp Med*, 207, 12, pp. 2537-2541.

Kiel, M.J., Yilmaz, O.H., Iwashita, T., Terhorst, C. & Morrison, S.J. (2005). SLAM family receptors distinguish hematopoietic stem and progenitor cells and reveal endothelial niches for stem cells. *Cell*, 121, 7, pp. 1109-1121.

Kim, J., Sif, S., Jones, B., Jackson, A., Koipally, J., Heller, E., Winandy, S., Viel, A., Sawyer, A., Ikeda, T., Kingston, R. & Georgopoulos, K. (1999). Ikaros DNA-binding proteins direct formation of chromatin remodeling complexes in lymphocytes. *Immunity*, 10, 3, pp. 345-355.

Kim, P.J., Pai, S.Y., Brigl, M., Besra, G.S., Gumperz, J. & Ho, I.C. (2006). GATA-3 regulates the development and function of invariant NKT cells. *J Immunol*, 177, 10, pp. 6650-6659.

Kirillov, A., Kistler, B., Mostoslavsky, R., Cedar, H., Wirth, T. & Bergman, Y. (1996). A role for nuclear NF-kappaB in B-cell-specific demethylation of the Igkappa locus. *Nat Genet*, 13, 4, pp. 435-441.

Kohn, D.B. (2010). Update on gene therapy for immunodeficiencies. *Clin Immunol*, 135, 2, pp. 247-254.

Koipally, J., Renold, A., Kim, J. & Georgopoulos, K. (1999). Repression by Ikaros and Aiolos is mediated through histone deacetylase complexes. *EMBO J*, 18, 11, pp. 3090-3100.

Kondo, M., Scherer, D.C., Miyamoto, T., King, A.G., Akashi, K., Sugamura, K. & Weissman, I.L. (2000). Cell-fate conversion of lymphoid-committed progenitors by instructive actions of cytokines. *Nature*, 407, 6802, pp. 383-386.

Kondo, M., Wagers, A.J., Manz, M.G., Prohaska, S.S., Scherer, D.C., Beilhack, G.F., Shizuru, J.A. & Weissman, I.L. (2003). Biology of hematopoietic stem cells and progenitors: implications for clinical application. *Annu Rev Immunol*, 21, pp. 759-806.

Kondo, M., Weissman, I.L. & Akashi, K. (1997). Identification of clonogenic common lymphoid progenitors in mouse bone marrow. *Cell*, 91, 5, pp. 661-672.

Koralov, S.B., Muljo, S.A., Galler, G.R., Krek, A., Chakraborty, T., Kanellopoulou, C., Jensen, K., Cobb, B.S., Merkenschlager, M., Rajewsky, N. & Rajewsky, K. (2008). Dicer ablation affects antibody diversity and cell survival in the B lymphocyte lineage. *Cell*, 132, 5, pp. 860-874.

Koschmieder, S., Halmos, B., Levantini, E. & Tenen, D.G. (2009). Dysregulation of the C/EBPalpha differentiation pathway in human cancer. *J Clin Oncol*, 27, 4, pp. 619-628.

Kovalovsky, D., Uche, O.U., Eladad, S., Hobbs, R.M., Yi, W., Alonzo, E., Chua, K., Eidson, M., Kim, H.J., Im, J.S., Pandolfi, P.P. & Sant'Angelo, D.B. (2008). The BTB-zinc finger transcriptional regulator PLZF controls the development of invariant natural killer T cell effector functions. *Nat Immunol*, 9, 9, pp. 1055-1064.

Kozmik, Z., Wang, S., Dorfler, P., Adams, B. & Busslinger, M. (1992). The promoter of the CD19 gene is a target for the B-cell-specific transcription factor BSAP. *Mol Cell Biol*, 12, 6, pp. 2662-2672.

Kreslavsky, T., Gleimer, M., Garbe, A.I. & von Boehmer, H. (2010). alphabeta versus gammadelta fate choice: counting the T-cell lineages at the branch point. *Immunol Rev*, 238, 1, pp. 169-181.

Kurschus, F.C., Croxford, A.L., Heinen, A.P., Wortge, S., Ielo, D. & Waisman, A. (2010). Genetic proof for the transient nature of the Th17 phenotype. *Eur J Immunol*, 40, 12, pp. 3336-3346.

Kwon, K., Hutter, C., Sun, Q., Bilic, I., Cobaleda, C., Malin, S. & Busslinger, M. (2008). Instructive role of the transcription factor E2A in early B lymphopoiesis and germinal center B cell development. *Immunity*, 28, 6, pp. 751-762.

Lacorazza, H.D., Miyazaki, Y., Di Cristofano, A., Deblasio, A., Hedvat, C., Zhang, J., Cordon-Cardo, C., Mao, S., Pandolfi, P.P. & Nimer, S.D. (2002). The ETS protein

MEF plays a critical role in perforin gene expression and the development of natural killer and NK-T cells. *Immunity,* 17, 4, pp. 437-449.

Laiosa, C.V., Stadtfeld, M., Xie, H., de Andres-Aguayo, L. & Graf, T. (2006). Reprogramming of committed T cell progenitors to macrophages and dendritic cells by C/EBP alpha and PU.1 transcription factors. *Immunity,* 25, 5, pp. 731-744.

Laslo, P., Pongubala, J.M., Lancki, D.W. & Singh, H. (2008). Gene regulatory networks directing myeloid and lymphoid cell fates within the immune system. *Semin Immunol,* 20, 4, pp. 228-235.

Laslo, P., Spooner, C.J., Warmflash, A., Lancki, D.W., Lee, H.J., Sciammas, R., Gantner, B.N., Dinner, A.R. & Singh, H. (2006). Multilineage transcriptional priming and determination of alternate hematopoietic cell fates. *Cell,* 126, 4, pp. 755-766.

Lauritsen, J.P., Wong, G.W., Lee, S.Y., Lefebvre, J.M., Ciofani, M., Rhodes, M., Kappes, D.J., Zuniga-Pflucker, J.C. & Wiest, D.L. (2009). Marked induction of the helix-loop-helix protein Id3 promotes the gammadelta T cell fate and renders their functional maturation Notch independent. *Immunity,* 31, 4, pp. 565-575.

Lazarevic, V., Chen, X., Shim, J.H., Hwang, E.S., Jang, E., Bolm, A.N., Oukka, M., Kuchroo, V.K. & Glimcher, L.H. (2011). T-bet represses T(H)17 differentiation by preventing Runx1-mediated activation of the gene encoding RORgammat. *Nat Immunol,* 12, 1, pp. 96-104.

Lee, C.H., Melchers, M., Wang, H., Torrey, T.A., Slota, R., Qi, C.F., Kim, J.Y., Lugar, P., Kong, H.J., Farrington, L., van der Zouwen, B., Zhou, J.X., Lougaris, V., Lipsky, P.E., Grammer, A.C. & Morse, H.C., 3rd. (2006). Regulation of the germinal center gene program by interferon (IFN) regulatory factor 8/IFN consensus sequence-binding protein. *J Exp Med,* 203, 1, pp. 63-72.

Lee, Y.K., Turner, H., Maynard, C.L., Oliver, J.R., Chen, D., Elson, C.O. & Weaver, C.T. (2009). Late developmental plasticity in the T helper 17 lineage. *Immunity,* 30, 1, pp. 92-107.

Lekstrom-Himes, J. & Xanthopoulos, K.G. (1998). Biological role of the CCAAT/enhancer-binding protein family of transcription factors. *J Biol Chem,* 273, 44, pp. 28545-28548.

Lekstrom-Himes, J. & Xanthopoulos, K.G. (1999). CCAAT/enhancer binding protein epsilon is critical for effective neutrophil-mediated response to inflammatory challenge. *Blood,* 93, 9, pp. 3096-3105.

Lekstrom-Himes, J.A., Dorman, S.E., Kopar, P., Holland, S.M. & Gallin, J.I. (1999). Neutrophil-specific granule deficiency results from a novel mutation with loss of function of the transcription factor CCAAT/enhancer binding protein epsilon. *J Exp Med,* 189, 11, pp. 1847-1852.

Li, L., Leid, M. & Rothenberg, E.V. (2010). An early T cell lineage commitment checkpoint dependent on the transcription factor Bcl11b. *Science,* 329, 5987, pp. 89-93.

Li, Q.J., Chau, J., Ebert, P.J., Sylvester, G., Min, H., Liu, G., Braich, R., Manoharan, M., Soutschek, J., Skare, P., Klein, L.O., Davis, M.M. & Chen, C.Z. (2007). miR-181a is an intrinsic modulator of T cell sensitivity and selection. *Cell,* 129, 1, pp. 147-161.

Liao, R., Sun, J., Zhang, L., Lou, G., Chen, M., Zhou, D., Chen, Z. & Zhang, S. (2008). MicroRNAs play a role in the development of human hematopoietic stem cells. *J Cell Biochem,* 104, 3, pp. 805-817.

Lin, C.S., Lim, S.K., D'Agati, V. & Costantini, F. (1996). Differential effects of an erythropoietin receptor gene disruption on primitive and definitive erythropoiesis. *Genes Dev,* 10, 2, pp. 154-164.

Lin, H. & Grosschedl, R. (1995). Failure of B-cell differentiation in mice lacking the transcription factor EBF. *Nature,* 376, 6537, pp. 263-267.

Lin, K.I., Angelin-Duclos, C., Kuo, T.C. & Calame, K. (2002). Blimp-1-dependent repression of Pax-5 is required for differentiation of B cells to immunoglobulin M-secreting plasma cells. *Mol Cell Biol,* 22, 13, pp. 4771-4780.

Lin, Y.C., Jhunjhunwala, S., Benner, C., Heinz, S., Welinder, E., Mansson, R., Sigvardsson, M., Hagman, J., Espinoza, C.A., Dutkowski, J., Ideker, T., Glass, C.K. & Murre, C. (2010). A global network of transcription factors, involving E2A, EBF1 and Foxo1, that orchestrates B cell fate. *Nat Immunol,* 11, 7, pp. 635-643.

Linch, D.C., Winfield, D., Goldstone, A.H., Moir, D., Hancock, B., McMillan, A., Chopra, R., Milligan, D. & Hudson, G.V. (1993). Dose intensification with autologous bone-marrow transplantation in relapsed and resistant Hodgkin's disease: results of a BNLI randomised trial. *Lancet,* 341, 8852, pp. 1051-1054.

Liu, F., Wu, H.Y., Wesselschmidt, R., Kornaga, T. & Link, D.C. (1996). Impaired production and increased apoptosis of neutrophils in granulocyte colony-stimulating factor receptor-deficient mice. *Immunity,* 5, 5, pp. 491-501.

Long, M., Park, S.G., Strickland, I., Hayden, M.S. & Ghosh, S. (2009). Nuclear factor-kappaB modulates regulatory T cell development by directly regulating expression of Foxp3 transcription factor. *Immunity,* 31, 6, pp. 921-931.

Lu, J., Guo, S., Ebert, B.L., Zhang, H., Peng, X., Bosco, J., Pretz, J., Schlanger, R., Wang, J.Y., Mak, R.H., Dombkowski, D.M., Preffer, F.I., Scadden, D.T. & Golub, T.R. (2008). MicroRNA-mediated control of cell fate in megakaryocyte-erythrocyte progenitors. *Dev Cell,* 14, 6, pp. 843-853.

Lyon, M.F., Peters, J., Glenister, P.H., Ball, S. & Wright, E. (1990). The scurfy mouse mutant has previously unrecognized hematological abnormalities and resembles Wiskott-Aldrich syndrome. *Proc Natl Acad Sci U S A,* 87, 7, pp. 2433-2437.

Mansfield, J.H., Harfe, B.D., Nissen, R., Obenauer, J., Srineel, J., Chaudhuri, A., Farzan-Kashani, R., Zuker, M., Pasquinelli, A.E., Ruvkun, G., Sharp, P.A., Tabin, C.J. & McManus, M.T. (2004). MicroRNA-responsive 'sensor' transgenes uncover Hox-like and other developmentally regulated patterns of vertebrate microRNA expression. *Nat Genet,* 36, 10, pp. 1079-1083.

Mantel, P.Y., Ouaked, N., Ruckert, B., Karagiannidis, C., Welz, R., Blaser, K. & Schmidt-Weber, C.B. (2006). Molecular mechanisms underlying FOXP3 induction in human T cells. *J Immunol,* 176, 6, pp. 3593-3602.

Manz, M.G., Traver, D., Miyamoto, T., Weissman, I.L. & Akashi, K. (2001). Dendritic cell potentials of early lymphoid and myeloid progenitors. *Blood,* 97, 11, pp. 3333-3341.

Matsuda, J.L., Zhang, Q., Ndonye, R., Richardson, S.K., Howell, A.R. & Gapin, L. (2006). T-bet concomitantly controls migration, survival, and effector functions during the development of Valpha14i NKT cells. *Blood,* 107, 7, pp. 2797-2805.

McArthur, G.A., Rohrschneider, L.R. & Johnson, G.R. (1994). Induced expression of c-fms in normal hematopoietic cells shows evidence for both conservation and lineage restriction of signal transduction in response to macrophage colony-stimulating factor. *Blood,* 83, 4, pp. 972-981.

Melichar, H.J., Narayan, K., Der, S.D., Hiraoka, Y., Gardiol, N., Jeannet, G., Held, W., Chambers, C.A. & Kang, J. (2007). Regulation of gammadelta versus alphabeta T lymphocyte differentiation by the transcription factor SOX13. *Science,* 315, 5809, pp. 230-233.

Metcalf, D. (2008). Hematopoietic cytokines. *Blood,* 111, 2, pp. 485-491.

Morceau, F., Schnekenburger, M., Dicato, M. & Diederich, M. (2004). GATA-1: friends, brothers, and coworkers. *Ann N Y Acad Sci,* 1030, pp. 537-554.

Moreau, P., Avet-Loiseau, H., Harousseau, J.L. & Attal, M. (2011). Current trends in autologous stem-cell transplantation for myeloma in the era of novel therapies. *J Clin Oncol,* 29, 14, pp. 1898-1906.

Mosmann, T.R., Cherwinski, H., Bond, M.W., Giedlin, M.A. & Coffman, R.L. (1986). Two types of murine helper T cell clone. I. Definition according to profiles of lymphokine activities and secreted proteins. *J Immunol,* 136, 7, pp. 2348-2357.

Mowen, K.A. & Glimcher, L.H. (2004). Signaling pathways in Th2 development. *Immunol Rev,* 202, pp. 203-222.

Muljo, S.A., Ansel, K.M., Kanellopoulou, C., Livingston, D.M., Rao, A. & Rajewsky, K. (2005). Aberrant T cell differentiation in the absence of Dicer. *J Exp Med,* 202, 2, pp. 261-269.

Nagai, Y., Garrett, K.P., Ohta, S., Bahrun, U., Kouro, T., Akira, S., Takatsu, K. & Kincade, P.W. (2006). Toll-like receptors on hematopoietic progenitor cells stimulate innate immune system replenishment. *Immunity,* 24, 6, pp. 801-812.

Naik, S.H., Sathe, P., Park, H.Y., Metcalf, D., Proietto, A.I., Dakic, A., Carotta, S., O'Keeffe, M., Bahlo, M., Papenfuss, A., Kwak, J.Y., Wu, L. & Shortman, K. (2007). Development of plasmacytoid and conventional dendritic cell subtypes from single precursor cells derived in vitro and in vivo. *Nat Immunol,* 8, 11, pp. 1217-1226.

Nishinakamura, R., Miyajima, A., Mee, P.J., Tybulewicz, V.L. & Murray, R. (1996). Hematopoiesis in mice lacking the entire granulocyte-macrophage colony-stimulating factor/interleukin-3/interleukin-5 functions. *Blood,* 88, 7, pp. 2458-2464.

Nishinakamura, R., Wiler, R., Dirksen, U., Morikawa, Y., Arai, K., Miyajima, A., Burdach, S. & Murray, R. (1996). The pulmonary alveolar proteinosis in granulocyte macrophage colony-stimulating factor/interleukins 3/5 beta c receptor-deficient mice is reversed by bone marrow transplantation. *J Exp Med,* 183, 6, pp. 2657-2662.

Nozad Charoudeh, H., Tang, Y., Cheng, M., Cilio, C.M., Jacobsen, S.E. & Sitnicka, E. (2010). Identification of an NK/T cell-restricted progenitor in adult bone marrow contributing to bone marrow- and thymic-dependent NK cells. *Blood,* 116, 2, pp. 183-192.

Nurieva, R.I., Chung, Y., Martinez, G.J., Yang, X.O., Tanaka, S., Matskevitch, T.D., Wang, Y.H. & Dong, C. (2009). Bcl6 mediates the development of T follicular helper cells. *Science,* 325, 5943, pp. 1001-1005.

Nutt, S.L., Heavey, B., Rolink, A.G. & Busslinger, M. (1999). Commitment to the B-lymphoid lineage depends on the transcription factor Pax5. *Nature,* 401, 6753, pp. 556-562.

Nutt, S.L., Morrison, A.M., Dorfler, P., Rolink, A. & Busslinger, M. (1998). Identification of BSAP (Pax-5) target genes in early B-cell development by loss- and gain-of-function experiments. *Embo J,* 17, 8, pp. 2319-2333.

Nutt, S.L., Urbanek, P., Rolink, A. & Busslinger, M. (1997). Essential functions of Pax5 (BSAP) in pro-B cell development: difference between fetal and adult B lymphopoiesis and reduced V- to DJ recombination at the IgH locus. *Genes Dev.*, 11, pp. 476-491.

Nutt, S.L., Urbanek, P., Rolink, A. & Busslinger, M. (1997). Essential functions of Pax5 (BSAP) in pro-B cell development: difference between fetal and adult B lymphopoiesis and reduced V-to-DJ recombination at the IgH locus. *Genes Dev*, 11, 4, pp. 476-491.

O'Riordan, M. & Grosschedl, R. (1999). Coordinate regulation of B cell differentiation by the transcription factors EBF and E2A. *Immunity*, 11, 1, pp. 21-31.

Onai, N., Obata-Onai, A., Schmid, M.A., Ohteki, T., Jarrossay, D. & Manz, M.G. (2007). Identification of clonogenic common Flt3+M-CSFR+ plasmacytoid and conventional dendritic cell progenitors in mouse bone marrow. *Nat Immunol*, 8, 11, pp. 1207-1216.

Orford, K., Kharchenko, P., Lai, W., Dao, M.C., Worhunsky, D.J., Ferro, A., Janzen, V., Park, P.J. & Scadden, D.T. (2008). Differential H3K4 methylation identifies developmentally poised hematopoietic genes. *Dev Cell*, 14, 5, pp. 798-809.

Park, J.H., Adoro, S., Guinter, T., Erman, B., Alag, A.S., Catalfamo, M., Kimura, M.Y., Cui, Y., Lucas, P.J., Gress, R.E., Kubo, M., Hennighausen, L., Feigenbaum, L. & Singer, A. (2010). Signaling by intrathymic cytokines, not T cell antigen receptors, specifies CD8 lineage choice and promotes the differentiation of cytotoxic-lineage T cells. *Nat Immunol*, 11, 3, pp. 257-264.

Park, K., He, X., Lee, H.O., Hua, X., Li, Y., Wiest, D. & Kappes, D.J. (2010). TCR-mediated ThPOK induction promotes development of mature (CD24-) gammadelta thymocytes. *EMBO J*, 29, 14, pp. 2329-2341.

Patrick, D.M., Zhang, C.C., Tao, Y., Yao, H., Qi, X., Schwartz, R.J., Jun-Shen Huang, L. & Olson, E.N. (2010). Defective erythroid differentiation in miR-451 mutant mice mediated by 14-3-3zeta. *Genes Dev*, 24, 15, pp. 1614-1619.

Person, R.E., Li, F.Q., Duan, Z., Benson, K.F., Wechsler, J., Papadaki, H.A., Eliopoulos, G., Kaufman, C., Bertolone, S.J., Nakamoto, B., Papayannopoulou, T., Grimes, H.L. & Horwitz, M. (2003). Mutations in proto-oncogene GFI1 cause human neutropenia and target ELA2. *Nat Genet*, 34, 3, pp. 308-312.

Peschon, J.J., Morrissey, P.J., Grabstein, K.H., Ramsdell, F.J., Maraskovsky, E., Gliniak, B.C., Park, L.S., Ziegler, S.F., Williams, D.E., Ware, C.B., Meyer, J.D. & Davison, B.L. (1994). Early lymphocyte expansion is severely impaired in interleukin 7 receptor-deficient mice. *J Exp Med*, 180, 5, pp. 1955-1960.

Petrie, H.T. & Zuniga-Pflucker, J.C. (2007). Zoned out: functional mapping of stromal signaling microenvironments in the thymus. *Annu Rev Immunol*, 25, pp. 649-679.

Philip, T., Guglielmi, C., Hagenbeek, A., Somers, R., Van der Lelie, H., Bron, D., Sonneveld, P., Gisselbrecht, C., Cahn, J.Y., Harousseau, J.L. & et al. (1995). Autologous bone marrow transplantation as compared with salvage chemotherapy in relapses of chemotherapy-sensitive non-Hodgkin's lymphoma. *N Engl J Med*, 333, 23, pp. 1540-1545.

Pongubala, J.M., Northrup, D.L., Lancki, D.W., Medina, K.L., Treiber, T., Bertolino, E., Thomas, M., Grosschedl, R., Allman, D. & Singh, H. (2008). Transcription factor EBF restricts alternative lineage options and promotes B cell fate commitment independently of Pax5. *Nat Immunol*, 9, 2, pp. 203-215.

Pronk, C.J., Rossi, D.J., Mansson, R., Attema, J.L., Norddahl, G.L., Chan, C.K., Sigvardsson, M., Weissman, I.L. & Bryder, D. (2007). Elucidation of the phenotypic, functional, and molecular topography of a myeloerythroid progenitor cell hierarchy. *Cell Stem Cell*, 1, 4, pp. 428-442.

Pulikkan, J.A., Peramangalam, P.S., Dengler, V., Ho, P.A., Preudhomme, C., Meshinchi, S., Christopeit, M., Nibourel, O., Muller-Tidow, C., Bohlander, S.K., Tenen, D.G. & Behre, G. (2010). C/EBPalpha regulated microRNA-34a targets E2F3 during granulopoiesis and is down-regulated in AML with CEBPA mutations. *Blood*, 116, 25, pp. 5638-5649.

Rasmussen, K.D., Simmini, S., Abreu-Goodger, C., Bartonicek, N., Di Giacomo, M., Bilbao-Cortes, D., Horos, R., Von Lindern, M., Enright, A.J. & O'Carroll, D. (2010). The miR-144/451 locus is required for erythroid homeostasis. *J Exp Med*, 207, 7, pp. 1351-1358.

Rieger, M.A., Hoppe, P.S., Smejkal, B.M., Eitelhuber, A.C. & Schroeder, T. (2009). Hematopoietic cytokines can instruct lineage choice. *Science*, 325, 5937, pp. 217-218.

Riera-Sans, L. & Behrens, A. (2007). Regulation of alphabeta/gammadelta T cell development by the activator protein 1 transcription factor c-Jun. *J Immunol*, 178, 9, pp. 5690-5700.

Robb, L. (2007). Cytokine receptors and hematopoietic differentiation. *Oncogene*, 26, 47, pp. 6715-6723.

Roessler, S., Gyory, I., Imhof, S., Spivakov, M., Williams, R.R., Busslinger, M., Fisher, A.G. & Grosschedl, R. (2007). Distinct promoters mediate the regulation of Ebf1 gene expression by interleukin-7 and Pax5. *Mol Cell Biol*, 27, 2, pp. 579-594.

Romania, P., Lulli, V., Pelosi, E., Biffoni, M., Peschle, C. & Marziali, G. (2008). MicroRNA 155 modulates megakaryopoiesis at progenitor and precursor level by targeting Ets-1 and Meis1 transcription factors. *Br J Haematol*, 143, 4, pp. 570-580.

Roncarolo, M.G., Gregori, S., Lucarelli, B., Ciceri, F. & Bacchetta, R. (2011). Clinical tolerance in allogeneic hematopoietic stem cell transplantation. *Immunol Rev*, 241, 1, pp. 145-163.

Ruan, Q., Kameswaran, V., Tone, Y., Li, L., Liou, H.C., Greene, M.I., Tone, M. & Chen, Y.H. (2009). Development of Foxp3(+) regulatory t cells is driven by the c-Rel enhanceosome. *Immunity*, 31, 6, pp. 932-940.

Saran, N., Lyszkiewicz, M., Pommerencke, J., Witzlau, K., Vakilzadeh, R., Ballmaier, M., von Boehmer, H. & Krueger, A. (2010). Multiple extrathymic precursors contribute to T-cell development with different kinetics. *Blood*, 115, 6, pp. 1137-1144.

Savage, A.K., Constantinides, M.G., Han, J., Picard, D., Martin, E., Li, B., Lantz, O. & Bendelac, A. (2008). The transcription factor PLZF directs the effector program of the NKT cell lineage. *Immunity*, 29, 3, pp. 391-403.

Schebesta, M., Pfeffer, P.L. & Busslinger, M. (2002). Control of pre-BCR signaling by Pax5-dependent activation of the BLNK gene. *Immunity*, 17, 4, pp. 473-485.

Schmitt, T.M., Ciofani, M., Petrie, H.T. & Zuniga-Pflucker, J.C. (2004). Maintenance of T cell specification and differentiation requires recurrent notch receptor-ligand interactions. *J Exp Med*, 200, 4, pp. 469-479.

Sciammas, R., Shaffer, A.L., Schatz, J.H., Zhao, H., Staudt, L.M. & Singh, H. (2006). Graded expression of interferon regulatory factor-4 coordinates isotype switching with plasma cell differentiation. *Immunity*, 25, 2, pp. 225-236.

Scott, E.W., Simon, M.C., Anastasi, J. & Singh, H. (1994). Requirement of transcription factor PU.1 in the development of multiple hematopoietic lineages. *Science*, 265, 5178, pp. 1573-1577.

Seet, C.S., Brumbaugh, R.L. & Kee, B.L. (2004). Early B cell factor promotes B lymphopoiesis with reduced interleukin 7 responsiveness in the absence of E2A. *J Exp Med*, 199, 12, pp. 1689-1700.

Semerad, C.L., Poursine-Laurent, J., Liu, F. & Link, D.C. (1999). A role for G-CSF receptor signaling in the regulation of hematopoietic cell function but not lineage commitment or differentiation. *Immunity*, 11, 2, pp. 153-161.

Serwold, T., Ehrlich, L.I. & Weissman, I.L. (2009). Reductive isolation from bone marrow and blood implicates common lymphoid progenitors as the major source of thymopoiesis. *Blood*, 113, 4, pp. 807-815.

Shaffer, A.L., Lin, K.I., Kuo, T.C., Yu, X., Hurt, E.M., Rosenwald, A., Giltnane, J.M., Yang, L., Zhao, H., Calame, K. & Staudt, L.M. (2002). Blimp-1 orchestrates plasma cell differentiation by extinguishing the mature B cell gene expression program. *Immunity*, 17, 1, pp. 51-62.

Shaffer, A.L., Shapiro-Shelef, M., Iwakoshi, N.N., Lee, A.H., Qian, S.B., Zhao, H., Yu, X., Yang, L., Tan, B.K., Rosenwald, A., Hurt, E.M., Petroulakis, E., Sonenberg, N., Yewdell, J.W., Calame, K., Glimcher, L.H. & Staudt, L.M. (2004). XBP1, downstream of Blimp-1, expands the secretory apparatus and other organelles, and increases protein synthesis in plasma cell differentiation. *Immunity*, 21, 1, pp. 81-93.

Shaffer, A.L., Yu, X., He, Y., Boldrick, J., Chan, E.P. & Staudt, L.M. (2000). BCL-6 represses genes that function in lymphocyte differentiation, inflammation, and cell cycle control. *Immunity*, 13, 2, pp. 199-212.

Sharrocks, A.D. (2001). The ETS-domain transcription factor family. *Nat Rev Mol Cell Biol*, 2, 11, pp. 827-837.

Shen, W.F., Hu, Y.L., Uttarwar, L., Passegue, E. & Largman, C. (2008). MicroRNA-126 regulates HOXA9 by binding to the homeobox. *Mol Cell Biol*, 28, 14, pp. 4609-4619.

Shi, G., Cox, C.A., Vistica, B.P., Tan, C., Wawrousek, E.F. & Gery, I. (2008). Phenotype switching by inflammation-inducing polarized Th17 cells, but not by Th1 cells. *J Immunol*, 181, 10, pp. 7205-7213.

Sigvardsson, M., O'Riordan, M. & Grosschedl, R. (1997). EBF and E47 collaborate to induce expression of the endogenous immunoglobulin surrogate light chain genes. *Immunity*, 7, 1, pp. 25-36.

Silva-Santos, B., Pennington, D.J. & Hayday, A.C. (2005). Lymphotoxin-mediated regulation of gammadelta cell differentiation by alphabeta T cell progenitors. *Science*, 307, 5711, pp. 925-928.

Sivakumar, V., Hammond, K.J., Howells, N., Pfeffer, K. & Weih, F. (2003). Differential requirement for Rel/nuclear factor kappa B family members in natural killer T cell development. *J Exp Med*, 197, 12, pp. 1613-1621.

Smith, E.M., Gisler, R. & Sigvardsson, M. (2002). Cloning and characterization of a promoter flanking the early B cell factor (EBF) gene indicates roles for E-proteins and autoregulation in the control of EBF expression. *J Immunol*, 169, 1, pp. 261-270.

Smith, L.T., Hohaus, S., Gonzalez, D.A., Dziennis, S.E. & Tenen, D.G. (1996). PU.1 (Spi-1) and C/EBP alpha regulate the granulocyte colony-stimulating factor receptor promoter in myeloid cells. *Blood*, 88, 4, pp. 1234-1247.

Smithgall, T.E., Briggs, S.D., Schreiner, S., Lerner, E.C., Cheng, H. & Wilson, M.B. (2000). Control of myeloid differentiation and survival by Stats. *Oncogene*, 19, 21, pp. 2612-2618.

Soligo, M., Camperio, C., Caristi, S., Scotta, C., Del Porto, P., Costanzo, A., Mantel, P.Y., Schmidt-Weber, C.B. & Piccolella, E. (2011). CD28 costimulation regulates FOXP3 in a RelA/NF-kappaB-dependent mechanism. *Eur J Immunol*, 41, 2, pp. 503-513.

Souabni, A., Cobaleda, C., Schebesta, M. & Busslinger, M. (2002). Pax5 promotes B lymphopoiesis and blocks T cell development by repressing Notch1. *Immunity*, 17, 6, pp. 781-793.

Spooner, C.J., Cheng, J.X., Pujadas, E., Laslo, P. & Singh, H. (2009). A recurrent network involving the transcription factors PU.1 and Gfi1 orchestrates innate and adaptive immune cell fates. *Immunity*, 31, 4, pp. 576-586.

Sridharan, R. & Smale, S.T. (2007). Predominant interaction of both Ikaros and Helios with the NuRD complex in immature thymocytes. *J Biol Chem*, 282, 41, pp. 30227-30238.

Stanic, A.K., Bezbradica, J.S., Park, J.J., Matsuki, N., Mora, A.L., Van Kaer, L., Boothby, M.R. & Joyce, S. (2004). NF-kappa B controls cell fate specification, survival, and molecular differentiation of immunoregulatory natural T lymphocytes. *J Immunol*, 172, 4, pp. 2265-2273.

Sullivan, K.M., Muraro, P. & Tyndall, A. (2010). Hematopoietic cell transplantation for autoimmune disease: updates from Europe and the United States. *Biol Blood Marrow Transplant*, 16, 1 Suppl, pp. S48-56.

Szabo, S.J., Sullivan, B.M., Peng, S.L. & Glimcher, L.H. (2003). Molecular mechanisms regulating Th1 immune responses. *Annu Rev Immunol*, 21, pp. 713-758.

Szalai, G., LaRue, A.C. & Watson, D.K. (2006). Molecular mechanisms of megakaryopoiesis. *Cell Mol Life Sci*, 63, 21, pp. 2460-2476.

Tadokoro, Y., Ema, H., Okano, M., Li, E. & Nakauchi, H. (2007). De novo DNA methyltransferase is essential for self-renewal, but not for differentiation, in hematopoietic stem cells. *J Exp Med*, 204, 4, pp. 715-722.

Taghon, T., Yui, M.A. & Rothenberg, E.V. (2007). Mast cell lineage diversion of T lineage precursors by the essential T cell transcription factor GATA-3. *Nat Immunol*, 8, 8, pp. 845-855.

Takahashi, K., Tanabe, K., Ohnuki, M., Narita, M., Ichisaka, T., Tomoda, K. & Yamanaka, S. (2007). Induction of pluripotent stem cells from adult human fibroblasts by defined factors. *Cell*, 131, 5, pp. 861-872.

Takahashi, K. & Yamanaka, S. (2006). Induction of pluripotent stem cells from mouse embryonic and adult fibroblast cultures by defined factors. *Cell*, 126, 4, pp. 663-676.

Taniuchi, I., Osato, M., Egawa, T., Sunshine, M.J., Bae, S.C., Komori, T., Ito, Y. & Littman, D.R. (2002). Differential requirements for Runx proteins in CD4 repression and epigenetic silencing during T lymphocyte development. *Cell*, 111, 5, pp. 621-633.

Terszowski, G., Waskow, C., Conradt, P., Lenze, D., Koenigsmann, J., Carstanjen, D., Horak, I. & Rodewald, H.R. (2005). Prospective isolation and global gene expression analysis of the erythrocyte colony-forming unit (CFU-E). *Blood*, 105, 5, pp. 1937-1945.

Theilgaard-Monch, K., Jacobsen, L.C., Borup, R., Rasmussen, T., Bjerregaard, M.D., Nielsen, F.C., Cowland, J.B. & Borregaard, N. (2005). The transcriptional program of terminal granulocytic differentiation. *Blood*, 105, 4, pp. 1785-1796.

Treiber, T., Mandel, E.M., Pott, S., Gyory, I., Firner, S., Liu, E.T. & Grosschedl, R. (2010). Early B cell factor 1 regulates B cell gene networks by activation, repression, and transcription- independent poising of chromatin. *Immunity*, 32, 5, pp. 714-725.

Trifari, S., Kaplan, C.D., Tran, E.H., Crellin, N.K. & Spits, H. (2009). Identification of a human helper T cell population that has abundant production of interleukin 22 and is distinct from T(H)-17, T(H)1 and T(H)2 cells. *Nat Immunol*, 10, 8, pp. 864-871.

Trowbridge, J.J., Snow, J.W., Kim, J. & Orkin, S.H. (2009). DNA methyltransferase 1 is essential for and uniquely regulates hematopoietic stem and progenitor cells. *Cell Stem Cell*, 5, 4, pp. 442-449.

Tsapogas, P., Zandi, S., Ahsberg, J., Zetterblad, J., Welinder, E., Jonsson, J.I., Mansson, R., Qian, H. & Sigvardsson, M. (2011). IL-7 mediates Ebf-1-dependent lineage restriction in early lymphoid progenitors. *Blood*, 118, 5, pp. 1283-1290.

Tunyaplin, C., Shaffer, A.L., Angelin-Duclos, C.D., Yu, X., Staudt, L.M. & Calame, K.L. (2004). Direct repression of prdm1 by Bcl-6 inhibits plasmacytic differentiation. *J Immunol*, 173, 2, pp. 1158-1165.

Van de Walle, I., De Smet, G., De Smedt, M., Vandekerckhove, B., Leclercq, G., Plum, J. & Taghon, T. (2009). An early decrease in Notch activation is required for human TCR-alphabeta lineage differentiation at the expense of TCR-gammadelta T cells. *Blood*, 113, 13, pp. 2988-2998.

Vanvalkenburgh, J., Albu, D.I., Bapanpally, C., Casanova, S., Califano, D., Jones, D.M., Ignatowicz, L., Kawamoto, S., Fagarasan, S., Jenkins, N.A., Copeland, N.G., Liu, P. & Avram, D. (2011). Critical role of Bcl11b in suppressor function of T regulatory cells and prevention of inflammatory bowel disease. *J Exp Med*, pp.

Veldhoen, M., Uyttenhove, C., van Snick, J., Helmby, H., Westendorf, A., Buer, J., Martin, B., Wilhelm, C. & Stockinger, B. (2008). Transforming growth factor-beta 'reprograms' the differentiation of T helper 2 cells and promotes an interleukin 9-producing subset. *Nat Immunol*, 9, 12, pp. 1341-1346.

Velu, C.S., Baktula, A.M. & Grimes, H.L. (2009). Gfi1 regulates miR-21 and miR-196b to control myelopoiesis. *Blood*, 113, 19, pp. 4720-4728.

Ventura, A., Young, A.G., Winslow, M.M., Lintault, L., Meissner, A., Erkeland, S.J., Newman, J., Bronson, R.T., Crowley, D., Stone, J.R., Jaenisch, R., Sharp, P.A. & Jacks, T. (2008). Targeted deletion reveals essential and overlapping functions of the miR-17 through 92 family of miRNA clusters. *Cell*, 132, 5, pp. 875-886.

Verbeek, W., Lekstrom-Himes, J., Park, D.J., Dang, P.M., Vuong, P.T., Kawano, S., Babior, B.M., Xanthopoulos, K. & Koeffler, H.P. (1999). Myeloid transcription factor C/EBPepsilon is involved in the positive regulation of lactoferrin gene expression in neutrophils. *Blood*, 94, 9, pp. 3141-3150.

Vire, E., Brenner, C., Deplus, R., Blanchon, L., Fraga, M., Didelot, C., Morey, L., Van Eynde, A., Bernard, D., Vanderwinden, J.M., Bollen, M., Esteller, M., Di Croce, L., de Launoit, Y. & Fuks, F. (2006). The Polycomb group protein EZH2 directly controls DNA methylation. *Nature*, 439, 7078, pp. 871-874.

Walter, K., Bonifer, C. & Tagoh, H. (2008). Stem cell-specific epigenetic priming and B cell-specific transcriptional activation at the mouse Cd19 locus. *Blood*, 112, 5, pp. 1673-1682.

Walunas, T.L., Wang, B., Wang, C.R. & Leiden, J.M. (2000). Cutting edge: the Ets1 transcription factor is required for the development of NK T cells in mice. *J Immunol*, 164, 6, pp. 2857-2860.

Wang, L., Wildt, K.F., Zhu, J., Zhang, X., Feigenbaum, L., Tessarollo, L., Paul, W.E., Fowlkes, B.J. & Bosselut, R. (2008). Distinct functions for the transcription factors GATA-3 and ThPOK during intrathymic differentiation of CD4(+) T cells. *Nat Immunol*, 9, 10, pp. 1122-1130.

Wang, Q., Huang, Z., Xue, H., Jin, C., Ju, X.L., Han, J.D. & Chen, Y.G. (2008). MicroRNA miR-24 inhibits erythropoiesis by targeting activin type I receptor ALK4. *Blood*, 111, 2, pp. 588-595.

Wang, W., Wang, X., Ward, A.C., Touw, I.P. & Friedman, A.D. (2001). C/EBPalpha and G-CSF receptor signals cooperate to induce the myeloperoxidase and neutrophil elastase genes. *Leukemia*, 15, 5, pp. 779-786.

Warr, M.R., Pietras, E.M. & Passegue, E. (2011). Mechanisms controlling hematopoietic stem cell functions during normal hematopoiesis and hematological malignancies. *Wiley Interdiscip Rev Syst Biol Med*, pp.

Weaver, C.H., Buckner, C.D., Longin, K., Appelbaum, F.R., Rowley, S., Lilleby, K., Miser, J., Storb, R., Hansen, J.A. & Bensinger, W. (1993). Syngeneic transplantation with peripheral blood mononuclear cells collected after the administration of recombinant human granulocyte colony-stimulating factor. *Blood*, 82, 7, pp. 1981-1984.

Weber, B.N., Chi, A.W., Chavez, A., Yashiro-Ohtani, Y., Yang, Q., Shestova, O. & Bhandoola, A. (2011). A critical role for TCF-1 in T-lineage specification and differentiation. *Nature*, 476, 7358, pp. 63-68.

Weishaupt, H., Sigvardsson, M. & Attema, J.L. (2010). Epigenetic chromatin states uniquely define the developmental plasticity of murine hematopoietic stem cells. *Blood*, 115, 2, pp. 247-256.

Weissman, I.L. & Shizuru, J.A. (2008). The origins of the identification and isolation of hematopoietic stem cells, and their capability to induce donor-specific transplantation tolerance and treat autoimmune diseases. *Blood*, 112, 9, pp. 3543-3553.

Wernig, M., Meissner, A., Foreman, R., Brambrink, T., Ku, M., Hochedlinger, K., Bernstein, B.E. & Jaenisch, R. (2007). In vitro reprogramming of fibroblasts into a pluripotent ES-cell-like state. *Nature*, 448, 7151, pp. 318-324.

Wildin, R.S., Ramsdell, F., Peake, J., Faravelli, F., Casanova, J.L., Buist, N., Levy-Lahad, E., Mazzella, M., Goulet, O., Perroni, L., Bricarelli, F.D., Byrne, G., McEuen, M., Proll, S., Appleby, M. & Brunkow, M.E. (2001). X-linked neonatal diabetes mellitus, enteropathy and endocrinopathy syndrome is the human equivalent of mouse scurfy. *Nat Genet*, 27, 1, pp. 18-20.

Wilson, A. & Trumpp, A. (2006). Bone-marrow haematopoietic-stem-cell niches. *Nat Rev Immunol*, 6, 2, pp. 93-106.

Wilson, N.J., Boniface, K., Chan, J.R., McKenzie, B.S., Blumenschein, W.M., Mattson, J.D., Basham, B., Smith, K., Chen, T., Morel, F., Lecron, J.C., Kastelein, R.A., Cua, D.J., McClanahan, T.K., Bowman, E.P. & de Waal Malefyt, R. (2007). Development, cytokine profile and function of human interleukin 17-producing helper T cells. *Nat Immunol*, 8, 9, pp. 950-957.

Wu, H., Liu, X., Jaenisch, R. & Lodish, H.F. (1995). Generation of committed erythroid BFU-E and CFU-E progenitors does not require erythropoietin or the erythropoietin receptor. *Cell*, 83, 1, pp. 59-67.

Wu, S.M. & Hochedlinger, K. (2011). Harnessing the potential of induced pluripotent stem cells for regenerative medicine. *Nat Cell Biol*, 13, 5, pp. 497-505.

Xiao, C., Calado, D.P., Galler, G., Thai, T.H., Patterson, H.C., Wang, J., Rajewsky, N., Bender, T.P. & Rajewsky, K. (2007). MiR-150 controls B cell differentiation by targeting the transcription factor c-Myb. *Cell*, 131, 1, pp. 146-159.

Xie, H., Ye, M., Feng, R. & Graf, T. (2004). Stepwise reprogramming of B cells into macrophages. *Cell*, 117, 5, pp. 663-676.

Xu, L., Kitani, A., Fuss, I. & Strober, W. (2007). Cutting edge: regulatory T cells induce CD4+CD25-Foxp3- T cells or are self-induced to become Th17 cells in the absence of exogenous TGF-beta. *J Immunol*, 178, 11, pp. 6725-6729.

Yamanaka, R., Barlow, C., Lekstrom-Himes, J., Castilla, L.H., Liu, P.P., Eckhaus, M., Decker, T., Wynshaw-Boris, A. & Xanthopoulos, K.G. (1997). Impaired granulopoiesis, myelodysplasia, and early lethality in CCAAT/enhancer binding protein epsilon-deficient mice. *Proc Natl Acad Sci U S A*, 94, 24, pp. 13187-13192.

Yekta, S., Shih, I.H. & Bartel, D.P. (2004). MicroRNA-directed cleavage of HOXB8 mRNA. *Science*, 304, 5670, pp. 594-596.

Yi, T., Chen, Y., Wang, L., Du, G., Huang, D., Zhao, D., Johnston, H., Young, J., Todorov, I., Umetsu, D.T., Chen, L., Iwakura, Y., Kandeel, F., Forman, S. & Zeng, D. (2009). Reciprocal differentiation and tissue-specific pathogenesis of Th1, Th2, and Th17 cells in graft-versus-host disease. *Blood*, 114, 14, pp. 3101-3112.

Yu, D., Rao, S., Tsai, L.M., Lee, S.K., He, Y., Sutcliffe, E.L., Srivastava, M., Linterman, M., Zheng, L., Simpson, N., Ellyard, J.I., Parish, I.A., Ma, C.S., Li, Q.J., Parish, C.R., Mackay, C.R. & Vinuesa, C.G. (2009). The transcriptional repressor Bcl-6 directs T follicular helper cell lineage commitment. *Immunity*, 31, 3, pp. 457-468.

Zandi, S., Mansson, R., Tsapogas, P., Zetterblad, J., Bryder, D. & Sigvardsson, M. (2008). EBF1 is essential for B-lineage priming and establishment of a transcription factor network in common lymphoid progenitors. *J Immunol*, 181, 5, pp. 3364-3372.

Zarebski, A., Velu, C.S., Baktula, A.M., Bourdeau, T., Horman, S.R., Basu, S., Bertolone, S.J., Horwitz, M., Hildeman, D.A., Trent, J.O. & Grimes, H.L. (2008). Mutations in growth factor independent-1 associated with human neutropenia block murine granulopoiesis through colony stimulating factor-1. *Immunity*, 28, 3, pp. 370-380.

Zhan, M., Miller, C.P., Papayannopoulou, T., Stamatoyannopoulos, G. & Song, C.Z. (2007). MicroRNA expression dynamics during murine and human erythroid differentiation. *Exp Hematol*, 35, 7, pp. 1015-1025.

Zhang, P., Iwasaki-Arai, J., Iwasaki, H., Fenyus, M.L., Dayaram, T., Owens, B.M., Shigematsu, H., Levantini, E., Huettner, C.S., Lekstrom-Himes, J.A., Akashi, K. & Tenen, D.G. (2004). Enhancement of hematopoietic stem cell repopulating capacity and self-renewal in the absence of the transcription factor C/EBP alpha. *Immunity*, 21, 6, pp. 853-863.

Zheng, S.G., Wang, J., Wang, P., Gray, J.D. & Horwitz, D.A. (2007). IL-2 is essential for TGF-beta to convert naive CD4+CD25- cells to CD25+Foxp3+ regulatory T cells and for expansion of these cells. *J Immunol*, 178, 4, pp. 2018-2027.

Zhuang, Y., Soriano, P. & Weintraub, H. (1994). The helix-loop-helix gene E2A is required for B cell formation. *Cell*, 79, 5, pp. 875-884.

2

The Role of EMT Modulators in Hematopoiesis and Leukemic Transformation

Goossens Steven and Haigh J. Jody
VIB and Ghent University
Belgium

1. Introduction

Mature blood cells arise from hematopoietic stem cells (HSCs) capable of generating every hematopoietic cell type; including the various lymphoid and myeloid lineages. To maintain the steady state levels of hematopoietic cells in the circulation, each HSC has the capacity to generate large numbers of mature cells daily via various multi- and oligopotent lineage-committed progenitors (Kondo et al., 2003; Orkin, 2000). Finely tuned self-renewal and differentiation programs, controlled by essential transcriptional regulatory networks (Miranda-Saavedra & Gottgens, 2008), determine the HSC and progenitor pool sizes in adults. These regulatory networks include both positive and negative transcriptional regulators that control lineage specific gene expression and ensure normal hematopoietic cell differentiation. Deregulation of these transcriptional networks caused by aberrant upstream signalling, point mutations as well as chromosomal translocations of key transcriptional regulators particularly within the HSC compartment (Bonnet & Dick, 1997) can lead to various blood related disorders including anemia and hematological malignancies or leukemia.

The origins of HSCs during the development of a mammalian embryo are only beginning to be understood. Tracing of the true stem cells via marker analysis is difficult and the 'gold standard' for identifying these cells is based on their ability to reconstitute lethally irradiated hosts over a long term. Various transplantation studies in the mouse (Dzierzak & Medvinsky, 2008) have revealed that HSCs arise in a complex developmental process during which multipotent progenitors sequentially migrate to several anatomical sites (Dzierzak & Speck, 2008; Orkin & Zon, 2008), including the yolk sac, the aorta-gonadomesonephros (AGM) region, placenta, fetal liver and finally the bone marrow in the adult (Palis et al., 2001). Lately, it is thought that the first definitive adult-type of HSCs are generated in the AGM region at embryonic day (E) 10.5 in the mouse (de Bruijn et al., 2002). It was demonstrated through fate mapping that the first HSCs arise as part of the hematopoietic progenitor clusters that emerge from the hemogenic endothelium and subendothelial layers at the ventral part of the dorsal aorta and in the vitelline artery (Rybtsov et al., 2011; Yokomizo et al., 2011). These small cell clusters of hematopoietic progenitors are closely associated with the endothelium and originate from vascular remodelling and extravascular budding (Boisset et al., 2010; Robin et al., 2011; Zovein et al., 2010). This involves changes in endothelial cell shape and loss of cellular adhesion that have been likened to the changes in cell adhesion that epithelial cells undergo during epithelial to mesenchymal transition (**EMT**). EMT encompasses a series of events in which well-polarized epithelial cells round up in shape, lose their cell contacts and acquire the motile, migratory properties of mesenchymal cells (Greenburg & Hay, 1982). EMT is essential for many developmental processes including mesoderm formation during gastrulation and neural crest delamination and migration (Kalluri & Weinberg, 2009; Thiery et al., 2009). Similar EMT-like changes in cellular morphology can be observed during tumor progression and allow tumor cells to acquire the capacity to invade into the surrounding tissue and ultimately metastasize to a distant site (Berx et al., 2007). Subsequent tissue colonization occurs via a reverse transitional mechanism, called mesenchymal to epithelial transition (MET) (Kalluri, 2009). Significant cross talk and interactions between members of the Snai family and Zeb family of transcription factors have been documented to be involved in the regulation of these EMT/MET processes (Thiery & Sleeman, 2006). More recently, it has been suggested that the expression of the EMT regulators are also involved in the formation/acquisition of (cancer) stem cell properties (Gupta et al., 2009). In addition to their roles in epithelial/mesenchymal biology there is accumulating evidence that these EMT inducers may be involved in several aspects of hematopoietic differentiation and hematological malignancies that is the main focus of this chapter and are reviewed below.

2. EMT regulators of the Snai family

Members of Snai family encode for transcription factors with a common structural organization consisting of a highly conserved C-terminal region with four to six C_2H_2 zinc-fingers (Knight & Shimeld, 2001) and a more divergent N-terminal region (Fig. 1). This zinc-finger domain serves as a sequence-specific DNA binding domain that recognizes consensus E2-box type elements C/A(CAGGTG) (Batlle et al., 2000; Cano et al., 2000; Mauhin et al., 1993). All vertebrate Snai family members share as well an evolutionary conserved 7-9 AA N-terminus, the SNAG (Snail/Gfi) domain (Grimes et al., 1996). This domain was originally identified as a repressor domain in the zinc-finger protein Gfi1 that acts as a molecular hook to recruit co-regulators and/or demethylases and is essential for their Snai transcriptional repressive function (Lin et al., 2010).

Snail (also known as Snai1, Sna, Snah, Slugh2, Snail1.) represents the founding member of the superfamily (Manzanares et al., 2001; Nieto, 2002) and was first described in *Drosophila melanogaster* (Grau et al., 1984). In mammals, besides Snail two other Snail family members were identified **Slug** (aka Snai2, Slugh1, Slugh, Snail2) and **Smuc** (aka Snai3, Zfp293, Znf293). Snail and Slug are the best characterized and have been implicated in the formation of the mesoderm (Boulay et al., 1987; Sefton et al., 1998) and neural crest cell migration (del Barrio & Nieto, 2002; LaBonne & Bronner-Fraser, 2000) as well as with the loss of epithelial features associated with the acquisition of a fibroblast-like motile and invasive phenotype of tumor cells. Induced expression of Snail or Slug in various epithelial cancer cell lines either by FGF, Wnt, Notch or TGFβ administration (De Craene et al., 2005) or directly via ectopic expression of the repressors is sufficient to adopt a more mesenchymal morphology (Cano et al., 2000). This phenotypic switch is characterized by the downregulation of a number of epithelial marker genes (E-cadherin, desmoplakin, Muc-1, cytokeratin-18) (Batlle et al., 2000; Cano et al., 2000) and the induction of various mesenchymal marker genes (vimentin, fibronectin) (Cano et al., 2000), which can vary dependent on the cellular context. Several lines of evidence indicated that Snail family members not only regulate cellular adhesion and motility or invasion but as well can bind and regulate genes that participate in other processes (Wu Y. & Zhou, 2010) like proliferation (CyclinD1) (Liu J. et al. 2010), cell survival/apoptosis (BID, caspase-6) (Kajita et al., 2004), inflammation (Lyons et al., 2008; Yang & Wolf, 2009) and angiogenesis (Gill et al. 2011).

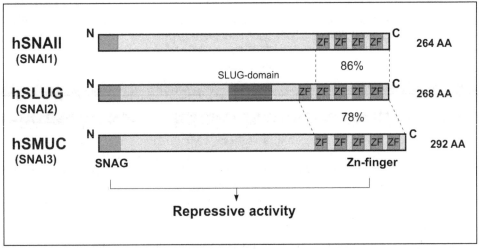

Fig. 1. Schematic diagram of conserved functional domains of the three members of the Snai family of transcription factors. All members contain an N-terminal SNAG domain and a C-terminal zinc-finger (ZF) domain. The central SLUG-domain is unique for Slug (Figure based on Cobaleda et al., 2007)

Besides this, Snai gain-of-function is correlated with the acquisition of (cancer) stem cell properties (Gupta et al., 2009). Studies of various neoplastic tissues have demonstrated the existence of cancer stem cells (CSC) or tumor-initiating-cells with self-renewal capacity that exhibit an ability to induce new tumors when transplated into nude and/or syngeneic mouse strains (Schatton et al., 2009). The existence of CSCs was initially discovered in leukemia samples (Bonnet & Dick, 1997), but subsequently they have been identified in various solid tumor types as well (Al-Hajj et al., 2003; Ricci-Vitiani et al., 2007; Singh et al., 2004). The origin of these stem cells is until now unclear but compelling results from Mani and colleagues (Mani et al., 2008) now link EMT processes with the formation of CSCs. Ectopic expression of Snail in an immortalized human mammary epithelial cell line resulted in the acquisition of mesenchymal traits, expression of stem cell markers and enhanced capacity to form mammospheres, a property previously and exclusively associated with mammary epithelial stem cells. For now it is unclear whether this is restricted to cancer stem cells of an epithelial origin or can be generalized to all (cancer) stem cells. Somewhat contradictory to this, is the recent findings that suppression of EMT inducers and the expression of E-cadherin is one of the first essential steps during the reprogramming of fibroblasts for the generating induced pluripotent stem cells (Li et al., 2010; Redmer et al., 2011; Wang et al., 2010). This may reflect the fact that stemness properties and totipotency are not equivalent and may be controlled by divergent molecular mechanisms.

Recently, the *in vivo* functions of Snail and Slug could be further analyzed by the generation of novel gain/loss-of-function mouse models. Here we shall focus more on the hematopoietic phenotypes observed in these mouse models.

2.1 Slug is an important downstream mediator of SCF/cKit signaling and plays pivotal roles in stress-induced hematopoietic stem/progenitor cell survival and self-renewal

The first evidence of an important role for Slug in hematopoiesis and leukemia came from study by Inukai et al. (1999) in which Slug was identified as a downstream target of the E2A-HLF oncogene in leukemic B-cells. The E2A-HLF fusion gene transforms human pro-B lymphocytes by interfering with the apoptotic signaling pathway at an early step. Moreover, Slug expression in IL3-dependent Baf-3 cells prolonged the survival of these cells significantly after deprivation of the cytokine. These initial data suggested a pivotal role for Slug in the cell survival pathway of lymphocyte progenitor cells and possibly as well in other hematopoietic progenitors, based on its expression profile. Endogenous Slug is normally expressed in both long- and short-term repopulating HSCs and in committed progenitors of the myeloid lineage but not in differentiated myeloid cells or pro-B or pro-T cells. Its role in other lineages was further investigated *in vivo* by the generation of Slug deficient mice. Mice lacking Slug survive and are fertile, but display postnatal growth retardation phenotypes (Inoue et al., 2002). Upon loss of Slug, normal circulating blood cell counts were observed but the number of hematopoietic colony-forming progenitors in the bone marrow and spleen were significantly (2-4-fold) increased. This suggested that in the absence of Slug, hematopoietic progenitor pools must expand to maintain normal levels of differentiated blood cells in the circulation. In addition, Slug deficient mice are more radio-sensitive; these mice not only died earlier upon γ-irradiation, but as well showed accentuated decreases in peripheral blood cell counts and marked increases in apoptotic (TUNEL+) bone marrow progenitors cells compared to their control littermates. These data implicated an important role for Slug in protecting hematopoietic progenitor cells from apoptosis after DNA damage (Inoue et al., 2002). By crossing the Slug knockout mice with various other mouse models it was demonstrated that Slug directly represses the proapoptotic factor Puma and in this way is able to antagonize the p53-mediated upregulation of Puma in γ-irradiated myeloid progenitor cells, allowing them to survive (Wu W.S. et al., 2005). All together these data suggest that Slug governs a pivotal checkpoint that controls cell survival/apoptosis decisions upon exposure to genotoxic stress.

The role of Slug in the regulation of the bone marrow stem cell compartment was further investigated under both normal steady-state and stress conditions via competitive repopulating assays and serial bone marrow transplants (Sun et al., 2010). Under normal conditions, Slug deficiency seems to have no effect on proliferation or differentiation of HSC or progenitors. However, if transplanted, Slug null HSCs demonstated increased repopulating potential that was not a result of altered differentiation nor homing ability, suggesting Slug deficiency alters HSC self-renewal. Indeed this was confirmed under the stress conditions of serial bone marrow transplantation. Consistently, 5-FU treatment of Slug knockout mice showed an expansion of the Lin-Sca1+ cell population, not by changing their cell survival capacity but by increasing their proliferation rates (Sun et al., 2010).

More detailed analysis of Slug deficient mice revealed macrocytic anemia as well as pigmentation deficiency and gonadal defects (Perez-Losada et al., 2002). These phenotypes are very similar to the defects reported in the white-spotting (W) and Steel (Sl) mutant mice with mutations in the c-Kit receptor (Chabot et al., 1988; Geissler et al., 1988) and its Stem Cell Factor (SCF) ligand (Copeland et al., 1990; Huang et al., 1990; Zsebo et al., 1990). The SCF/c-Kit signaling pathway has pleiotrophic functions in hematopoiesis and beyond. The primary function of SCF/c-Kit in early hematopoiesis seems to induce the growth of quiescent progenitor/stem cells through synergistic interactions with other early-acting cytokines (Migliaccio et al., 1991; Williams N. et al., 1992). Ample evidence indicates that in the absence of other cytokines, SCF selectively promotes viability rather than proliferation of primitive murine progenitor cells (Fleming et al., 1993) and confirms previous findings of Slug playing a role in both cell cycle/proliferation and cell survival/apoptosis. Next to its role in hematopoiesis, SCF/c-Kit signaling has been implicated in the development/migration of melanocytes (Nishikawa et al., 1991). In human piebaldism patients, c-Kit signaling has been demonstrated to be involved in congenital depigmented patches and poliosis, (Giebel & Spritz, 1991). Interestingly in some piebaldism patients, also heterozygous SLUG deletions could be detected, providing further genetic evidence that Slug may play crucial roles in the SCF/c-Kit signaling pathway (Sanchez-Martin et al., 2003). The importance of Slug as a putative downstream mediator of c-Kit signaling was further tested by means of a complementation study in which transduction with TAT-Slug protein was sufficient to rescue the radio-sensitivity of c-Kit deficient mice. Taken together these data clearly demonstrate that Slug is an important mediator downstream of c-Kit receptor activation (Perez-Losada et al., 2003).

The observed macrocytic anemia observed in the Slug mutant mice resemble in some ways human congenital anemias such as Diamond-Blackfan anemia (Perez-Losada et al., 2002), however more research is necessary to explore the involvement of Slug in this disease.

2.2 Snail and Smuc in normal hematopoiesis

Mice deficient for Snail are embryonic lethal at E7.5-8.5 due to defects in mesoderm formation (Carver et al., 2001) as well as vascular defects (Lomeli et al., 2009). Consequently, due to the early embryonic lethality, the effects of Snail loss on hematopoiesis could not be further investigated in these mice. Although some evidence exists that Snail is expressed in the hematopoietic system, more detailed research is necessary and final proof of its potential role in hematpoiesis will come from breeding the conditional floxed Snail mice (Murray S.A. et al., 2006) to mice with hematopoietic-specific transgenic Cre lines.

Based upon the fact that *in vitro* Snail binds similar E-box binding domains and in general shows more drastic phenotypes both *in vitro* as *in vivo* compared to Slug, Snail may also play crucial roles in hematopoiesis. Interestingly, Snail and Slug in most cases can complement each other and differences in phenotypes can be explained by differences in expression patterns as exemplified by the aggravated phenotypes of the Snail/Slug double knockouts (Murray S.A. et al., 2007). In addition, loss of one Snai family member often induces or increases the expression of the other(s). In this way hematopoietic-specific double knockouts may reveal even more functions for Snail and Slug in normal hematopoiesis.

More recently a third family member of the Snail family was identified in vertebrates, Smuc. Until now, little is known about its functions but it is abundantly expressed in thymocytes (Zhuge et al., 2005), specifically in the early CD4-CD8- double negative (DN) and

CD4+CD8+ double positive (DP) stages of thymocyte maturation and then solely expressed in the CD8+ T lymphocyte lineage both in the thymus and peripheral immune system. In macrophages, Smuc is able to interact with PU.1, a master regulator of myeloid differentiation, and binds the negative regulatory element within the Pactolus promoter. These data suggests that Smuc is modulating the PU.1 transcriptional activity and lack of Smuc leads to aberrant PU.1 transactivation (Hale et al., 2006).

2.3 Overexpression of Snail or Slug induces leukemia

Based on the prominent roles of Snail and Slug in stress-induced hematopoiesis, and their roles in the progression of solid tumours, as well as acquisition of cancer stem cell characteristics, it is therefore surprising that only a limited number of studies have addressed the roles of Snai family members in hematopoietic malignancies.

Nevertheless, strong evidence that Snail and Slug are involved in leukemia formation and/or progression comes from the gain-of-function mouse models that were previously developed. CombiTA-Snail mice, carrying a hypermorphic tetracycline-repressible Snail transgene, showed increased Snail expression up to 20% above normal levels (Perez-Mancera et al., 2005b). These mice survive and are fertile and although no morphological alterations were observed, their thymus were smaller and showed reduced differentiation towards CD4+CD8+ DP thymocytes. From 5-7 months onwards, CombiTA-Snail mice started to develop various types of epithelial and non-epithelial cancers especially lymphomas and acute leukemias (> 75% in two separate transgenic lines). Suppression of the Snail transgene expression by tetracycline administration did not ameliorate the malignant phenotype, suggesting that the effect of Snail overexpression is irreversible. As well, CombiTA-Snail transgene expression resulted in increased *in vivo* radioprotection, suggesting similar roles for Snail in hematopoietic cell survival upon genotoxic stress as was previously shown for Slug.

Similar experiments were performed for *in vivo* overexpression of Slug. In a similar setup as described above for Snail, CombiTA-Slug mice were generated. To prove transgene functionality, these mice were crossed with Slug deficient mice, which rescued the null phenotype. Again these mice were born without overt morphological abnormalities (Perez-Mancera et al., 2006). Only after 6-8 months 20% of the transgenic mice died as a consequence of congestive heart failure. The surviving mice started to develop various tumors from 9 months of age with highest incidence of (90%) acute leukemias (Perez-Mancera et al., 2005a). Similar as to the CombiTA-Snail mice this malignant phenotype was irreversible after tetracycline administration. As well, c-Kit signaling has been implicated both in solid tumors as well as leukemias, e.g. constitutive activating mutations of the receptor have been described in AML (Jung et al., 2011) Furthermore, the BCR–ABL oncogene did not induce leukaemia in Slug-deficient mice, implicating Slug in BCR–ABL leukemogenesis *in vivo* (Perez-Mancera et al., 2005a). As well, in an independent study it was shown that the increased Slug expression upon Bcr-Abl mutations is involved in the prolonged survival of chronic myeloid leukemia cells (Mancini et al., 2010).

From the Slug knockout mice it appears that it is governing a pivotal role in cell survival upon DNA damage by repressing the pro-apoptotic factor Puma. These results may be highly relevant for cancer therapy. Analyzing or controlling Slug levels before or during treatment may be useful as a prognostic marker for sensitivity to genotoxic agents and can be helpful for limiting therapeutic doses or increasing the efficiency of radiation or chemotherapy.

3. EMT regulators of the Zeb family

The Zinc finger E-Box binding (**ZEB**) family of DNA-binding transcriptional regulators consists of two structurally related proteins (Fortini et al., 1991)(Fig. 2): **Zeb1** (also known as δEF-1, TCF8, BZP, ZEB, AREB6, NIL-2-A, Zfhep, and Zfhx1a) and **Zeb2** (also known as Sip1, KIAA0569 and Zfhx1b). Both genes have a very similar genomic structures (Fortini et al., 1991; Vandewalle et al., 2009) and encode for large multi-domain proteins that possess N-terminal and C-terminal zinc finger DNA binding domains along with more centrally located homeo (HD), Smad protein binding (SBD) and CtBP interaction (CID) domains; and in the case of Zeb2, an N-terminal NuRD interaction domain (Verstappen et al., 2008). ¶

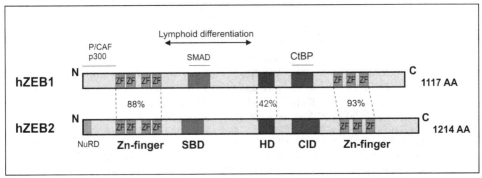

Fig. 2. Schematic diagram of conserved functional domains of the two members of the Zeb family of transcription factors. Both possess 2 zinc-finger domains, a homeodomain (HD), Smad (SBD) and CtBP (CID) binding domain (Figure based on Vandewalle et al., 2009)

Especially within the Zn-finger domains there exists a high degree of sequence similarity/identity between the two Zeb proteins, suggesting they bind similar target sequences (Verschueren et al., 1999). Each Zn-finger cluster independently can bind a 5'-CACCT(G)-3' sequence located in the target promotor region (Remacle et al., 1999). The domains outside the Zn-finger clusters seem less conserved and may be essential for the recruitment of various co-repressors, like CtBP (Grooteclaes & Frisch, 2000;Postigo & Dean, 1999b; van Grunsven et al., 2007) or co-activators like p300 or P/CAF (van Grunsven et al., 2006). Still a lot of controversy exists over whether Zeb proteins can only act as transcriptional repressors or as well as activators. The molecular mechanism underlying the choice between repression or activation are currently unknown and may include cell-type specific differences and/or posttranslational modifications (Costantino et al., 2002). Similarly, the roles of Zeb proteins in TGFβ/BMP signaling are not well understood; both Zebs have been shown to be able to bind receptor activated R-Smads (Postigo, 2003; Verschueren et al., 1999). Postigo et al. (Postigo, 2003) postulated Zeb proteins as putative important downstream mediators of this signaling pathway however with opposing effects. While Zeb1 would synergize with Smad proteins to activate transcription of TGFβ responsive reporter constructs, the structurally very similar Zeb2 would inhibit transcriptional activation donwstream of TGFβ (Postigo, 2003). These antagonistic effects were hypothesized to result from differential recruitment of co-activators and co-repressors to the Smads by Zeb1 or Zeb2 respectively (Postigo et al., 2003).

The Zeb family of zinc finger/homeodomain proteins genes was first idenfied in *Drosphila melanogaster* (Fortini et al., 1991) and shown to be essential for myogenesis (Postigo et al., 1999) and the organization of the central nervous system (Clark & Chiu, 2003). As well in vertebrates a vast number of muscle master regulatory genes have been shown to be repressed directly by Zeb1/2 (α7 integrin, δ crystalin enhancer, Mef2c) (Postigo & Dean, 1997, 1999a) as well as genes essential for cartilage and bone formation (Col2α1) (Murray D. et al., 2000). The first functional studies in Xenopus proved Zeb1 to be essential for the expression of XBra (Xenopus Brachyury) (Papin et al., 2002), a member of T-box family of transcription factor essential for mesoderm formation and notochord differentiation and previously been implicated in EMT processes. Subsequently various *in vitro* studies using multiple epithelial cancer cell lines, it was demonstrated that both Zeb1/2 are able to bind and downregulate E-cadherin (Comijn et al., 2001; Eger et al., 2005) and other epithelial-specific marker genes via binding bipartite E-boxes in their promotor regions. Exogeneous Zeb1/2 overexpression results in EMT-like phenotypes similarly as described above for the Snai family members of EMT inducers (Comijn et al., 2001; Vandewalle et al., 2005). Increased *in vivo* Zeb1/2 expression has been correlated in various tumor types with increased invasion, metastasis, dedifferentiation, cancer stem cell characteristics, recurrence and bad prognosis (Spaderna et al., 2006; Spoelstra et al., 2006; Wellner et al., 2009; Yoshihara et al., 2009).

Besides their roles in suppression of epithelial marker genes more and more studies revealed their participation in other cellular processes like cell division (Mejlvang et al., 2007), apoptosis and senescence (Liu Y. et al., 2008; Ozturk et al., 2006; Sayan et al., 2009) and inflammation (Chua et al., 2007).

From expression analysis it was clear that both Zeb proteins are also expressed in the hematopoietic system. Actually, Zeb1 has been demonstrated to be more expressed during T-lymphocyte development, while Zeb2 expression has been seen more in splenic B cells (Postigo & Dean, 2000). Using various novel mouse models recent data clearly indicated that this family of EMT inducers also plays pivotal roles in various steps of hematopoietic differentiation and progression of hematopoietic malignancies, which are discussed in detail below.

3.1 Role of Zeb2 in hematopoietic stem/progenitor differentiation and mobilization

Moderate to high Zeb2 expression is reported in all hematopoietic cells with highest levels in stem (HSC) and progenitor (HPC) populations (Goossens et al., 2011) and lowest expression in mature T cells (Postigo & Dean, 2000). Through the use of a conditional Zeb2 knockout mouse (Higashi et al., 2002) model we could show that it is not essential for the initial formation of HSCs in the embryo but it is crucial for HSC differentiation and mobilization/homing (Goossens et al., 2011). Hematopoietic-specific Zeb2 loss-of-function resulted in embryonic lethality resulting from bleedings occurring in the developing brain. The observed phenotype is very reminiscent of the phenotypes associated with ubiquitous loss of the hematopoietic transcriptional regulators AML/Runx1 (Okuda et al., 1996). Runx1 knockout embryos are deficient in AGM HSCs and lack intra-arterial hematopoietic clusters, suggesting that Zeb2 deletion may also affect hematopoietic cluster formation. However, no changes in the number of hematopoietic progenitor clusters was detected for the Zeb2 null AGM regions (Goossens et al., 2011) indicating that the formed stem cells are not functional at later stages of development. Zeb2 seems to be more involved in stem/progenitor differentiation properties as isolated progenitors from various developing hematopoietic organs were unable to differentiate *in vitro*. As well, significant decreases in fully differentiated hematopoietic cells were observed. Next to this differentiation block, an increased adhesion/clustering of hematopoietic cells in the fetal liver and less mobile progenitors in the peripheral blood were observed. It was hypothesized that the increased levels of Cxcr4 within the Zeb2 null progenitors lead to their retention in the fetal liver that resulted in less progenitors in the embryonic circulation. This decreased mobilization of hematopoietic progenitors likely contributed to the decreased levels of angiogenic factors (like Ang1) within the circulation, thereby resulting in less maturation and pericyte recruitment towards the newly formed vessels in the developing brain. Most probably this defect contributed to the observed cephalic bleeding phenotype. From this initial data it has become clear that Zeb2 is not only a crucial transcriptional regulator of hematopoietic differentiation but as well plays pivotal roles in the mobilization and homing of HSCs within the embryo (Goossens et al., 2011). More experiments need to be performed to analyze whether this also holds true in adult haematopoiesis.

3.2 Role of Zeb1 in T cell development

Neonatal Zeb1 total knockout mice die shortly after birth. Drastic skeletal abnormalities (Takagi et al., 1998) and serious thymic atrophy were observed. Through the use of a second Zeb1 loss-of-function mouse model, expressing a C-terminal zinc finger truncation allowed survival to adulthood, it was feasible to further investigate the *in vivo* role of Zeb1 in adult hematopoiesis (Higashi et al., 1997). In these ΔC-fin mice no skeletal phenotypes were observed. On the other hand T lymphocyte differentiation was drastically impaired. This observation points towards the hypothesis that different domains of Zeb1 are responsible for alternative/synergistic functions, which as well was hypothesized previously by Postigo and colleagues via their *in vitro* approaches described above (Postigo & Dean, 1999a). More detailed FACS analysis of Zeb1 ΔC-fin mutant thymocytes revealed a block at a very early stage in the cKit+ CD4-CD8-DN population, before rearrangements of the T cell receptor (TCR) locus (Higashi et al., 1997). Only a very small proportion of the intrathymic T cell precursors (<1%compared of the normal T cell development) was able to differentiate further and expressed differentiated T cell markers. These differentiated cells were skewed mainly towards CD4+CD8-SP cells, indicated that also at later stages of T cell development Zeb1 expression may play essential roles. More recently it was shown that Zeb1 binds the 5′ E-boxes in the proximal enhancer of the CD4 promoter and competes with the transcriptional activators E12 and HEB for DNA binding. Therefore it was concluded that overexpression of Zeb1 in T cells converts the CD4 proximal enhancer into a silencer element leading to a reduction of CD4 expression. This data shows that the CD4 gene is a direct target of the transcriptional repressor Zeb1 and can explain the increased proportion of CD4+CD8-SP mature T cells in Zeb1 mutant mice (Brabletz et al., 1999).

Another known downstream target of Zeb1 during myogenesis is α4-integrin. Also in hematopoietic differentiation of various lineages α4-integrin is known to play crucial roles through its interaction with fibronectin and V-CAM in the stromal matrix and stromal cells of the bone marrow and fetal liver. α4-integrin is highly expressed in stem and progenitor cells and upon further differentiation its expression is restricted to lymphocytes and myeloid subpopulations. Zeb1 binds and directly represses α4-integrin expression (Postigo & Dean, 1999a). Previously it was shown that α4 integrin expression depends on C-Myb and Ets family of transcription factors. Based on *in vitro* α4-intregrin promotor analysis, Postigo (Postigo & Dean, 1997) concluded that Zeb1 blocks activity of c-Myb and Ets individually but together these synergize to overcome Zeb1 repression. Next to CD4 and α4 integrin, Zeb1 has been suggested to repress a number of other genes implicated in proper T cell differentiation like Gata3 (Gregoire & Romeo, 1999), immunoglobin heavy chain enhancer (Genetta et al.,1994) and interleukin-2 (Williams T.M. et al., 1991; Yasui et al., 1998).

Within B-lymphocytes a functional cooperation between FoxO transcription factors and Zeb1 has been revealed. Zeb1 binds and activates two promotors of known FoxO target genes cyclin G2 and retinoblastoma-like 2. Both have been implicated in cell cycle arrest and Foxo-dependent quiescence in fibroblasts (Chen et al., 2006). However a role of Zeb1 in B-cell development has not been reported

3.3 Role of Zeb1/2 in T and B cell acute lymphoblastic leukemia

Using the same ΔC-fin Zeb1 mutant mice described above it was demonstrated that expression of the truncated Zeb1 protein resulted in the development of spontaneous CD4[+] T-cell lymphomas with a median onset at 30 weeks of age. This is consistent with the fact that ZEB1 expression is frequently lost in human adult T-cell leukemia/lymphoma (T-ALL) patients (Hidaka et al., 2008; Vermeer et al., 2008). In T-ALL cell lines it was demonstrated that the tumour cell's resistance to TGF-β mediated growth suppression is via up-regulation of the inhibitory Smad7 (Nakahata et al., 2010). Here the role of Zeb proteins in the regulation of Smad7 remains needs to be better understood. Similarly the actual role of the other above described Zeb1 targets remains to be determined in T cell lymphomas.

The role of Zeb1 in B-Cell leukemia has not been reported. However, in terms of hematological malignancy, some independent genome-wide retroviral insertional mutagenesis screens have identified Zeb2 and not Zeb1 as a possible gene involved in mouse B-cell lymphoma progression (Lund et al., 2002; Mikkers et al., 2002; Shin et al., 2004). From these initial studies it was not clear if Zeb2 expression is lost due to retroviral integration and translocation events or enhanced during the transformation process. More recently in CALM-AF10 transgenic mice, enhanced Zeb2 expression was found to correlate with increased leukemia progression (Caudell et al., 2010). Additionally, knockdown of Zeb2 in a B-ALL cell line resulted in decreased proliferation rates. However *in vivo* Zeb2 overexpression studies are missing to be conclusive concerning the role of Zeb2 in leukemogenesis. Nevertheless, ZEB2 genomic locus rearrangements are commonly associated with aggressive B cell lymphomas in humans as well (Matteucci et al., 2008).

4. Conclusions

From the above literature survey it is clear that EMT inducers of the Snai and Zeb families play crucial and yet specific roles during various stages of hematopoiesis and leukemic transformation. These specific roles are in some way surprising given that they all bind similar E box-containing DNA sequences and a significant overlap in target genes has been reported. This can in some ways be explained by differences in their expression patterns and/or the recruitment of other cell-specific co-repressors and/or activators.

As well, the above reviewed data clearly indicate crucial roles for the EMT inducers of the Zeb and Snai family in different aspects of hematopoiesis: differentiation, proliferation, apoptosis/survival, mobilization, stemness, as well as quiescence. All of this suggests that these two family of proteins might be excellent targets for developing novel and improved cancer therapies not only as was suggested before for solid tumours but as well for blood-borne cancers and other haematological defects associated with improper lineage differentiation.

5. Acknowledgment

This work was partially supported by the European Hematology Association (EHA Young Investigator Fellowship 2009/26 to SG). SG is a postdoctoral fellow of the Basic Science Research Foundation-Flanders (FWO).

6. References

Al-Hajj, M., Wicha, M.S., Benito-Hernandez, A., Morrison, S.J. & Clarke, M.F. (2003) Prospective identification of tumorigenic breast cancer cells. *Proceedings of the National Academy of Sciences of the United States of America,* Vol.100, No.7, pp. 3983-3988

Batlle, E., Sancho, E., Franci, C., Dominguez, D., Monfar, M., Baulida, J. & Garcia De Herreros, A. (2000) The transcription factor snail is a repressor of e-cadherin gene expression in epithelial tumour cells. *Nature cell biology,* Vol.2, No.2, pp. 84-89

Berx, G., Raspe, E., Christofori, G., Thiery, J.P. & Sleeman, J.P. (2007) Pre-emting metastasis? Recapitulation of morphogenetic processes in cancer. *Clinical & experimental metastasis,* Vol.24, No.8, pp. 587-597

Boisset, J.C., van Cappellen, W., Andrieu-Soler, C., Galjart, N., Dzierzak, E. & Robin, C. In vivo imaging of haematopoietic cells emerging from the mouse aortic endothelium. *Nature,* Vol.464, No.7285, pp. 116-120

Bonnet, D. & Dick, J.E. (1997) Human acute myeloid leukemia is organized as a hierarchy that originates from a primitive hematopoietic cell. *Nature medicine,* Vol.3, No.7, pp. 730-737

Boulay, J.L., Dennefeld, C. & Alberga, A. (1987) The drosophila developmental gene snail encodes a protein with nucleic acid binding fingers. *Nature,* Vol.330, No.6146, pp. 395-398

Brabletz, T., Jung, A., Hlubek, F., Lohberg, C., Meiler, J., Suchy, U. & Kirchner, T. (1999) Negative regulation of cd4 expression in t cells by the transcriptional repressor zeb. *International immunology,* Vol.11, No.10, pp. 1701-1708

Cano, A., Perez-Moreno, M.A., Rodrigo, I., Locascio, A., Blanco, M.J., del Barrio, M.G., Portillo, F. & Nieto, M.A. (2000) The transcription factor snail controls epithelial-mesenchymal transitions by repressing e-cadherin expression. *Nature cell biology,* Vol.2, No.2, pp. 76-83

Carver, E.A., Jiang, R., Lan, Y., Oram, K.F. & Gridley, T. (2001) The mouse snail gene encodes a key regulator of the epithelial-mesenchymal transition. *Molecular and cellular biology*, Vol.21, No.23, pp. 8184-8188

Caudell, D., Harper, D.P., Novak, R.L., Pierce, R.M., Slape, C., Wolff, L. & Aplan, P.D. (2010) Retroviral insertional mutagenesis identifies zeb2 activation as a novel leukemogenic collaborating event in calm-af10 transgenic mice. *Blood*, Vol.115, No.6, pp. 1194-1203

Chabot, B., Stephenson, D.A., Chapman, V.M., Besmer, P. & Bernstein, A. (1988) The proto-oncogene c-kit encoding a transmembrane tyrosine kinase receptor maps to the mouse w locus. *Nature*, Vol.335, No.6185, pp. 88-89

Chen, J., Yusuf, I., Andersen, H.M. & Fruman, D.A. (2006) Foxo transcription factors cooperate with delta ef1 to activate growth suppressive genes in b lymphocytes. *Journal of immunology*, Vol.176, No.5, pp. 2711-2721

Chua, H.L., Bhat-Nakshatri, P., Clare, S.E., Morimiya, A., Badve, S. & Nakshatri, H. (2007) Nf-kappab represses e-cadherin expression and enhances epithelial to mesenchymal transition of mammary epithelial cells: Potential involvement of zeb-1 and zeb-2. *Oncogene*, Vol.26, No.5, pp. 711-724

Clark, S.G. & Chiu, C. (2003) C. Elegans zag-1, a zn-finger-homeodomain protein, regulates axonal development and neuronal differentiation. *Development*, Vol.130, No.16, pp. 3781-3794

Cobaleda, C., Perez-Caro, M., Vicente-Duenas, C. & Sanchez-Garcia, I. (2007) Function of the zinc-finger transcription factor snai2 in cancer and development. *Annual review of genetics*, Vol.41, pp. 41-61

Comijn, J., Berx, G., Vermassen, P., Verschueren, K., van Grunsven, L., Bruyneel, E., Mareel, M., Huylebroeck, D. & van Roy, F. (2001) The two-handed e box binding zinc finger protein sip1 downregulates e-cadherin and induces invasion. *Molecular Cell*, Vol.7, No.6, pp. 1267-1278

Copeland, N.G., Gilbert, D.J., Cho, B.C., Donovan, P.J., Jenkins, N.A., Cosman, D., Anderson, D., Lyman, S.D. & Williams, D.E. (1990) Mast cell growth factor maps near the steel locus on mouse chromosome 10 and is deleted in a number of steel alleles. *Cell*, Vol.63, No.1, pp. 175-183

Costantino, M.E., Stearman, R.P., Smith, G.E. & Darling, D.S. (2002) Cell-specific phosphorylation of zfhep transcription factor. *Biochemical and biophysical research communications*, Vol.296, No.2, pp. 368-373

de Bruijn, M.F., Ma, X., Robin, C., Ottersbach, K., Sanchez, M.J. & Dzierzak, E. (2002) Hematopoietic stem cells localize to the endothelial cell layer in the midgestation mouse aorta. *Immunity*, Vol.16, No.5, pp. 673-683

De Craene, B., van Roy, F. & Berx, G. (2005) Unraveling signalling cascades for the snail family of transcription factors. *Cellular signalling*, Vol.17, No.5, pp. 535-547

del Barrio, M.G. & Nieto, M.A. (2002) Overexpression of snail family members highlights their ability to promote chick neural crest formation. *Development*, Vol.129, No.7, pp. 1583-1593

Dzierzak, E. & Medvinsky, A. (2008) The discovery of a source of adult hematopoietic cells in the embryo. *Development*, Vol.135, No.14, pp. 2343-2346

Dzierzak, E. & Speck, N.A. (2008) Of lineage and legacy: The development of mammalian hematopoietic stem cells. *Nature immunology*, Vol.9, No.2, pp. 129-136

Eger, A., Aigner, K., Sonderegger, S., Dampier, B., Oehler, S., Schreiber, M., Berx, G., Cano, A., Beug, H. & Foisner, R. (2005) Deltaef1 is a transcriptional repressor of e-cadherin and regulates epithelial plasticity in breast cancer cells. *Oncogene,* Vol.24, No.14, pp. 2375-2385

Fleming, W.H., Alpern, E.J., Uchida, N., Ikuta, K. & Weissman, I.L. (1993) Steel factor influences the distribution and activity of murine hematopoietic stem cells in vivo. *Proceedings of the National Academy of Sciences of the United States of America,* Vol.90, No.8, pp. 3760-3764

Fortini, M.E., Lai, Z.C. & Rubin, G.M. (1991) The drosophila zfh-1 and zfh-2 genes encode novel proteins containing both zinc-finger and homeodomain motifs. *Mechanisms of development,* Vol.34, No.2-3, pp. 113-122

Geissler, E.N., Ryan, M.A. & Housman, D.E. (1988) The dominant-white spotting (w) locus of the mouse encodes the c-kit proto-oncogene. *Cell,* Vol.55, No.1, pp. 185-192

Genetta, T., Ruezinsky, D. & Kadesch, T. (1994) Displacement of an e-box-binding repressor by basic helix-loop-helix proteins: Implications for b-cell specificity of the immunoglobulin heavy-chain enhancer. *Molecular and cellular biology,* Vol.14, No.9, pp. 6153-6163

Giebel, L.B. & Spritz, R.A. (1991) Mutation of the kit (mast/stem cell growth factor receptor) protooncogene in human piebaldism. *Proceedings of the National Academy of Sciences of the United States of America,* Vol.88, No.19, pp. 8696-8699

Gill, J.G., Langer, E.M., Lindsley, R.C., Cai, M., Murphy, T.L. & Murphy, K.M. (2011) Snail promotes the cell-autonomous generation of flk1+ endothelial cells through the repression of the mir-200 family. *Stem cells and development,* in press.

Goossens, S., Janzen, V., Bartunkova, S., Yokomizo, T., Drogat, B., Crisan, M., Haigh, K., Seuntjens, E., Umans, L., Riedt, T., Bogaert, P., Haenebalcke, L., Berx, G., Dzierzak, E., Huylebroeck, D. & Haigh, J.J. (2011) The emt regulator zeb2/sip1 is essential for murine embryonic hematopoietic stem/progenitor cell differentiation and mobilization. *Blood,* Vol.117, No.21, pp. 5620-5630

Grau, Y., Carteret, C. & Simpson, P. (1984) Mutations and chromosomal rearrangements affecting the expression of snail, a gene involved in embryonic patterning in drosophila melanogaster. *Genetics,* Vol.108, No.2, pp. 347-360

Greenburg, G. & Hay, E.D. (1982) Epithelia suspended in collagen gels can lose polarity and express characteristics of migrating mesenchymal cells. *The Journal of cell biology,* Vol.95, No.1, pp. 333-339

Gregoire, J.M. & Romeo, P.H. (1999) T-cell expression of the human gata-3 gene is regulated by a non-lineage-specific silencer. *The Journal of biological chemistry,* Vol.274, No.10, pp. 6567-6578

Grimes, H.L., Chan, T.O., Zweidler-McKay, P.A., Tong, B. & Tsichlis, P.N. (1996) The gfi-1 proto-oncoprotein contains a novel transcriptional repressor domain, snag, and inhibits g1 arrest induced by interleukin-2 withdrawal. *Molecular and cellular biology,* Vol.16, No.11, pp. 6263-6272

Grooteclaes, M.L. & Frisch, S.M. (2000) Evidence for a function of ctbp in epithelial gene regulation and anoikis. *Oncogene,* Vol.19, No.33, pp. 3823-3828

Gupta, P.B., Chaffer, C.L. & Weinberg, R.A. (2009) Cancer stem cells: Mirage or reality? *Nature medicine,* Vol.15, No.9, pp. 1010-1012

Hale, J.S., Dahlem, T.J., Margraf, R.L., Debnath, I., Weis, J.J. & Weis, J.H. (2006) Transcriptional control of pactolus: Evidence of a negative control region and comparison with its evolutionary paralogue, cd18 (beta2 integrin). *Journal of leukocyte biology*, Vol.80, No.2, pp. 383-398

Hidaka, T., Nakahata, S., Hatakeyama, K., Hamasaki, M., Yamashita, K., Kohno, T., Arai, Y., Taki, T., Nishida, K., Okayama, A., Asada, Y., Yamaguchi, R., Tsubouchi, H., Yokota, J., Taniwaki, M., Higashi, Y. & Morishita, K. (2008) Down-regulation of tcf8 is involved in the leukemogenesis of adult t-cell leukemia/lymphoma. *Blood*, Vol.112, No.2, pp. 383-393

Higashi, Y., Moribe, H., Takagi, T., Sekido, R., Kawakami, K., Kikutani, H. & Kondoh, H. (1997) Impairment of t cell development in deltaef1 mutant mice. *The Journal of experimental medicine*, Vol.185, No.8, pp. 1467-1479

Higashi, Y., Maruhashi, M., Nelles, L., Van de Putte, T., Verschueren, K., Miyoshi, T., Yoshimoto, A., Kondoh, H. & Huylebroeck, D. (2002) Generation of the floxed allele of the sip1 (smad-interacting protein 1) gene for cre-mediated conditional knockout in the mouse. *Genesis*, Vol.32, No.2, pp. 82-84

Huang, E., Nocka, K., Beier, D.R., Chu, T.Y., Buck, J., Lahm, H.W., Wellner, D., Leder, P. & Besmer, P. (1990) The hematopoietic growth factor kl is encoded by the sl locus and is the ligand of the c-kit receptor, the gene product of the w locus. *Cell*, Vol.63, No.1, pp. 225-233

Inoue, A., Seidel, M.G., Wu, W., Kamizono, S., Ferrando, A.A., Bronson, R.T., Iwasaki, H., Akashi, K., Morimoto, A., Hitzler, J.K., Pestina, T.I., Jackson, C.W., Tanaka, R., Chong, M.J., McKinnon, P.J., Inukai, T., Grosveld, G.C. & Look, A.T. (2002) Slug, a highly conserved zinc finger transcriptional repressor, protects hematopoietic progenitor cells from radiation-induced apoptosis in vivo. *Cancer cell*, Vol.2, No.4, pp. 279-288

Inukai, T., Inoue, A., Kurosawa, H., Goi, K., Shinjyo, T., Ozawa, K., Mao, M., Inaba, T. & Look, A.T. (1999) Slug, a ces-1-related zinc finger transcription factor gene with antiapoptotic activity, is a downstream target of the e2a-hlf oncoprotein. *Molecular Cell*, Vol.4, No.3, pp. 343-352

Jung, C.L., Kim, H.J., Kim, D.H., Huh, H., Song, M.J. & Kim, S.H. (2011) Ckit mutation in therapy-related acute myeloid leukemia with mllt3/mll chimeric transcript from t(9;11)(p22;q23). *Annals of clinical and laboratory science*, Vol.41, No.2, pp. 193-196

Kajita, M., McClinic, K.N. & Wade, P.A. (2004) Aberrant expression of the transcription factors snail and slug alters the response to genotoxic stress. *Molecular and cellular biology*, Vol.24, No.17, pp. 7559-7566

Kalluri, R. (2009) Emt: When epithelial cells decide to become mesenchymal-like cells. *The Journal of clinical investigation*, Vol.119, No.6, pp. 1417-1419

Kalluri, R. & Weinberg, R.A. (2009) The basics of epithelial-mesenchymal transition. *The Journal of clinical investigation*, Vol.119, No.6, pp. 1420-1428

Knight, R.D. & Shimeld, S.M. (2001) Identification of conserved c2h2 zinc-finger gene families in the bilateria. *Genome biology*, Vol.2, No.5, pp. RESEARCH0016

Kondo, M., Wagers, A.J., Manz, M.G., Prohaska, S.S., Scherer, D.C., Beilhack, G.F., Shizuru, J.A. & Weissman, I.L. (2003) Biology of hematopoietic stem cells and progenitors: Implications for clinical application. *Annual review of immunology*, Vol.21, pp. 759-806

LaBonne, C. & Bronner-Fraser, M. (2000) Snail-related transcriptional repressors are required in xenopus for both the induction of the neural crest and its subsequent migration. *Developmental biology,* Vol.221, No.1, pp. 195-205

Li, R., Liang, J., Ni, S., Zhou, T., Qing, X., Li, H., He, W., Chen, J., Li, F., Zhuang, Q., Qin, B., Xu, J., Li, W., Yang, J., Gan, Y., Qin, D., Feng, S., Song, H., Yang, D., Zhang, B., Zeng, L., Lai, L., Esteban, M.A. & Pei, D. (2010) A mesenchymal-to-epithelial transition initiates and is required for the nuclear reprogramming of mouse fibroblasts. *Cell stem cell,* Vol.7, No.1, pp. 51-63

Lin, Y., Wu, Y., Li, J., Dong, C., Ye, X., Chi, Y.I., Evers, B.M. & Zhou, B.P. (2010) The snag domain of snail1 functions as a molecular hook for recruiting lysine-specific demethylase 1. *The EMBO journal,* Vol.29, No.11, pp. 1803-1816

Liu, J., Uygur, B., Zhang, Z., Shao, L., Romero, D., Vary, C., Ding, Q. & Wu, W.S. (2010) Slug inhibits proliferation of human prostate cancer cells via downregulation of cyclin d1 expression. *The Prostate,* Vol.70, No.16, pp. 1768-1777

Liu, Y., El-Naggar, S., Darling, D.S., Higashi, Y. & Dean, D.C. (2008) Zeb1 links epithelial-mesenchymal transition and cellular senescence. *Development,* Vol.135, No.3, pp. 579-588

Lomeli, H., Starling, C. & Gridley, T. (2009) Epiblast-specific snail1 deletion results in embryonic lethality due to multiple vascular defects. *BMC research notes,* Vol.2, pp. 22

Lund, A.H., Turner, G., Trubetskoy, A., Verhoeven, E., Wientjens, E., Hulsman, D., Russell, R., DePinho, R.A., Lenz, J. & van Lohuizen, M. (2002) Genome-wide retroviral insertional tagging of genes involved in cancer in cdkn2a-deficient mice. *Nature genetics,* Vol.32, No.1, pp. 160-165

Lyons, J.G., Patel, V., Roue, N.C., Fok, S.Y., Soon, L.L., Halliday, G.M. & Gutkind, J.S. (2008) Snail up-regulates proinflammatory mediators and inhibits differentiation in oral keratinocytes. *Cancer research,* Vol.68, No.12, pp. 4525-4530

Mancini, M., Petta, S., Iacobucci, I., Salvestrini, V., Barbieri, E. & Santucci, M.A. (2010) Zinc-finger transcription factor slug contributes to the survival advantage of chronic myeloid leukemia cells. *Cellular signalling,* Vol.22, No.8, pp. 1247-1253

Mani, S.A., Guo, W., Liao, M.J., Eaton, E.N., Ayyanan, A., Zhou, A.Y., Brooks, M., Reinhard, F., Zhang, C.C., Shipitsin, M., Campbell, L.L., Polyak, K., Brisken, C., Yang, J. & Weinberg, R.A. (2008) The epithelial-mesenchymal transition generates cells with properties of stem cells. *Cell,* Vol.133, No.4, pp. 704-715

Manzanares, M., Locascio, A. & Nieto, M.A. (2001) The increasing complexity of the snail gene superfamily in metazoan evolution. *Trends in genetics,* Vol.17, No.4, pp. 178-181

Matteucci, C., Bracci, M., Barba, G., Carbonari, M., Casato, M., Visentini, M., Pulsoni, A., Varasano, E., Roti, G., La Starza, R., Crescenzi, B., Martelli, M.F., Fiorilli, M. & Mecucci, C. (2008) Different genomic imbalances in low- and high-grade hcv-related lymphomas. *Leukemia,* Vol.22, No.1, pp. 219-222

Mauhin, V., Lutz, Y., Dennefeld, C. & Alberga, A. (1993) Definition of the DNA-binding site repertoire for the drosophila transcription factor snail. *Nucleic acids research,* Vol.21, No.17, pp. 3951-3957

Mejlvang, J., Kriajevska, M., Vandewalle, C., Chernova, T., Sayan, A.E., Berx, G., Mellon, J.K. & Tulchinsky, E. (2007) Direct repression of cyclin d1 by sip1 attenuates cell cycle progression in cells undergoing an epithelial mesenchymal transition. *Molecular biology of the cell*, Vol.18, No.11, pp. 4615-4624

Migliaccio, G., Migliaccio, A.R., Valinsky, J., Langley, K., Zsebo, K., Visser, J.W. & Adamson, J.W. (1991) Stem cell factor induces proliferation and differentiation of highly enriched murine hematopoietic cells. *Proceedings of the National Academy of Sciences of the United States of America*, Vol.88, No.16, pp. 7420-7424

Mikkers, H., Allen, J., Knipscheer, P., Romeijn, L., Hart, A., Vink, E. & Berns, A. (2002) High-throughput retroviral tagging to identify components of specific signaling pathways in cancer. *Nature genetics*, Vol.32, No.1, pp. 153-159

Miranda-Saavedra, D. & Gottgens, B. (2008) Transcriptional regulatory networks in haematopoiesis. *Current opinion in genetics & development*, Vol.18, No.6, pp. 530-535

Murray, D., Precht, P., Balakir, R. & Horton, W.E., Jr. (2000) The transcription factor deltaef1 is inversely expressed with type ii collagen mrna and can repress col2a1 promoter activity in transfected chondrocytes. *The Journal of biological chemistry*, Vol.275, No.5, pp. 3610-3618

Murray, S.A., Carver, E.A. & Gridley, T. (2006) Generation of a snail1 (snai1) conditional null allele. *Genesis*, Vol.44, No.1, pp. 7-11

Murray, S.A., Oram, K.F. & Gridley, T. (2007) Multiple functions of snail family genes during palate development in mice. *Development*, Vol.134, No.9, pp. 1789-1797

Nakahata, S., Yamazaki, S., Nakauchi, H. & Morishita, K. (2010) Downregulation of zeb1 and overexpression of smad7 contribute to resistance to tgf-beta1-mediated growth suppression in adult t-cell leukemia/lymphoma. *Oncogene*, Vol.29, No.29, pp. 4157-4169

Nieto, M.A. (2002) The snail superfamily of zinc-finger transcription factors. *Nature reviews*, Vol.3, No.3, pp. 155-166

Nishikawa, S., Kusakabe, M., Yoshinaga, K., Ogawa, M., Hayashi, S., Kunisada, T., Era, T., Sakakura, T. & Nishikawa, S. (1991) In utero manipulation of coat color formation by a monoclonal anti-c-kit antibody: Two distinct waves of c-kit-dependency during melanocyte development. *The EMBO journal*, Vol.10, No.8, pp. 2111-2118

Okuda, T., van Deursen, J., Hiebert, S.W., Grosveld, G. & Downing, J.R. (1996) Aml1, the target of multiple chromosomal translocations in human leukemia, is essential for normal fetal liver hematopoiesis. *Cell*, Vol.84, No.2, pp. 321-330

Orkin, S.H. (2000) Diversification of haematopoietic stem cells to specific lineages. *Nature reviews*, Vol.1, No.1, pp. 57-64

Orkin, S.H. & Zon, L.I. (2008) Hematopoiesis: An evolving paradigm for stem cell biology. *Cell*, Vol.132, No.4, pp. 631-644

Ozturk, N., Erdal, E., Mumcuoglu, M., Akcali, K.C., Yalcin, O., Senturk, S., Arslan-Ergul, A., Gur, B., Yulug, I., Cetin-Atalay, R., Yakicier, C., Yagci, T., Tez, M. & Ozturk, M. (2006) Reprogramming of replicative senescence in hepatocellular carcinoma-derived cells. *Proceedings of the National Academy of Sciences of the United States of America*, Vol.103, No.7, pp. 2178-2183

Palis, J., Chan, R.J., Koniski, A., Patel, R., Starr, M. & Yoder, M.C. (2001) Spatial and temporal emergence of high proliferative potential hematopoietic precursors during murine embryogenesis. *Proceedings of the National Academy of Sciences of the United States of America*, Vol.98, No.8, pp. 4528-4533

Papin, C., van Grunsven, L.A., Verschueren, K., Huylebroeck, D. & Smith, J.C. (2002) Dynamic regulation of brachyury expression in the amphibian embryo by xsip1. *Mechanisms of development*, Vol.111, No.1-2, pp. 37-46

Perez-Losada, J., Sanchez-Martin, M., Rodriguez-Garcia, A., Sanchez, M.L., Orfao, A., Flores, T. & Sanchez-Garcia, I. (2002) Zinc-finger transcription factor slug contributes to the function of the stem cell factor c-kit signaling pathway. *Blood*, Vol.100, No.4, pp. 1274-1286

Perez-Losada, J., Sanchez-Martin, M., Perez-Caro, M., Perez-Mancera, P.A. & Sanchez-Garcia, I. (2003) The radioresistance biological function of the scf/kit signaling pathway is mediated by the zinc-finger transcription factor slug. *Oncogene*, Vol.22, No.27, pp. 4205-4211

Perez-Mancera, P.A., Gonzalez-Herrero, I., Perez-Caro, M., Gutierrez-Cianca, N., Flores, T., Gutierrez-Adan, A., Pintado, B., Sanchez-Martin, M. & Sanchez-Garcia, I. (2005a) Slug in cancer development. *Oncogene*, Vol.24, No.19, pp. 3073-3082

Perez-Mancera, P.A., Perez-Caro, M., Gonzalez-Herrero, I., Flores, T., Orfao, A., de Herreros, A.G., Gutierrez-Adan, A., Pintado, B., Sagrera, A., Sanchez-Martin, M. & Sanchez-Garcia, I. (2005b) Cancer development induced by graded expression of snail in mice. *Human Molecular Genetics*, Vol.14, No.22, pp. 3449-3461

Perez-Mancera, P.A., Gonzalez-Herrero, I., Maclean, K., Turner, A.M., Yip, M.Y., Sanchez-Martin, M., Garcia, J.L., Robledo, C., Flores, T., Gutierrez-Adan, A., Pintado, B. & Sanchez-Garcia, I. (2006) Slug (snai2) overexpression in embryonic development. *Cytogenetic and Genome Research*, Vol.114, No.1, pp. 24-29

Postigo, A.A. & Dean, D.C. (1997) Zeb, a vertebrate homolog of drosophila zfh-1, is a negative regulator of muscle differentiation. *The EMBO journal*, Vol.16, No.13, pp. 3935-3943

Postigo, A.A. & Dean, D.C. (1999a) Independent repressor domains in zeb regulate muscle and t-cell differentiation. *Molecular and cellular biology*, Vol.19, No.12, pp. 7961-7971

Postigo, A.A. & Dean, D.C. (1999b) Zeb represses transcription through interaction with the corepressor ctbp. *Proceedings of the National Academy of Sciences of the United States of America*, Vol.96, No.12, pp. 6683-6688

Postigo, A.A., Ward, E., Skeath, J.B. & Dean, D.C. (1999) Zfh-1, the drosophila homologue of zeb, is a transcriptional repressor that regulates somatic myogenesis. *Molecular and cellular biology*, Vol.19, No.10, pp. 7255-7263

Postigo, A.A. & Dean, D.C. (2000) Differential expression and function of members of the zfh-1 family of zinc finger/homeodomain repressors. *Proceedings of the National Academy of Sciences of the United States of America*, Vol.97, No.12, pp. 6391-6396

Postigo, A.A. (2003) Opposing functions of zeb proteins in the regulation of the tgfbeta/bmp signaling pathway. *The EMBO journal*, Vol.22, No.10, pp. 2443-2452

Postigo, A.A., Depp, J.L., Taylor, J.J. & Kroll, K.L. (2003) Regulation of smad signaling through a differential recruitment of coactivators and corepressors by zeb proteins. *The EMBO journal*, Vol.22, No.10, pp. 2453-2462

Redmer, T., Diecke, S., Grigoryan, T., Quiroga-Negreira, A., Birchmeier, W. & Besser, D. (2011) E-cadherin is crucial for embryonic stem cell pluripotency and can replace oct4 during somatic cell reprogramming. *EMBO reports*, Vol.12, No.7, pp. 720-726

Remacle, J.E., Kraft, H., Lerchner, W., Wuytens, G., Collart, C., Verschueren, K., Smith, J.C. & Huylebroeck, D. (1999) New mode of DNA binding of multi-zinc finger transcription factors: Deltaef1 family members bind with two hands to two target sites. *The EMBO journal*, Vol.18, No.18, pp. 5073-5084

Ricci-Vitiani, L., Lombardi, D.G., Pilozzi, E., Biffoni, M., Todaro, M., Peschle, C. & De Maria, R. (2007) Identification and expansion of human colon-cancer-initiating cells. *Nature*, Vol.445, No.7123, pp. 111-115

Robin, C., Ottersbach, K., Boisset, J.C., Oziemlak, A. & Dzierzak, E. (2011) Cd41 is developmentally regulated and differentially expressed on mouse hematopoietic stem cells. *Blood*, Vol.117, No.19, pp. 5088-5091

Rybtsov, S., Sobiesiak, M., Taoudi, S., Souilhol, C., Senserrich, J., Liakhovitskaia, A., Ivanovs, A., Frampton, J., Zhao, S. & Medvinsky, A. (2011) Hierarchical organization and early hematopoietic specification of the developing hsc lineage in the agm region. *The Journal of experimental medicine*, Vol.208, No.6, pp. 1305-1315

Sanchez-Martin, M., Perez-Losada, J., Rodriguez-Garcia, A., Gonzalez-Sanchez, B., Korf, B.R., Kuster, W., Moss, C., Spritz, R.A. & Sanchez-Garcia, I. (2003) Deletion of the slug (snai2) gene results in human piebaldism. *American journal of medical genetics*, Vol.122A, No.2, pp. 125-132

Sayan, A.E., Griffiths, T.R., Pal, R., Browne, G.J., Ruddick, A., Yagci, T., Edwards, R., Mayer, N.J., Qazi, H., Goyal, S., Fernandez, S., Straatman, K., Jones, G.D., Bowman, K.J., Colquhoun, A., Mellon, J.K., Kriajevska, M. & Tulchinsky, E. (2009) Sip1 protein protects cells from DNA damage-induced apoptosis and has independent prognostic value in bladder cancer. *Proceedings of the National Academy of Sciences of the United States of America*, Vol.106, No.35, pp. 14884-14889

Schatton, T., Frank, N.Y. & Frank, M.H. (2009) Identification and targeting of cancer stem cells. *BioEssays*, Vol.31, No.10, pp. 1038-1049

Sefton, M., Sanchez, S. & Nieto, M.A. (1998) Conserved and divergent roles for members of the snail family of transcription factors in the chick and mouse embryo. *Development*, Vol.125, No.16, pp. 3111-3121

Shin, M.S., Fredrickson, T.N., Hartley, J.W., Suzuki, T., Akagi, K. & Morse, H.C., 3rd (2004) High-throughput retroviral tagging for identification of genes involved in initiation and progression of mouse splenic marginal zone lymphomas. *Cancer research*, Vol.64, No.13, pp. 4419-4427

Singh, S.K., Clarke, I.D., Hide, T. & Dirks, P.B. (2004) Cancer stem cells in nervous system tumors. *Oncogene*, Vol.23, No.43, pp. 7267-7273

Spaderna, S., Schmalhofer, O., Hlubek, F., Berx, G., Eger, A., Merkel, S., Jung, A., Kirchner, T. & Brabletz, T. (2006) A transient, emt-linked loss of basement membranes indicates metastasis and poor survival in colorectal cancer. *Gastroenterology*, Vol.131, No.3, pp. 830-840

Spoelstra, N.S., Manning, N.G., Higashi, Y., Darling, D., Singh, M., Shroyer, K.R., Broaddus, R.R., Horwitz, K.B. & Richer, J.K. (2006) The transcription factor zeb1 is aberrantly expressed in aggressive uterine cancers. *Cancer research*, Vol.66, No.7, pp. 3893-3902

Sun, Y., Shao, L., Bai, H., Wang, Z.Z. & Wu, W.S. (2010) Slug deficiency enhances self-renewal of hematopoietic stem cells during hematopoietic regeneration. *Blood*, Vol.115, No.9, pp. 1709-1717

Takagi, T., Moribe, H., Kondoh, H. & Higashi, Y. (1998) Deltaef1, a zinc finger and homeodomain transcription factor, is required for skeleton patterning in multiple lineages. *Development*, Vol.125, No.1, pp. 21-31

Thiery, J.P. & Sleeman, J.P. (2006) Complex networks orchestrate epithelial-mesenchymal transitions. *Nature reviews*, Vol.7, No.2, pp. 131-142

Thiery, J.P., Acloque, H., Huang, R.Y. & Nieto, M.A. (2009) Epithelial-mesenchymal transitions in development and disease. *Cell*, Vol.139, No.5, pp. 871-890

van Grunsven, L.A., Taelman, V., Michiels, C., Opdecamp, K., Huylebroeck, D. & Bellefroid, E.J. (2006) Deltaef1 and sip1 are differentially expressed and have overlapping activities during xenopus embryogenesis. *Developmental dynamics*, Vol.235, No.6, pp. 1491-1500

van Grunsven, L.A., Taelman, V., Michiels, C., Verstappen, G., Souopgui, J., Nichane, M., Moens, E., Opdecamp, K., Vanhomwegen, J., Kricha, S., Huylebroeck, D. & Bellefroid, E.J. (2007) Xsip1 neuralizing activity involves the co-repressor ctbp and occurs through bmp dependent and independent mechanisms. *Developmental biology*, Vol.306, No.1, pp. 34-49

Vandewalle, C., Comijn, J., De Craene, B., Vermassen, P., Bruyneel, E., Andersen, H., Tulchinsky, E., Van Roy, F. & Berx, G. (2005) Sip1/zeb2 induces emt by repressing genes of different epithelial cell-cell junctions. *Nucleic acids research*, Vol.33, No.20, pp. 6566-6578

Vandewalle, C., Van Roy, F. & Berx, G. (2009) The role of the zeb family of transcription factors in development and disease. *Cellular and molecular life sciences*, Vol.66, No.5, pp. 773-787

Vermeer, M.H., van Doorn, R., Dijkman, R., Mao, X., Whittaker, S., van Voorst Vader, P.C., Gerritsen, M.J., Geerts, M.L., Gellrich, S., Soderberg, O., Leuchowius, K.J., Landegren, U., Out-Luiting, J.J., Knijnenburg, J., Ijszenga, M., Szuhai, K., Willemze, R. & Tensen, C.P. (2008) Novel and highly recurrent chromosomal alterations in sezary syndrome. *Cancer research*, Vol.68, No.8, pp. 2689-2698

Verschueren, K., Remacle, J.E., Collart, C., Kraft, H., Baker, B.S., Tylzanowski, P., Nelles, L., Wuytens, G., Su, M.T., Bodmer, R., Smith, J.C. & Huylebroeck, D. (1999) Sip1, a novel zinc finger/homeodomain repressor, interacts with smad proteins and binds to 5'-cacct sequences in candidate target genes. *The Journal of biological chemistry*, Vol.274, No.29, pp. 20489-20498

Verstappen, G., van Grunsven, L.A., Michiels, C., Van de Putte, T., Souopgui, J., Van Damme, J., Bellefroid, E., Vandekerckhove, J. & Huylebroeck, D. (2008) Atypical mowat-wilson patient confirms the importance of the novel association between zfhx1b/sip1 and nurd corepressor complex. *Human Molecular Genetics*, Vol.17, No.8, pp. 1175-1183

Wang, Y., Mah, N., Prigione, A., Wolfrum, K., Andrade-Navarro, M.A. & Adjaye, J. (2010) A transcriptional roadmap to the induction of pluripotency in somatic cells. *Stem cell reviews*, Vol.6, No.2, pp. 282-296

Wellner, U., Schubert, J., Burk, U.C., Schmalhofer, O., Zhu, F., Sonntag, A., Waldvogel, B., Vannier, C., Darling, D., zur Hausen, A., Brunton, V.G., Morton, J., Sansom, O., Schuler, J., Stemmler, M.P., Herzberger, C., Hopt, U., Keck, T., Brabletz, S. & Brabletz, T. (2009) The emt-activator zeb1 promotes tumorigenicity by repressing stemness-inhibiting micrornas. *Nature cell biology*, Vol.11, No.12, pp. 1487-1495

Williams, N., Bertoncello, I., Kavnoudias, H., Zsebo, K. & McNiece, I. (1992) Recombinant rat stem cell factor stimulates the amplification and differentiation of fractionated mouse stem cell populations. *Blood*, Vol.79, No.1, pp. 58-64

Williams, T.M., Moolten, D., Burlein, J., Romano, J., Bhaerman, R., Godillot, A., Mellon, M., Rauscher, F.J., 3rd & Kant, J.A. (1991) Identification of a zinc finger protein that inhibits il-2 gene expression. *Science,* Vol.254, No.5039, pp. 1791-1794

Wu, W.S., Heinrichs, S., Xu, D., Garrison, S.P., Zambetti, G.P., Adams, J.M. & Look, A.T. (2005) Slug antagonizes p53-mediated apoptosis of hematopoietic progenitors by repressing puma. *Cell,* Vol.123, No.4, pp. 641-653

Wu, Y. & Zhou, B.P. (2010) Snail: More than emt. *Cell adhesion & migration,* Vol.4, No.2, pp. 199-203

Yang, C.C. & Wolf, D.A. (2009) Inflamed snail speeds metastasis. *Cancer cell,* Vol.15, No.5, pp. 355-357

Yasui, D.H., Genetta, T., Kadesch, T., Williams, T.M., Swain, S.L., Tsui, L.V. & Huber, B.T. (1998) Transcriptional repression of the il-2 gene in th cells by zeb. *Journal of immunology,* Vol.160, No.9, pp. 4433-4440

Yokomizo, T., Ng, C.E., Osato, M. & Dzierzak, E. (2011) Three-dimensional imaging of whole midgestation murine embryos shows an intravascular localization for all hematopoietic clusters. *Blood,* Vol.117, No.23, pp. 6132-6134

Yoshihara, K., Tajima, A., Komata, D., Yamamoto, T., Kodama, S., Fujiwara, H., Suzuki, M., Onishi, Y., Hatae, M., Sueyoshi, K., Fujiwara, H., Kudo, Y., Inoue, I. & Tanaka, K. (2009) Gene expression profiling of advanced-stage serous ovarian cancers distinguishes novel subclasses and implicates zeb2 in tumor progression and prognosis. *Cancer science,* Vol.100, No.8, pp. 1421-1428

Zhuge, X., Kataoka, H., Tanaka, M., Murayama, T., Kawamoto, T., Sano, H., Togi, K., Yamauchi, R., Ueda, Y., Xu, Y., Nishikawa, S., Kita, T. & Yokode, M. (2005) Expression of the novel snai-related zinc-finger transcription factor gene smuc during mouse development. *International journal of molecular medicine,* Vol.15, No.6, pp. 945-948

Zovein, A.C., Turlo, K.A., Ponec, R.M., Lynch, M.R., Chen, K.C., Hofmann, J.J., Cox, T.C., Gasson, J.C. & Iruela-Arispe, M.L. (2010) Vascular remodeling of the vitelline artery initiates extravascular emergence of hematopoietic clusters. *Blood,* Vol.116, No.18, pp. 3435-3444

Zsebo, K.M., Williams, D.A., Geissler, E.N., Broudy, V.C., Martin, F.H., Atkins, H.L., Hsu, R.Y., Birkett, N.C., Okino, K.H., Murdock, D.C. & et al. (1990) Stem cell factor is encoded at the sl locus of the mouse and is the ligand for the c-kit tyrosine kinase receptor. *Cell,* Vol.63, No.1, pp. 213-224

3

Negative Regulation of Haematopoiesis: Role of Inhibitory Adaptors

Laura Velazquez

UMR U978 Inserm/Université Paris 13, UFR SMBH, Bobigny
France

1. Introduction

Cytokine signalling is initiated through ligand interaction with specific members of the cytokine receptor superfamily. The subsequent receptor oligomerization and conformational change result in activation of either an intrinsic kinase domain or receptor associated kinases, notably the Janus (JAK) family of cytoplasmic tyrosine kinases. The activated JAKs phosphorylate tyrosine residues in the receptor and subsequently downstream substrates, such as the signal transducers and activators of transcription (STAT) proteins. Once recruited to the receptor complex, STAT proteins are themselves phosphorylated on tyrosine, dimerize and translocate into the nucleus, where they activate the transcription of genes mediating cytokine-induced responses (Ortmann et al., 2000). Cytokines also activate other signaling cascades, such as the Ras/Mitogen-Activated Protein Kinase (MAPK) and the Phosphoinositide 3-kinase (PI3K)/Akt pathways. These cascades have been implicated in the proliferation, survival, and differentiation of several cell types in the haematopoietic system (Geest and Coffer, 2009; Leevers et al., 1999. However, all these signalling pathways require precise cellular control and their deregulation has been implicated in haematopoietic disorders, autoimmune and chronic inflammatory diseases and cancer, making it important to understand the mechanisms by which these cytokine-mediated signalling pathways are controlled (Schade et al., 2006; Khwaja, 2006).

It is therefore not surprising that multiple levels of control have evolved to finely modulate the threshold, magnitude and specific responses elicited by cytokine stimulation. This regulation is achieved through both positive and negative mechanisms. The aim of the present chapter is to review the current advances in the regulation of haematopoiesis, with special interest on inhibitory pathways. Understanding how haematopoiesis is modulated is essential to provide useful information on its physiological functioning, the pathological origin of many related haematological disorders and to yield potential therapeutic targets.

2. Regulation of cytokine signalling pathways: Role of adaptor proteins

Cytokine binding to their receptors results in tyrosine autophosphorylation of the associated tyrosine kinase and of the receptor cytoplasmic domain at sites where specific signalling molecules can bind. In this way, the cytoplasmic domain of these cytokine receptors serves to initially localize the signalling response to the plasma membrane. It is the combination of the signalling proteins that are recruited to the receptor that then determines the quality of the response that is generated. Indeed, the location of the proteins inside the cell and the kinetics of their activation are important features of signal-transduction pathways. How the signalling molecules are localized in the cell and how the strength and quality of the signal is regulated is an area of intense research, and increasing attention has focused on the so-called adaptor proteins as key molecules controlling these more complex aspects of signal transduction.

Adaptor proteins lack enzymatic activity or other direct effector function. Adaptors can be transmembrane proteins, reside in the cytoplasm under resting conditions and be recruited to the membrane upon activation, or be localized by specific interactions in intracellular compartments. Regardless of their cellular localization, they possess an array of binding sites and modules that allow them to mediate specific protein-protein and protein-lipid interactions. Examples of binding domains in adaptors include Src-homology 2 (SH2) and Phosphotyrosine-binding (PTB) domains that bind to phosphotyrosine motifs, SH3 domains that bind to proline-rich sequences and Pleckstrin homology (PH) domain that recognizes phospholipids (Pawson and Scott, 1996). With an assemblage of modules and binding sequences, a single adaptor can serve as a scaffold protein for the binding of multiple proteins into complexes, bringing in this way effectors into close proximity to their targets. However, the general ability of adaptor proteins to amplify or inhibit signalling, highly depends on their cell-specific expression and level, as well as on that of their binding partners, their location in the cell, the stability of the interactions between the adaptor and its targets and in certain conditions, on the basal kinase/phosphatase activity in the cell.

Lastly, it should be noted that the domains and motifs found in adaptors are also frequently present in enzymatically active molecules, such as tyrosine phosphatases of the SH2-containing phosphatase (SHP) family and the ubiquitin ligases Casitas B-cell lineage lymphoma (c-Cbl) proteins, where they can mediate true adaptor-like functions and also orchestrate signalling complex formation.

3. Inhibitory adaptors in cytokine signalling regulation

New insights into the biology of adaptor protein function have been possible with the use of a variety of biochemical, cellular and imaging techniques, as well as *in vivo* genetic approaches. All these techniques have helped establish that adaptor proteins can affect the thresholds and the dynamics of signalling reactions by coordinating positive and negative feedback signals. Over the years, the majority of investigations on cytokine signalling pathways have mainly focused on the mechanisms of cytokine-receptor activation, whereas our knowledge of negative regulation has been less explored. However, the most recent research has placed increasing emphasis on the mechanisms by which cytokine signals are attenuated or terminated. Indeed, stringent mechanisms of signal attenuation are essential for ensuring an appropriate, controlled cellular response following cytokine stimulation. One could imagine how the aberrant assembly of macromolecular active signalling complexes could lead to disease: excess positive signalling or insufficient negative signalling may lead to autoimmunity, chronic inflammation or malignant transformation, while excess negative signalling or insufficient positive signalling may lead to immunodeficiency or certain haematological disorders.

A number of mechanisms have been proposed to regulate the initiation, duration, magnitude and specificity of cytokine signalling at multiple levels: 1) receptor internalization and inhibition mediated by soluble receptor antagonists and/or specific inhibitors (such as the Lnk and Dok adaptor proteins); 2) tyrosine dephosphorylation of the receptor and signalling intermediates mediated by tyrosine phosphatases; 3) proteosomal degradation of signalling molecules mediated by the suppressors of cytokine signalling (SOCS) proteins and the Cbl E3 ubiquitin ligases proteins; and lastly 4) transcriptional suppression mediated by specific inhibitors such as the protein inhibitors of activated STATs (PIAS) proteins. In this section, we review what is currently known about the function and regulation of four families of inhibitory adaptor proteins that are key players in some of the regulatory mechanisms mentioned above. These families are the DOK, the Lnk/SH2B3, the Cbl and the SOCS proteins. We first discuss the adaptors without catalytic activity (DOK and Lnk), followed by those possessing an enzymatic function (Cbl and SOCS). The latter ones are also known as scaffold proteins; however we will refer to them as adaptors in hopes that this distinction provides a clear picture on the different properties of each.

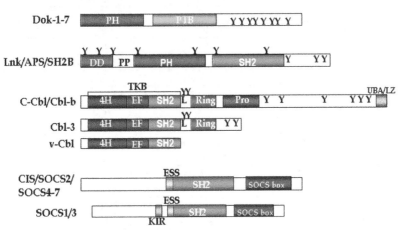

Fig. 1. Schematic representation of the domain structure of inhibitory adaptors

3.1 The DOK family

3.1.1 Structure and cell expression

The Dok (Downstream Of Tyrosine Kinases) family of adaptor proteins consists of seven members, Dok 1 to Dok-7, that differ in the length of their C-terminal region. They are all characterized by an N-terminal PH domain, a central PTB domain and multiple SH2 and SH3 binding motifs in the C-terminal region (Figure 1). Dok-1 (p62[dok]), Dok-2 (p56[dok-2], also called Dok-R, or FRIP) and Dok-3 (also called DokL) are preferentially expressed in the haematopoietic compartment, as well as co-expressed in haematopoietic progenitors (Carpino et al., 1997; Yamanashi et al., 1997; Di Cristofano et al., 1998; Lemay et al., 2000). All three Dok proteins are expressed in myeloid cells, but differ in their lymphoid lineage expression. While Dok-1 and Dok-2 are highly expressed in T cells, Dok-3 is little or not detected at all. In contrast, Dok-1 and Dok-3 are expressed in B cells, while Dok-2 is not normally detected in these cells. Moreover, several studies have demonstrated that Dok-1 and Dok-2 expression was up or down-regulated, respectively, by different signalling pathways in immune cells. Dok-1 expression was upregulated in response to the glucocorticoid dexamethasone in RBL-2H3 mast cells (Hiragun et al., 2005). By contrast, its expression was downregulated in bone marrow-derived macrophages in response to lipopolysaccharide (LPS) [Shinohara et al., 2005]. As for Dok-2, its expression increased in response to cytokines such as M-CSF, granulocyte–macrophage colony stimulating factor (GM-CSF), and interleukin-3 (IL-3) in NFS-60 myeloid leukemia cells, suggesting its implication in a negative feedback loop for the regulation of these cytokine pathways (Suzu et al., 2000). The other Dok proteins, Dok-4 (IRS5), Dok-5 (IRS6), Dok-6 and Dok-7 are mainly expressed in non-haematopoietic cells, notably in neural cells. However, Dok-4 was reported to function as negative regulator in human T cells (Favre et al., 2003).

Dok protein	Binding domain	Binding partner	Signalling Receptor
Dok-1	PTB	Abl	BCR
		SHIP-1	FcγRIIB
		Dok-1, Dok-2	CD2
		TCRε	idem
	pY	CD3ε	idem
		p120RasGap	BCR, CD2+CD28, FcεRI
		Abl, Lyn	BCR
		Nck	FcεRI
		SHIP-1	FcγRIIB, FcεRI
Dok-2	PTB	SHIP-1	FcγRIIB
		Dok-1, Dok-2	CD2
		TCRε, CD3ε	idem
	pY	p120RasGAP,Abl	BCR
		Nck	TCR
Dok-3	PTB	SHIP-1, Abl	FcγRIIB
		Dok-3	BCR
	pY	Grb2	BCR
		SHIP-1	FcγRIIB

Table 1. Signalling partners bound to the different domains and motifs of Dok proteins

3.1.2 Signalling partners

The biological functions of the Dok proteins have been defined with the identification and functional analysis of their binding partners, as well as of their subcellular localization. Dok-1 was the first member of this family identified as a tyrosine-phosphorylated 62 kDa substrate of both v-ABL and BCR-ABL and associated with p120RasGap, a negative regulator of Ras. Several studies have later shown that Dok-1/2/3 can be tyrosine phosphorylated by a variety of growth factors, cytokines and immuno receptors, providing multiple docking sites for SH2 and PTB-containing proteins such as Nck, SHP-1, SHIP-1 and p120RasGap (Table 1). The interaction between p120RasGap and Dok-1/2 has been the most extensively studied and the one likely responsible for the negative regulation of the Ras/Erk pathway mediated by the Dok adaptors. It involves the SH2 domain of p120RasGap and its binding motifs present in the C-terminal moiety of Dok-1/2 (Songyang et al., 2001). In contrast, Dok-3 protein has no YxxP motifs and therefore is unable to associate with p120 RasGap. However, it can negatively regulate Erk activation through its binding with Grb2 (Honma et al., 2006). Fewer signalling molecules have been reported to associate with the PTB domain of Dok-1/2/3 (Table 1). Interestingly, these Dok proteins show homotypic and heterotypic (for Dok-1/2) oligomerization that is dependent on their tyrosine phosphorylation and PTB domains. Moreover, this oligomerization appears crucial to their function, at least for Dok-1/2 (Boulay et al., 2005). Instead, the functional relevance of Dok-3 oligomerization is not yet clear (Stork et al., 2007). The presence of a PH domain in the structure of Dok proteins suggests an important role for this domain in the localization or translocation of the Dok adaptors to cellular membranes. Indeed, it seems that Dok-1 and PI3K activity are required for the recruitment of the adaptor to the membrane and its negative effect on PDGF-mediated ERK activation. Furthermore, Dok-1/2 PH domain can bind tightly to PI(5)P and modulate the negative function and tyrosine phosphorylation of the adaptors in T-cells (Guittard et al., 2009). Conversely, the PH domain of Dok-3 is important for its localization to the membrane in B cells (Stork et al., 2007).

3.1.3 Signalling pathways in immune cells

Studies with Dok-1/2/3 deficient mice and/or cells have helped demonstrate the physiological importance of these inhibitory adaptors to the function and development of immune cells. Using *Dok-1*-deficient splenic B cells, Yamanashi et al. demonstrated a negative role of Dok-1 in antigen receptor-mediated signalling through suppression of MAPK activity and cell proliferation (Yamanashi et al., 2000). Moreover, co-cross-linking of the B-cell receptor (BCR) and FcγRIIB receptor induces the tyrosine phosphorylation of Dok-1 and its subsequent association with RasGap (Vuica et al., 1997). In FcγRIIB signalling, Dok-1 is recruited to the receptor complex at the membrane via SHIP, and in this way, contributes to the negative regulation of the Erk pathway [Figure 2.] (Tamir et al., 2000). On the other hand, Dok-3 is also expressed in B cells and therefore, one can expect a functional redundancy between Dok-1/3 in these cells. Indeed, it was reported that Dok-3 can function as a negative regulator of BCR-mediated responses (Ng et al., 2007). Furthermore, both Dok-1 and Dok-3 were shown to be phosphorylated by Lyn kinase after stimulation of the BCR, suggesting that Lyn can activate these Dok proteins to then function as negative regulators in B cells (Yamanashi et al., 2000; Stork et al., 2007). However, B cells from *Dok-3*-deficient mice exhibited augmented proliferation and Ca^{2+} influx upon BCR stimulation (Ng et al., 2007), while these responses are not observed in the absence of Dok-1 (Yamanashi et al., 2000). These phenotypic differences could be attributed to Dok-1, but not Dok-3, recruiting p120RasGAP, which can inhibit Ras/Erk signalling; by contrast, Dok-3, but not Dok-1, can recruit Grb2, which can then inhibit Ca^{2+} signalling in B cells.

Dok-1 and Dok-2 adaptor proteins have been also shown to play a role in the maintenance of T-cell homeostasis. In some cell line systems, Dok-1 is phosphorylated by Lck kinase and associates with RasGap upon CD2 and CD28 stimulation, but not CD3-TCR engagement, indicating a possible role of Dok-1 in T cell signalling (Nemorin & Duplay, 2000). Furthermore, overexpression of Dok-2 results in a dramatic reduction in both thymocytes and splenic T-cell numbers, suggesting a negative role of Dok-2 in T-cell development

(Gugasyan et al., 2002). Although the molecular mechanisms underlying the Dok-mediated inhibition are unclear, Dok proteins can bind to the ITAM motifs of TCRζ and CD3ε through their PTB domain. As these ITAMs are essential for the binding and activation of ZAP-70, interference between the Dok proteins and ZAP-70 might occur through their binding to the ITAMs (Figure 2). Recently, Nunès and colleagues reported that the PH domain of Dok-1 and Dok-2 is necessary for the tyrosine phosphorylation of these Dok proteins and their negative functions in T cells (Guittard et al., 2009). These results demonstrate the functional relevance of the membrane localization of the Dok adaptors.

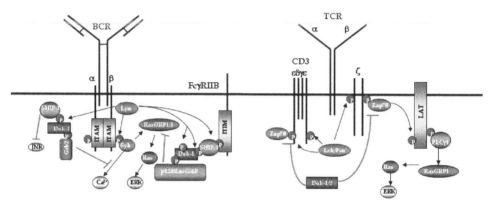

Fig. 2. Dok-mediated signalling pathways in immune cells

Unlike lymphoid cells, myeloid cells express all the immune cell Dok proteins. However, the loss of Dok-1 and Dok-2 causes mainly neoplastic abnormalities in myeloid cells, suggesting an important role in immune and cytokine receptor signalling in these cells. Analysis of *Dok-1* and *Dok-2* deficient myeloid cells showed enhanced proliferation and survival in response to Stem Cell Factor (SCF), IL-3, macrophage-colony stimulating factor (M-CSF), and granulocyte-monocyte-colony stimulating factor (GM-CSF), which are cytokines crucial for myelopoiesis. These findings indicate that Dok-1 and Dok-2 act as key negative regulators of signalling downstream of these cytokine receptors. Indeed, the activation of Erk and Akt in macrophages deficient for *Dok-1* and *Dok-2* was strongly augmented compared with that in wild type controls upon M-CSF receptor stimulation, confirming the role of Dok adaptors as negative regulators for these pathways. On the other hand, the role of Dok-1 and Dok-2 was examined in innate immune signalling in macrophages. Stimulation of macrophages by LPS induces rapid tyrosine phosphorylation of Dok-1 and Dok-2, suggesting the involvement of these adaptors in TLR4 signalling (Shinohara et al., 2005). In addition, the stimulation of *Dok-1* or *Dok-2*-deficient macrophages promoted the activation of Erk and hyperproduction of TNF-α and nitric oxide, two major signalling mediators of innate immunity, indicating that the Dok proteins are key negative regulators of TLR4 signalling in macrophages. The Dok adaptors are also expressed in mast cells where they have been shown to interact exclusively with negative regulators of FcεRI signalling. FcεRI stimulation leads to the tyrosine phosphorylation of only Dok-1 and Dok-2. Nevertheless, Dok-3 associates with tyrosine-phosphorylated proteins upon FcεRI stimulation, implicating a yet undefined function for this adaptor protein downstream of the receptor (Abramson et al., 2003). A complex of Dok-1, RasGAP, and SHIP-1, similar to the one described in B cells after co-aggregation of the BCR with FcγRIIB, was also described in mast cells after FcεRI and FcγRIIB co-aggregation (Ott et al., 2002). Moreover, Dok-1 has also been involved downstream of activating receptors, like FcεRI, by associating with and negatively regulating signals without the involvement of inhibitory receptors (Ott et al., 2002; Abramson et al., 2003). However, Dok-1-deficiency did not affect mast cell activation, suggesting a possible functional redundancy among the different isoforms expressed in these cells.

Recently, two groups have reported the expression and function of the Dok proteins in human platelets. Using a proteomic approach in these cells, it was shown that Dok proteins are tyrosine phosphorylated downstream of main platelet activation receptors (Garcia et al., 2004; Hughan et al., 2007; Senis et al., 2009). Tyrosine phosphorylation of Dok-1 and Dok-3 was primarily Src kinase-independent downstream of the integrin pathway, whereas it was Src-dependent downstream of glycoprotein VI (GPVI) pathway. Both proteins interact in an inducible-fashion with Grb-2 and SHIP-1 in fibrinogen-spread platelets, suggesting that the formation of a multi-molecular negative signalling complex may be a mechanism of down-regulating αIIbβ3 outside-in signalling.

3.2 The Lnk/SH2B family

3.2.1 Structure, origin and cell expression

The Lnk (or SH2B) family of adaptor proteins is composed of 3 members, SH2-B [also known as PSM (proline-rich, PH and SH2 domain-containing signalling mediator) or SH2B1], APS (for Adaptor protein with PH and SH2 domain, also known as SH2B2) and Lnk (SH2B3). They all possess a dimerization (DD) domain and proline-rich motifs at the N-terminus, followed by a PH and SH2 domains, and several potential tyrosine phosphorylation sites, notably a conserved tyrosine residue at the C-terminus [Figure 1](Rudd, 2001). The SH2B1 gene encodes four isoforms (α, β, γ, δ) resulting from alternative mRNA splicing at their 3' terminus giving rise to proteins differing at their C-terminus (Nelms et al., 1999). SH2-Bα and β isoforms were originally cloned from yeast tribrid and two-hybrid systems screening, respectively, using different proteins as baits (Osborne et al., 1995; Riedel et al, 1997; Rui et al., 1997). Despite its initial identification in immune cells, SH2-B isoforms are mainly expressed and functional, as shown by gene inactivation in mice, in non-haematopoietic tissues. The APS/SH2B2 gene encodes for two isoforms, SH2B2α and recently identified SH2B2β (Li et al., 2007). The APS protein was also identified in a two-hybrid system screening of human B cells or adipocytes (Yokouchi et al., 1997; Moodie et al., 1999). Like SH2-B, APS adaptor protein is also highly expressed in non-haematopoietic tissues. However, it is also expressed in haematopoietic cells, notably in mature B and mast cells. As for Lnk, it has only one form in mammalians and one invertebrate orthologue in Drosophila melanogaster (D-Lnk) to date (Werz et al., 2009). The Lnk adaptor protein was the first member of this family identified (Huang et al., 1995; Takaki et al., 1997). However, it was later found that the Lnk protein was much larger than initially reported (Li et al., 2000; Takaki et al., 2000; Velazquez et al., 2002). In contrast to SH2-B and APS, Lnk is mainly expressed in haematopoietic cells, notably in haematopoietic stem cells (HSC), and haematopoietic (lymphoid and myeloid) progenitors. Moreover, Lnk expression is up-regulated by certain cytokines important for the development and function of these haematopoietic cells, such as SCF, thrombopoietin [TPO], and erythropoietin [EPO] (Kent et al., 2008; Buza-Vidas et al., 2006; Gerry et al., 2009a, 2009b; Baran-Marszak et al., 2010). Interestingly, Lnk is also highly expressed in endothelial cells and its expression is also induced by Tumor Necrosis Factor (TNF)-α (Fitau et al., 2006; Kwon et al., 2009). These findings suggest the implication of Lnk adaptor in a negative feedback loop for the regulation of these cytokine pathways.

3.2.2 Signalling partners

Over the last years, much effort has gone into understanding the role of the Lnk family as signalling regulators through the identification of the molecules binding to their different functional domains and motifs, as well as their signalling pathways (Table. 2). The SH2 domain of the Lnk adaptor proteins is implicated in most of the key molecular interactions between the adaptors and their partners/effectors and their biological functions. The fist identified binding partner of the Lnk protein was the SCF receptor, Kit. The primary Kit-binding site for Lnk SH2 domain has been identified as phosphotyrosine 567 (pTyr567), which resides in the juxtamembrane region of the receptor (Simon et al., 2008; Gueller et al., 2008). Similarly, the SH2 domain of APS was reported to bind to Y568 and Y936 in the human c-Kit receptor (Wollberg et al., 2003). Interestingly, this region of Kit contains critical tyrosine (Y) residues (Y567/69) for the recruitment of different regulatory signalling molecules (Chan et al., 2003). In this system, a proposed mode of action of Lnk is that once bound to the juxtamembrane region of Kit, it will then block the association of activators with the receptor, resulting in down-regulation of SCF-mediated pathways. Indeed, expression of an SH2-inactive Lnk protein abolishes Lnk-mediated negative regulation of SCF-induced cell proliferation and migration (Simon et al., 2008). Lnk has been also reported to bind through its SH2 domain to other tyrosine kinase receptors, such as the PDGFR and the M-CSF receptor (c-Fms); however the physiological implication of these associations is not yet clear (Gueller et al., 2010, 2011).

The JAK2 tyrosine kinase was the first characterized binding partner of SH2-B and APS, and subsequently of Lnk. This association results in activation of the kinase in the case of SH2-B and APS or in its inhibition when bound to Lnk. Different biochemical studies have shown that the interaction of the SH2 domains of SH2-B and APS occurs preferentially with kinase-active, tyrosyl phosphorylated JAK2 (Rui et al., 1997). The primary JAK2-binding site for the SH2 domain of the Lnk family has been identified as pTyr813, which resides within the regulatory JH2 pseudokinase domain of JAK2 (Kurzer et al., 2004, 2006). Crystallographic studies have demonstrated that the SH2 domain of APS dimerizes when binding to the insulin receptor, whereas the SH2 domain of SH2-B, binds JAK2 as a monomer (Hu et al., 2003; Hu & Hubbard, 2006). Less is known on how the Lnk SH2 domain binds JAK2. However, it has been shown that Lnk is capable of binding JAK2 wild-type form, as well as the constitutive active JAK2-V617F form present in myeloproliferative neoplasms (Bersenev et al., 2008; Gery et al., 2009; Baran-Marszak et al., 2010). In addition to the SH2-dependent interaction of the Lnk adaptor family with pTyr813 in JAK2, there appears to be one low-affinity interaction involving amino acids outside the SH2 domain in the adaptors and inactive JAK2 that might prevent abnormal activation of the kinase. (Rui et al., 2000; Kurzer et al., 2006; Baran-Marzak et al., 2010).

The N-terminal region of the Lnk adaptor family contains a dimerization domain whose crystal structure has revealed a "phenylalanine zipper" motif. This domain mediates SH2-B

Lnk proteins	Binding domain	Binding partner	Cells System
Lnk	N-term	Lnk	COS
	Inter PH-SH2	ABP-280	COS, T cells (TCR)
	SH2	Kit	Mast (SCF)
		JAK2	Myeloid (EPO, TPO)
		c-Fms	Myeloid (M-CSF)
		PDGFR	COS (PDGF)
APS	N-term	APS, SH2B	HEK293, CHO (In)
	PH	Vav3	NIH3T3
	SH2	Kit	Mast (SCF)
		JAK2	Myeloid (GH)
		IR	Adipocyte (In)
	pY618	Cbl	Adipocyte (In)
SH2B	N-term	SH2B, APS	CHO (In), COS
		Rac	CHO, COS (GH)
	SH2	JAK2	Myeloid (GH)
		GHR, IR	Adipocyte (GH, In)

GHR, growth hormone receptor; IR, insulin receptor; In, insulin

Table 2. Signalling partners bound to the different domains and motifs of Lnk proteins.

and APS homo and heterodimerization that appears crucial to their function (Dhe-Paganon et al., 2004). Instead, Lnk homodimerization has only been shown in an over-expressed system (Takizawa et al., 2006) and therefore, its functional relevance is not yet clear.

The presence of a PH domain in the structure of Lnk proteins suggests an important role for this domain in the localization or translocation of these adaptor proteins to cellular membranes. Indeed, previous reports showed that Lnk PH mutants (W191A or W270A) proteins moderately affected Lnk modulation of TPO-, EPO- or SCF-dependent biological responses (Tong & Lodish, 2004; Tong et al., 2005; Simon et al., 2008). Moreover, the Lnk PH domain seemed to display moderate affinity and little specificity to phosphoinositides *in vitro*. It is therefore possible that the Lnk PH domain may down-regulate membrane targeting of Lnk in the absence of docking site for the SH2 domain and increase binding stability to membrane receptors when the SH2 domain is engaged.

Association of Lnk, APS and SH2-B with growth factor, cytokine receptors or the JAK2 kinase allows phosphorylation of these adaptors and their proper localization at the signalling complex. The conserved C-terminal tyrosine residue present in all members of this family has been shown to be a main site for phosphorylation upon growth factor or cytokine stimulation. In Lnk, this residue, Y536, was suggested to be phosphorylated upon SCF stimulation in a mast cell line (Takaki et al., 2002). However, an Lnk form mutated at this tyrosine still gets phosphorylated upon Kit activation in primary mast cells (Simon et al., 2008). This result suggested that Lnk could be phosphorylated at sites other than Y536. Indeed, a similar result was reported with human Lnk mutated at this residue (Li et al., 2000). On the other hand, the biological relevance of Lnk Y536 seems to depend on the signalling pathway analyzed. Lnk Y536 is dispensable for lymphoid development, TPO- or SCF-dependent signalling pathways, but it might play a regulatory role in IL3- and EPO-mediated proliferation (Takaki et al., 2003; Tong & Lodish, 2004; Simon et al., 2008).

However, no Lnk binding partners for this site has so far been identified. In contrast, APS C-terminal tyrosine, Y618, has been shown to get phosphorylated by activated growth factor (IR), cytokine (EPO) and immune (BCR) receptors and then serve as binding site for the Cbl protein (Moodie et al., 1999; Yokouchi et al., 1997; Wakioka et al., 1999). The APS/Cbl association plays an important role in down-regulation of IR signalling (Kishi et al., 2007). Other binding proteins have been identified that associate with other regions of Lnk, APS and SH2-B that are involved in actin regulation. In particular, an amino acid sequence in the N-terminal region of SH2-B has been shown to bind to Rac, a mayor actin regulating protein, while a similar sequence in APS can associate with Vav3, a guanine nucleotide exchange factor for Rac (Diakonova et al., 2002; Yabana and Shibuya, 2002). Lnk was demonstrated to associate with the actin binding protein ABP-280 via a sequence between the PH and SH2 domains of human Lnk in Jurkat T cells (He et al., 2000). These findings suggest a role for the Lnk family members in the regulation of actin cytoskeleton and cell motility.

3.2.3 Signalling pathways in haematopoietic cells

The initial *in vitro* biochemical analysis was done on SH2-B and APS and showed that these adaptors were phosphorylated and became positive mediators of receptor and protein tyrosine kinases cascades. However, APS can also function as negative regulator in the BCR and JAK2 signalling pathways (Yokouchi et al., 1997; Wakioka et al., 1999). Conversely, Lnk is considered as a negative regulator of growth factor and cytokine receptor-induced proliferation and migration (Takaki et al., 2000, 2002; Velazquez et al., 2002; Tong & Lodish, 2004; Tong et al., 2005; Fitau et al., 2006; Simon et al., 2008; Gueller et al., 2010, 2011). Nonetheless, Lnk seems to play a positive role in mouse platelets for the stabilization of thrombus through the integrin $\alpha IIb\beta 3$ outside-in signalling and in human vascular endothelial cells via the PI3K/Akt pathway activated by TNF-α (Takizawa et al., 2010; Fitau et al., 2006). Together with data on *in vivo* ablation of these adaptors, these findings demonstrate that these adaptor proteins can function as positive and/or negative regulators depending on their cell expression and on the growth factor or cytokine receptor–mediated pathway.

The generation of mice and cell lines deficient for members of this family has confirmed Lnk and APS, but not SH2-B, specific function in the haematopoietic system, while establishing SH2-B implication in other tissues. As stated before, Lnk is highly expressed in HSC, so as expected, *Lnk-/-*-derived HSC show an increased capacity to proliferate and to self-renew together with an increase in the quiescent fraction. These effects on HSC homeostasis are due to abnormal TPO signalling in these cells, that results from an enhanced TPO hypersensibility, increased TPO-dependent activation of Akt, STAT5 and down-regulation of p38MAPK (Ema et al., 2005; Buza-Vidas et al., 2006; Seita et al., 2007; Bersenev et al., 2008). These findings therefore confirm that Lnk controls TPO-induced self-renewal, quiescence and proliferation of HSC. Moreover, *Lnk* deficiency enhances the ability of HSC and haematopoietic progenitors to reconstitute the haematopoietic system in irradiated hosts. Indeed, transient inhibition of endogenous Lnk significantly increased the repopulating capacity of the transduced cells and thereby, engraftment (Takizawa et al., 2006). Moreover, analysis of *Lnk-/-*-derived haematopoietic progenitors show an hypersensibility to several cytokines resulting in sustained MAPK, JAK/STAT activation and cell proliferation (Takaki et al., 2000; Velazquez et al., 2002; Tong, 2005; Takizawa et al., 2008).

Lnk-deficient mice have also revealed an essential role for Lnk in B cell lymphopoiesis with the selective expansion of pro-/pre-B and immature B cells in bone marrow and spleen. This abnormal proliferation is partly due to hypersensitivity to SCF and IL-7 (Takaki et al., 2000; Velazquez et al., 2002). Alternatively, Lnk over-expression in transgenic mice show impaired B production in an Lnk dose-dependent manner confirming the negative control mediated by this adaptor in B-lineage cell production (Takaki et al., 2003). However, no evident effect on mature B cells was observed in the absence of Lnk, suggesting either a lack of role for Lnk in this population or a functional compensation by APS in these cells. APS has also been shown to play a role in B cell development and function. Ablation of *APS* in mice caused an increase in B-1 cell number and an enhanced humoral immune response against a thymus-independent type 2 antigen, suggesting a role for APS in mature B cell proliferation (Iseki et al., 2004). Accordingly, APS transgenic mice showed reduced numbers of peritoneal B-1 and splenic B cells and impaired BCR-induced proliferation of mature B cells (Iseki et al., 2005). In these cells, APS co-localized with pre-activated capped BCR complexes and filamentous actin, indicating a negative regulatory role for APS in BCR signalling and actin reorganization.

Lnk has been also shown to control erythropoiesis and megakaryopoiesis. Studies on primary *Lnk*-/- erythrocytes and megakaryocytes indicate an abnormal proliferation due to the absence of negative regulation of EPO and TPO signalling pathways (Figure 3). Indeed, Lnk, through its SH2 domain, negatively modulates MPL, and EPO receptor (EPOR) signalling by attenuating three major signalling pathways: JAK2/STAT, MAPK and Akt (Tong et al., 2005; Tong & Lodish, 2004). Moreover, Lnk is capable of binding and regulating MPL-W515L and JAK2-V617F, the mutated forms expressed in Myeloproliferative Neoplasms [MPN] (Gery et al., 2007, 2009; Bersenev et al., 2008; Baran-Marszak et al., 2010). In addition, Lnk also regulates thrombopoiesis through control of crosstalk between integrin- and TPO-mediated pathways implicated in the megakaryocyte maturation and platelet release process (Takizawa et al., 2008). Furthermore, Lnk plays an important role in stabilizing thrombus formation through positive regulation of integrin signalling pathways. In this way, it contributes to platelet cytoskeleton rearrangement and spreading (Takizawa et al., 2010).

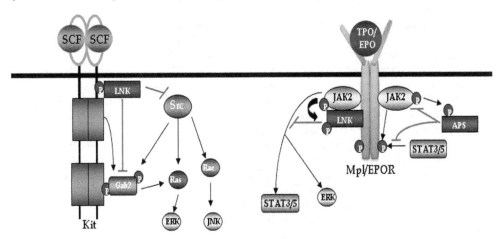

Fig. 3. Lnk family signalling pathways in haematopoietic cells

Studies on *Lnk*-/- and *APS*-/- mast cells demonstrated their physiological implication in mast-cell functions. Lnk regulates SCF-mediated signalling pathways controlling proliferation (MAPK and JNK) and migration (Rac and p38MAPK) in these cells (Takizawa et al., 2006; Simon et al., 2008). These functions are mainly mediated by binding of its SH2 domain to specific effectors involved in actin rearrangement. On the other hand, APS controls actin cytoskeleton and magnitude of degranulation induced by FcεRI receptor cross-linking (Kubo-Akashi et al., 2004). Besides its specific expression in the haematopoietic system, Lnk is also highly expressed in endothelial-like cells in the aorta-gonad-mesonephros (AGM) region and in endothelial progenitor (EPC) and mature cells [EC](Nobuhisa et al., 2003; Fitau et al., 2006; Kwon et al., 2009). Fitau *et al.* have shown that the pro-inflammatory cytokine TNF-α rapidly evokes Lnk phosphorylation together with down-regulation of vascular cell adhesion molecule 1 (VCAM-1) expression in activated vascular ECs. These results implicate Lnk as an important negative regulator of TNF-α signalling pathway (Fitau et al., 2006).

3.3 The Cbl family

3.3.1 Origin, cell expression and structure

The Cbl (for Casitas B-lineage Lymphoma) family comprises multidomain regulators with dual function, as E3 ubiquitin ligases and adaptor proteins. It consists of three mammalian homologues, c-Cbl, Cbl-b and Cbl-c/Cbl-3 (Blake et al., 1991; Keane et al., 1995, 1999), as well as invertebrate orthologues (Thien & Langdon, 2001). The first isoform of this family identified was the oncogenic protein v-Cbl, a Gag-fusion transforming protein of Cas NS-1 retrovirus, which induces pre- and pro-B lymphomas and the transformation of rodent fibroblasts (Langdon et al., 1989). The cellular form, c-Cbl was subsequently cloned and revealed that v-Cbl was a result of a large truncation of its C-terminal portion and that overexpression of c-Cbl did not promote tumorigenesis. The 120 kDa c-Cbl protein is ubiquitously expressed, primarily cytoplasmic, with highest expression levels in haematopoietic organs (thymus) and testis. In contrast, Cbl-3 is expressed mainly in epithelial cells of the gastrointestinal system.

All Cbl proteins share highly conserved N-terminal regions, but their C-terminal sequence differs and is less well-conserved (Figure 1). The N-terminal half encompasses two important domains: a tyrosine kinase-binding (TKB) and a C3HC4 zinc-binding RING finger domains, both separated by a small linker sequence. The TKB domain contains three distinct subdomains comprising a four-helix bundle (4H), a calcium-binding EF hand and a modified SH2 domain, all necessary for its function as phosphotyrosine-binding (PTB) module. The second conserved domain in the N-terminal region is a zinc-binding RING finger domain responsible for the E3 ubiquitin ligase activity of c-Cbl (Joazeiro et al., 1999). The C-terminal sequences are less homologous among Cbl proteins; however, they all have proline-rich regions that are involved in numerous SH3-domain interactions (Keane et al., 1995) and the major sites of tyrosine phosphorylation, which enable interactions of Cbl with SH2 domain containing proteins. The C-terminus of c-Cbl, Cbl-b contains a sequence homologous to both the leucine zipper (LZ) and the ubiquitin associated (UBA) domain. The LZ domain has been shown to mediate Cbl dimerization (Bartkiewicz et al., 1999; Liu et al., 2003), while only Cbl-b and not c-Cbl can bind to ubiquitin through its UBA domain (Davies et al., 2004).

3.3.2 Signalling binding partners

The TKB domain is unique to Cbl proteins and its feature role is to determine Cbl substrate specificity by engaging specific phosphorylated tyrosine residues on proteins that are to be ubiquitylated by Cbl. Some of Cbl TKB domain targets include: receptor tyrosine kinases (RTKs), non-receptor protein tyrosine kinases (PTKs) of the Syk family, several adaptors and regulatory proteins (Table 3). In contrast to SH2 binding motif, the TKB phosphotyrosine recognition consensus sequence displays an specificity conferred by amino acid residues C-terminal to the tyrosine (Lupher et al., 1997). These findings argue that interaction of the TKB domain with RTKs may then primarily be to ensure the appropriate orientation of the receptor such that Cbl's E3 ligase activity can promote the transfer of ubiquitin. TKB domain interactions may therefore determine the number of ubiquitin molecules transferred to the substrate and thus regulate the extent to which activated RTKs are ubiquitylated. Thus the TKB domain appears to have at least two important roles in regulating E3 ligase activity, and, as such, it is functionally more complex than classical SH2 or PTB domains.

Binding domain	Binding partner	Signalling receptor
TKB	Syk, Zap-70	AgR
	c-Src	AgR, GFR, CyR
	APS	HR
	EGFR, PDGFR	GFR
RING	E2s(Ub-conjugated enzyme)	GFR, AgR, CyR
Pro-rich	Grb2	GFR
	Nck	GFR, AgR
	Src kinases	GFR, AgR, CyR
pY	Vav, CrkL, Src kinases	AgR
	p85 (only with c-Cbl)	AgR, GFR
UBA	Ub (only with Cbl-b)	GFR
LZ	c-Cbl, Cbl-b	GFR, HR

AgR, antigen receptor; GFR, growth factor receptor; CyR, cytokine receptor; HR, hormone receptor.

Table 3. Signalling proteins bound to the different domains and motifs of c-Cbl/Cbl-b proteins.

Separating the TKB and the RING domains, a short linker sequence extends which has been shown crucial for Cbl ubiquitin ligase activity (Thien et al., 2001). The TKB domain makes intramolecular contacts with the linker α-helix and these contacts are centred on conserved residues Y368 and Y371 in human c-Cbl (Zheng et al., 2000). Interestingly, deletion of these tyrosines causes c-Cbl to become oncogenic (Thien et al., 2001). Molecular modelling data predicted that this structural alteration, in addition to loss of E3 activity, is required to activate fully the oncogenic potential of Cbl proteins. The second highly conserved domain among all Cbl proteins is the RING finger. *In vitro* ubiquitylation assays proved that the highly conserved Cbl RING finger has intrinsic E3 ligase activity and can independently recruit E2s or ubiquitin-conjugating (Ubc) enzymes for the transfer of ubiquitin to substrates (Joazeiro et al., 1999). The structural integrity of the RING finger domain is an absolute requirement for Cbl proteins to function as E3 ligases. Moreover, the RING finger domain acts in concert with the TKB domain to facilitate ubiquitylation and degradation of activated

PTKs, with the TKB domain conferring substrate specificity and the RING finger bringing in an E2 ubiquitin-conjugating enzyme. The carboxy-terminal half of c-Cbl is rich in proline residues, which contributes at least 15 and 17 potential SH3-domain-binding sites in c-Cbl and Cbl-b respectively, while Cbl-3 encodes five potential SH3-binding sites. Moreover, the proline-rich region in c-Cbl is also required for the ubiquitylation and proteasomal degradation of activated forms of Src (Yokouchi et al., 2001). In this case, the Cbl substrate is targeted by proline sequence interactions, rather than the TKB domain.

c-Cbl and Cbl-b are prominent substrates of RTKs and PTKs following stimulation of diverse cell surface receptors, as they possess major sites of tyrosine phosphorylation at their C-terminal part that enable them to interact with different SH2 domain containing proteins. Indeed, several studies have demonstrated the important role of tyrosine phosphorylation of Cbl proteins for their adaptor function, as well as for their E3 activity. The best-characterized phosphorylation sites are Y700, Y731 and Y774 in human c-Cbl and Y709 and Y665 in Cbl-b (Tsygankov et al., 1996; Keane et al., 1995). These residues are efficiently phosphorylated by Syk and the Src-family kinases Fyn, Yes and Lyn, but not by Lck or ZAP-70. An important difference between c-Cbl and Cbl-b is the unique presence of Y731 in c-Cbl which binds the SH2 domain of the p85 regulatory subunit of PI3K. Surprisingly, this association enables c-Cbl to function as a positive regulator by recruiting PI3K to the cell membrane (Hunter et al., 1999).

3.3.3 E3 ligase activity and adaptor function

The multi-domain nature of Cbl allows it to interact, directly or indirectly, with a wide range of signalling molecules. In this way, activated Cbl proteins act essentially as attenuators of cellular signals by exerting their function as E3 ubiquitin ligases or as adaptors/inhibitors proteins towards PTK pathways.

Cbl E3 ligase activity. Extensive biochemical studies have demonstrated Cbl-mediated ubiquitylation of its substrates (Figure 4). It is clear that ubiquitylation of a targeted receptor occurs in parallel to the onset of receptor internalization and continues to occur throughout the endosomal pathway. One of the best-studied examples of how Cbl-mediated ubiquitylation affects receptor trafficking, and helps terminate the signal from the activated receptor complex, is the EGF receptor (EGFR). This multistep process was initially described in *C. elegans*, where SLI-1 (the Cbl orthologue) was shown to negatively regulate signalling downstream of the LET-23 receptor [the EGFR orthologue] (reviewed in Thien and Langdon, 2001). This mechanism has become a model for the regulation of other RTKs by Cbl.

Cbl as an adaptor/inhibitor protein. An alternative way for Cbl to ubiquitylate EGFR is indirect and utilises its adaptor/inhibitor function by binding to the adaptor protein growth factor- receptor bound-2 (Grb2). One of the first proteins to be recruited into the complex is Grb2, which can recruit Cbl proteins from the cytoplasm to the plasma membrane through interactions between the proline-rich region of Cbl proteins and the N-terminal SH3 domain of Grb2. In this way, Cbl competes with the guanine-nucleotide-exchange factor son-of-sevenless (SOS) to bind Grb2, thereby blocking signalling through the Ras–mitogen-activated protein kinase (MAPK) pathway and inhibiting proliferation.

3.3.4 Signalling pathways in the haematopoietic and immune systems

Cbl gene deletions primarily affected the haematopoietic, immune and metabolic systems. A recent study on *c-Cbl*[-/-] HSC showed that the number and ability to reconstitute the haematopoietic system was increased in these cells compared to wild-type HSC. These results suggested that Cbl ubiquitin-mediated protein degradation is important for HSC homeostasis (Rathinam et al., 2008). Furthermore, it was shown that c-Cbl is capable of controlling HSC development and function through negative regulation of TPO-dependent STAT5 activation, an important pathway for HSC maintenance. Indeed, *c-Cbl*-deficient HSC displayed TPO hypersensibility, as well as increased levels of STAT5 and its activated form, phospho-STAT5. Thus, these findings underline the role of c-Cbl as important modulator of the TPO/Mpl/JAK/STAT5 signalling pathway in HSCs.

The importance of c-Cbl and Cbl-b in immunity and immune receptor signalling pathways has been demonstrated clearly by the phenotypes of their respective gene knockout mice. Both *c-Cbl*[-/-] and *Cbl-b*[-/-] mice display hyperactive signalling downstream of the TCR. Loss of either Cbl protein results in lower activation threshold for signalling through the TCR, hypersensitivity to low affinity/avidity engagement of the receptor, and activation of downstream signalling pathways without the normal requirement for co-receptor stimulation (Figure 4) (Murphy et al., 1998; Naramura et al., 1998; Bachmaier et al., 2000; Chiang et al., 2007). Interestingly, these c-Cbl and Cbl-b phenotypes are restricted to thymocytes and T-cells, respectively, reflecting a difference in tissue distribution with c-Cbl more prominent in the thymus and Cbl-b highly expressed in peripheral T-cells. Loss of Cbl-b dramatically increases T-cell activation threshold and uncouples T-cell activation from the requirement for CD28 co-stimulation, thus leading to spontaneous autoimmunity (Gronski et al., 2004).

Cbl proteins have been also shown to differentially modulate BCR-dependent signalling. Loss of c-Cbl in primary B cells showed a significant inhibition of BCR-mediated signalling mainly caused, not by down-regulation of Syk, but instead by up-regulation of Lyn kinase (Shao et al., 2004). In contrast, Cbl-b negatively regulates BCR-mediated signalling, this time, by down-regulating Syk in primary B cells (Sohn et al., 2003). Furthermore, the activity of Cbl proteins as adaptors was also implicated in the effect of Cbl proteins on B-cell activation. In this case, it has been shown that c-Cbl negatively regulates the phospholipase C-γ2 (PLC-γ2) pathway in B cells, while Cbl-b was shown to positively regulate this same pathway (Yasuda et al., 2002).

Studies carried out with cell lines have demonstrated that both c-Cbl and Cbl-b negatively regulated FcϵRI-mediated mast cell activation (Figure 4). However, experiments on primary mast cells derived from *c-Cbl* and *Cbl-b*-deficient mice revealed a more profound effect with the lack of Cbl-b than of c-Cbl (Zhang et al., 2004). Cbl-dependent FcϵRI down-regulation occurs mainly via Cbl E3 ubiquitin ligase activity that promotes receptor β and γ multiubiquitination, providing signals for receptor internalization and sorting into lysosomal compartments for degradation. Interestingly, Syk activity is required for c-Cbl-dependent ubiquitylation of FcϵRI receptor (Paolini et al., 2002). On the other hand, Cbl proteins can also down-modulate engaged FcϵRI through its adaptor function by interacting with molecules involved in clathrin-mediated endocytosis (Molfetta et al., 2005). Remarkably, Cbl proteins also negatively regulate mast cell activation by selectively ubiquitinating and degrading the activated kinase form of Lyn and Syk proteins (Paolini et al., 2002; Kyo et al., 2003; Qu et al., 2004).

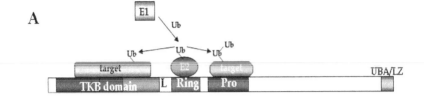

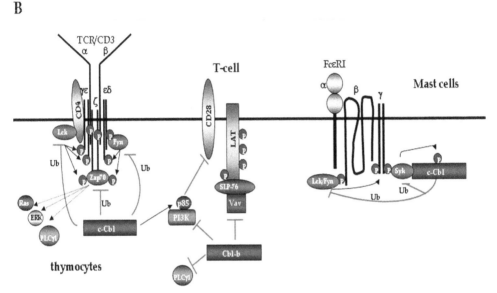

Fig. 4. A) Model of Cbl ligase activity. B) Schematic model of Cbl signalling pathways in T and mast cells

c-Cbl also participates in the modulation of monocyte/macrophage signalling mediated by Fcγ and Colony Stimulating Factor (CSF)-1 receptors through its adaptor functions. c-Cbl is capable of attenuating CSF-1-mediated signalling by binding to a phosphotyrosine residue of this receptor and then ubiquitylating and targeting it for degradation. Lastly, c-Cbl also appears to play a negative regulatory role in platelets as well. This is not so surprising considering that Syk kinase has a biological function in these cells, a known substrate of c-Cbl. The contribution of c-Cbl-dependent ubiquitylation of Syk to the negative effect of c-Cbl on platelet functions is not yet understood, however, it is possible that the biological role of c-Cbl in platelets consists in preventing unwanted platelet activation *in vivo* by increasing the threshold of platelet activation.

3.3.5 Regulation of Cbl function

Cbl proteins are potent regulators of cell function and development through their adaptor function and ligase activity. It is therefore necessary that the Cbl proteins are at their turn, subject to complex and sophisticated regulatory mechanisms that fine-tune the effects that these proteins have on signalling (Ryan et al., 2006). These include: *cis*-acting structural elements that prevent inappropriate E3 activity until the Cbl proteins interact with their substrate, degradation of the Cbl proteins, inhibition of Cbl protein function mediated by protein interactions, deubiquitination of the Cbl substrates, and negative regulation of trafficking of the ubiquitinated Cbl substrates. Therefore, abnormal Cbl regulation can lead to pathological conditions such as immunological and malignant diseases, thus underscoring the essential role of Cbl in normal homeostasis.

3.4 The SOCS family

3.4.1 Origin, structure and cellular expression

The SOCS (for Suppressors Of Cytokine Signalling) proteins are a family of intracellular molecules that negatively regulate the strength and duration of cytokine receptor signalling cascades, notably the JAK/STAT pathway. This family consists of eight members, CIS and SOCS1-7 that share structural and functional homology. The first family member identified was CIS (for Cytokine-Inducible SH2-containing protein) cloned as an early gene differentially induced following IL-3 and EPO exposure (Yoshimura et al., 1995). The second member identified, SOCS1 (also known as JAB for JAK-Binding protein or SSI for STAT-induced STAT Inhibitor) was identified simultaneously by three separate groups (Starr et al., 1997; Endo et al., 1997; Naka et al., 1997). SOCS-2 and SOCS-3 were cloned using distantly related expressed sequence tags [ESTs] and the rest of the members (SOCS4-7) were identified on the basis of a conserved C-terminal amino acid sequence using various DNA databases (Starr et al. 1997; Minamoto et al., 1997; Hilton et al., 1998). All members of the SOCS family have a similar tripartite domain organization composed of a variable N-terminal region, followed by a central SH2 domain and a conserved C-terminal SOCS box domain (Fig. 1). SOCS1 and SOCS3 differ from other family members in that they possess an extended SH2 domain at the N-terminus (for SOCS1 and SOCS3) or the C-terminus (for SOCS3) of this domain. Additionally, they also present at their N-terminal region and adjacent to their SH2 domain, a Kinase-Inhibitory Region (KIR) required for inhibition of JAK kinase activity (Yasukawa et al., 1999; Sasaki et al., 1999). Another exception is SOCS7 which is unique in its possession of a proline-rich N-terminus and a nuclear localisation signal.

SOCS molecules expression is controlled at the transcriptional, translational and post-translational levels. Many *SOCS* genes contain STAT-binding sequences in their promoter region and their STAT-dependent transcription can be differentially regulated in a factor- and tissue specific manner. SOCS proteins are often low or undetectable at the basal level in unstimulated cells and their expression is rapidly induced to a variable extent in different cell types and tissues by immunoregulatory cytokines, colony stimulating factors, growth factors and hormones that signal via JAK-STAT pathway or via RTK [Table 4] (Starr et al., 1997). Certain cytokines that do not signal via JAK kinases or RTKs, and a number of non-cytokine ligands can also induce *SOCS* gene expression, such as TNF signalling and bacterial products such as LPS and CpG DNA which signal via Toll-like receptors (TLR). Because *SOCS* genes are induced by cytokines and the corresponding proteins inhibit further cytokine-induced signalling, SOCS proteins are believed to form part of a classical negative feedback loop mechanism. Northern blot analysis of murine tissues has shown that *CIS* and *SOCS2* mRNA was ubiquitously expressed, with expression being particularly strong (CIS) or weak (SOCS2) in kidney, lung, liver, heart, testis and male spleen (Yoshimura et al., 1995; Starr et al., 1997). *SOCS1* and *SOCS3* mRNA was detected at different levels in adult haematopoietic organs such as the thymus and spleen and to some extent in other organs like lung, spleen and testis (Starr et al., 1997). However, *SOCS3* show high expression in fetal liver (Marine et al., 1999). Although some of the SOCS members appear to be co-expressed in only a few organs, the *in vivo* expression of *SOCS* genes may be more pronounced than is detectable by Northern hybridisation, since most cell types seem to depend on cytokine stimuli for SOCS induction.

3.4.2 Signalling targets

The different domains in the SOCS proteins allow them to bind to the cytokine receptors, associated JAKs or other signalling molecules and to attenuate signal transduction directly or indirectly by targeting the receptor complex for ubiquitin-mediated degradation in proteosomes. The N-terminal region of the SOCS proteins is variable in length and sequence. In SOCS1 and SOCS3, there is a 12 amino acid sequence adjacent to the SH2 domain that is essential for the inhibition of JAK2 kinase called KIR. This sequence is supposed to function via a conserved tyrosine residue as a pseudo-substrate, lodging in the catalytic cleft to block further JAK kinase activity. Removal of this tyrosine does not affect binding of the SOCS proteins to the kinase, but does abrogate its inhibition (Sasaki et al., 1999). Inded, a SOCS1-KIR mimetic peptide is sufficient to inhibit IFNγ-mediated JAK2 activity in primary cells (Waiboci et al., 2007). The role of the remaining N-terminal region among the SOCS family members has yet to be elucidated.

The central SH2 domain determines the target protein for degradation of each SOCS protein. It binds to distinct phosphorylated tyrosine motifs on SOCS target proteins (Table 4). Once the SH2 domain binds to its specific target, it brings other domains in proximity to the target protein, directing degradation of the appropriate protein. Mutagenesis studies allowed the identification of small regions at the N-termini of SOCS1 and SOCS3, and at the C-terminus of SOCS3 SH2 domains, critical for phosphotyrosine binding. These regions have been defined as an N- and C-extended SH2 domain (N-ESS and C-ESS, respectively). The solved structure of SOCS3 SH2 domain had shown that the N-ESS sequence directly contacts the phosphotyrosine-binding loop of the kinase and determines its orientation (Babon et al., 2006). The C-ESS of SOCS3 forms part of the SH2 domain that is spatially displaced by a 35 amino acid PEST [for Proline, Glutamic acid (E), Serine and Threonine rich sequence] insertion. This sequence is thought to signal for rapid proteolytic degradation. It is therefore not surprising that removal of this sequence lowers SOCS3 turnover without affecting the SH2 domain folding and function (Babon et al., 2006). Since other SOCS members contain putative PEST sequences, this may prove to be a common mechanism for regulation of SOCS protein levels.

The SOCS proteins are substrate recognition factors for an E3 ligase that targets their specific cargo for ubiquitin-mediated degradation. They serve this function by binding to the E3 complex via the highly conserved SOCS box domain at their C-terminus. The SOCS box is a 40 amino acid motif found not only in the SOCS family members, but also in a vast number of proteins. The SOCS box consists of a three-α-helical structure bound to an E3 ubiquitin ligase complex that in turn covalently binds ubiqutin to lysines in the target protein. The N-terminus of the SOCS box mediates interaction with Elongin C/B, while the C-terminus of

SOCS proteins	SH2 partner	Inducer system	Signalling system inhibited
CIS	EPOR, PRLR, Leptin R	EPO, IL-2/3/6, IFNα, PRL, GH, Leptin	EPO, PRL, IL-2/3, GH
SOCS1	JAK2, IFNGRI	EPO, TPO, GM-CSF, G-CSF,M-CSF,IL-2/4/6/7/9/10/13/15, PRL, LPS, TNFα, GH, In, CpG DNA	IL-2/4/6/7/12/15, IFNα/β/γ, LIF, TNFα, EPO, TPO, GH, PRL, In, Leptin
SOCS2	GHR, Leptin R	GH, IL-6, IFNα/γ, LIF	IL-6, GH, IGF-1
SOCS3	EPOR, gp130, G-CSFR, IL-12Rβ2, Leptin R	IL-1, TGF-β, IL-2/6/9/10/13, GH, LPS, EGF, IFNα/γ, LIF, EPO, GM-CSF, PRL, In, Leptin	IL-2/4/6/9/11, IFNα/β/γ, LIF, EPO, GH, PRL, In, Leptin
SOCS4, SOCS5	EGFR	EGF, IL-6	EGF, IL-4/6
SOCS6, SOCS7	IRS2/4, IR	In, IGF	In, IGF

In, insulin; PRL, prolacftin.

Table 4. Signalling partners, transduction pathways and factors regulating SOCS protein expression and function.

the SOCS box directs the SOCS/Elongin C/B association with Cullin 5 (Cul5) scaffold protein (Zhang et al., 1999). The latter one recruits the stabilizing RING finger protein Rbx and allows Cul5 to bind to an E2 ubiquitin-conjugating enzyme. The resulting complex SOCS/Elongin B/C/Cul5/Rbx/E2 forms a functional E3 ubiquitin ligase (Figure 5a). The SOCS1-SOCS box has been shown to be capable of driving the ubiquitination of specific proteins such as TEL-JAK2 fusion and Vav1, and only in very few cases the receptor complex for subsequent degradation through the proteosome (Frantsve et al., 2001; De Sepulveda et al., 2000; Irandoust et al., 2007; Verdier et al., 1998). The importance of the SOCS box has been further shown by *in vivo* targeted deletion of SOCS1 and SOCS3 in mice that resulted in partial loss of SOCS function with enhanced IFNγ and G-CSF signalling, respectively (Zhang et al., 2001).

3.4.3 Regulation of cytokine receptor signalling pathways

The structural analysis of the SOCS molecules revealed they can control cytokine receptor signalling by several mechanisms (Figure 5):

(1) Direct inhibition of intrinsic kinase activity by binding to JAKs. Immunoprecipitation assays revealed that both SOCS1 and SOCS3 were able to co-precipitate with JAK kinases upon cytokine stimulation, and that this association blocked JAK kinase activity, although with a different affinity and kinetics (Endo et al., 1997; Sasaki et al., 1999). Structure-function studies using truncated versions of SOCS1 identified the regions essential for SOCS-JAK association and for inhibition of JAK activity. SOCS1 inhibits tyrosine kinase activity upon interaction with phosphorylated tyrosine Y1007 located in the activation loop of JAK.

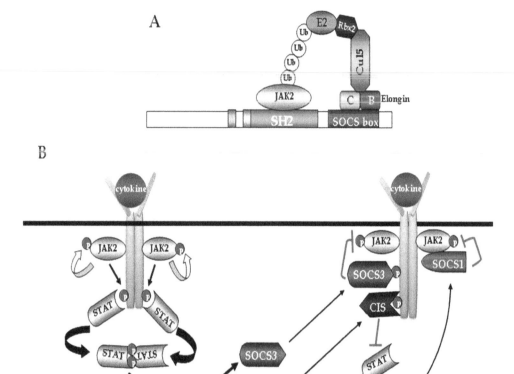

Fig. 5. A) Schematic representation of the SOCS box function, B) Mechanisms of suppression by the SOCS proteins.

However, complete inhibition of the kinase activity requires not only the SH2 domain but also the KIR region (Narazaki et al., 1998; Nicholson et al., 1999). The critical amino acids for the KIR region's function are conserved between SOCS1 and SOCS3, suggesting a common inhibitory mechanism for these two family members.

(2) Indirect inhibition of JAKs by binding to the receptor. As with SOCS1, the SOCS3 SH2 domain was initially shown to interact with Y1007 in JAK2, albeit with lower affinity than SOCS1. However, subsequent studies demonstrated that SOCS3 SH2 domain exhibited a higher affinity for phosphotyrosine residues located within the receptor subunits than for JAK2 (Sasaki et al., 1999). Accordingly, it was found that SOCS3 associated with higher affinity with phosphorylated residues in the IL-6 receptor subunit, gp130, notably Y759, than with the activation loop of JAKs (Nicholson et al., 2000). SOCS3, therefore, in contrast to SOCS1, has to be recruited to the receptor complex in order to inhibit IL-6 signal transduction (Schmitz et al., 2000). Subsequently, SOCS3 might inhibit the kinase activity of JAKs through the pseudo-substrate, KIR, in the same way as SOCS1, but only after recruitment and binding to critical phosphotyrosine residues in the cytokine receptor. Given that SOCS1 and SOCS3 can interact with both receptor and JAK, a two-step interaction model has been proposed, whereby the SOCS1/3 SH2 domains are first recruited to the receptor and subsequent bi-modal binding to nearby JAK through the SH2 domain and KIR region results in a high affinity interaction, inhibition of JAK kinase activity and potential proteosomal degradation.

(3) Blocking binding of downstream signalling molecules to the receptor. This mechanism has been shown for CIS and SOCS2 for EPO and GH signalling inhibition, respectively. Upon stimulation of the receptors, the SOCS proteins bind to tyrosine residues at the membrane distal region of receptor chains that are docking sites for downstream signalling molecules, such as STAT5 or SHP-2. By masking these phosphorylated residues, CIS/SOCS2 competes with STAT thereby down-modulating the signalling (Yoshimura et al., 1995; Ram & Waxman, 1999). On the other hand, SOCS3-mediated inhibition of signalling via EpoR, gp130 and LeptinR could partially result from competitive inhibition of SHP-2 binding to gp130, LeptinR, and EpoR, resulting in the blockade of SHP-2-mediated ERK activation (Schmitz et al., 2000; Bjorbaek et al., 2001; Sasaki et al., 2000).

(4) Ubiquitination and subsequent proteasomal degradation of JAKs and receptor. Studies on EPO receptor using proteasome inhibitors showed that these compounds protected the EpoR and STAT5 from the normal reduction in phosphorylation upon CIS expression, indicating proteasome involvement of both EPO-receptor and STAT5 inactivation (Verdier et al., 1998). These results allow proposing a model where the phosphorylated target molecules may become a substrate of the proteolytic machinery by binding to SOCS. In this situation, the SOCS box acts as an adaptor molecule, bringing into this complex the Elongin B/C/E3 ligase for ubiquitination of the target protein. Subsequently, the substrate and the associated SOCS proteins may be destroyed, and the cell is ready to respond again to stimulation. Therefore, targeting the signalling proteins for degradation by the SOCS box seems to be another mechanism by which cytokine signalling might be inhibited under physiological levels of SOCS proteins.

3.4.4 Regulation of SOCS proteins

Besides elaborate transcriptional regulation, another control point of the expression of SOCS molecules is their protein stability. SOCS proteins exhibit a rapid turnover rate, and the half lives of SOCS1, SOCS2 and SOCS3 have been estimated to be less than 2 h (Siewert et al., 1999). Several mechanisms have been proposed to regulate SOCS expression. The presence of a PEST sequence in SOCS3 appears to mediate non-proteosomal degradation, while SOCS box-dependent ubiquitination of SOCS3 on lysine 6, at least *in vitro*, contributes to proteosomal degradation of the SOCS3 protein (Sasaki et al., 2003). Furthermore, SOCS3 is uniquely phosphorylated within the SOCS box on Y204 and Y221 and this appears to have two consequences, interaction with the Elongin B/C complex is lost, destabilizing the SOCS3 protein, and signalling through the Ras/MAPK pathway can be potentiated (Haan et al., 2003; Cacalano et al., 2001). Nevertheless, the full implication of SOCS3 phosphorylation on its regulation remains to be explored.

4. Animal models of inhibitory adaptors: Definition of their physiological significance

Central to understanding the physiological role of families of inhibitory adaptors in the haematopoietic and immune systems, has been the generation of mice deficient for these proteins when possible. This has also helped dissect regulatory and/or compensatory mechanisms through the functional, complete or partial, reconstitution in these mice, in particular for members of multi-gene families. These approaches have allowed 1) analyse changes in the expression level of the adaptor that can also affect its signalling pathway; 2) establish how deficiency of an adaptor can have dramatically different effects in different cell lineages; 3) understand the functional synergy between members of the same family of adaptors; 4) identify null mutations leading to the complete absence of some cell types, while leaving others with no discernable defect and 5) define how some deficiencies are selective within a cell type, disrupting only particular pathways while leaving others intact. Mice deficient for the different families of inhibitory adaptors discussed in this chapter have certainly provided important new insights into the biology and function of these adaptors. However, in some cases, these animal models have also raised important questions regarding the mechanisms of action of these regulators and their potential therapeutic application.

4.1 *Dok* deficient mice

Although Dok-1, Dok-2, and Dok-3 have been shown to act as negative regulators downstream of a wide range of immunoreceptors, cytokine, and LPS receptors mediated signalling, insights into their physiological importance in immune cells have and will continue to come from studies with mice or cells lacking individually or in combination Dok-1, Dok-2, and Dok-3. *Dok-1* or *Dok-2*-deficient mice displayed normal steady-state haematopoiesis. By contrast, mice lacking both *Dok-1* and *Dok-2* succumbed to a myeloproliferative disease resembling human chronic myelogenous leukaemia (CML) and chronic myelomonocytic leukaemia (CMMoL) at around one year of age (Yasuda et al., 2004; Niki et al., 2004) [Table 5]. These animals displayed medullary and extramedullary hyperplasia of granulocyte/macrophage progenitors with leukemic potential, and their myeloid cells showed hyperproliferation and hypo-apoptosis upon treatment and deprivation of cytokines, respectively. Consistently, the mutant myeloid cells showed aberrant Ras/MAP kinase and Akt activation upon cytokine stimulation. Strikingly, ablation of *Dok-1* and *Dok-2* markedly accelerated leukaemia and blastic crisis onset in *bcr-abl* transgenic mice known to develop a CML-like disease. These results demonstrate the critical role of Dok-1 and Dok-2 in myeloid homeostasis and suppression of leukaemia. Interestingly, half of the double-deficient mice also developed histiocytic sarcoma (HS) of macrophage origin. These results suggest an involvement of additional genetic changes.

Similar to *Dok-1* and *Dok-2* deficiency, *Dok-3* inactivation did not result in development of aggressive tumors in haematopoietic cells (Ng et al., 2007). However, ablation of all three Dok proteins (Dok-1/2/3) in mice has recently shown drastic phenotypic consequences. These mice showed earlier mortality due to development of aggressive HS with multiple organ invasions, but no incidence of other types of tumors (Mashima et al., 2010). This disease is a haematological malignancy characterized by cells displaying a tissue macrophage-like (histiocytic) morphology (Grogan et al., 2008). Indeed, loss of *Dok-1/2/3* causes aberrant proliferation of macrophages in the lung, already detectable before the onset of morphologically recognizable HS. These cells displayed an exaggerated proliferative response to M-CSF or GM-CSF compared to wild type littermates. These results suggest that Dok proteins can mutually compensate and inhibit macrophage proliferation and therefore suppress the aggressive transformation of HS.

4.2 *Lnk/APS/SH2-B* deficient mice

Mice deficient for members of this family have demonstrated the positive (SH2-B) and negative (Lnk and APS) physiological role of these adaptors in growth factor, cytokine, and immune receptors signalling (Table 5). Deletion of the *SH2B1* gene resulted in severe obesity, hyperphagia and both leptin and insulin resistance as well as infertility, which might be a consequence of resistance to IGF-1 (Ohtsuka et al., 2002; Ren et al., 2005). Thus, SH2-B-deficient mice support a role for this adaptor as a positive regulator of JAK2 signalling pathways initiated by leptin, insulin and potentially, by IGF-1.

Interestingly, *APS*-deficient mice also displayed an insulin-related phenotype. They showed a hypersensibility to insulin and enhanced glucose tolerance, a finding that is consistent with APS playing a negative role in insulin signalling (Minami et al., 2003). Moreover, these mice present also a haematopoietic phenotype with defects in degranulation of mast cells and cytoskeleton rearrangement in both mast and B-1 cells (Kubo-Akashi et al, 2004; Iseki et

Gene	Approach	System	Mouse phenotype/Human disease
Dok-1 Dok-2	KO	mu	Impaired immunoreceptor signaling in lymphocytes, allergic responses in mast cells, enhanced ERK signaling, hyperresponsiveness to LPS
Dok-1/2	KO	mu	MPN, Lupus Renal disease/CML, CMMoL
Dok-1/2/3	KO	mu	HS
Lnk	KO	mu	MPN-like (ET/PMF), CML (aged mice)
	Tg	mu	Impaired lymphopoiesis
	Mu (SNP)	hu	MPN, autoimmune, cardiovascular and inflammatory diseases
APS	KO	mu	Insulin hypersensitivity, enhanced glucose tolerance, enhanced B1 cells proliferation
	Tg	mu	Reduced B1 and B2 cell number, impaired B-cell development and BCR-dependent proliferation, reduced mast cell degranulation and actin assembly
SH2B	KO	mu	Severe obesity, hyperphagia, increased leptin and insulin resistance, infertility
c-Cbl	KO	mu	Enlarged thymus, splenomegaly, extramedullar haematopoiesis, enhanced thymocyte function/ myeloid malignancies
	Mu	mu	Oncogenesis, mastocytosis, myeloid leukemia, tumourigenesis

Gene	Approach	System	Mouse phenotype/Human disease
c-Cbl	Mu	hu	AML, MPD/MPN, aCML, JMML
Cbl-b	KO	mu	Impaired immunological tolerance, autoimmune diseases with inflammatory organ and tissue damage, enhanced peripheral T-cell function, rejection of certain tumours
c-Cbl/ Cbl-b	KO	mu	Embryonic lethal
	T-cell KO	mu	Autoimmune-like vasculitis, SLE-like autoimmune disease
CIS	KO	mu	No specific phenotype
	Tg	mu	Fewer T-cells, NK, and NK-T cells, lactation deficiency, similar phenotype to STAT5 KO
SOCS1	KO	mu	perinatal lethality, enhanced IFNγ production and responsiveness, lymphopenia and inflammation with multi-organ infiltration
	Tg(Tcell)	mu	Inhibited T-cell response to IFNγ, IL-6 and IL-7, increased CD4+T-cells, reduced peripheral T-cell activation
		hu	Increased expression in Th-driven inflammatory diseases (RA, UC, Crohn, dermatitis), decreased expression and/or hyper-methylation in certain cancers
SOCS2	KO	mu	Gigantism, deregulated GH signalling
	Tg	mu	Gigantism
SOCS3	KO	mu	Embryonic lethality due to placental deficiency, erythrocytosis, deregulated LIF response
	Tg	mu	Embryonic lethality due to anemia
	Tg(Tcell)	mu	High TGFβ1 and IL-10 production
	Mu (SNP)	hu	Allergic diseases
		hu	Increased expression in Th2-driven asthma patients and inflammatory diseases, hyper-phosphorylation in MPN
SOCS5	KO	mu	No specific phenotype
	Tg	mu	Reduced IL-4-mediated STAT6 activation, reduced Th2 development and cytokine production
SOCS6	KO	mu	Mild growth retardation
SOCS7	KO	mu	Growth retardation (strain-dependent), hypoglucemia, hydrocephalus, altered glucose homeostasis, enlarged pancreatic islets

KO, knock out; Tg, transgenic; Mu, mutations; hu, human; mu, murine, RA, theumatoid arthritis; UC, ulcer colitis.

Table 5. Mouse phenotype and human diseases related to deficiencies in inhibitory adaptors.

al., 2004). These results suggest a negative role for APS in controlling actin dynamics in these cells. Furthermore, *APS*-deficient mice display an increase in B-1 cells in the peritoneal cavity and humoral responses to type-2 antigen, indicating a negative regulatory role for APS in BCR-mediated cell proliferation and cytoskeletal regulation.

By contrast, mice deficient for *Lnk* display a profound perturbation in haematopoiesis that confirmed its role as a key negative regulator of cytokine signalling in the haematopoietic system. Indeed, these mice exhibit splenomegaly together with fibrosis, expansion of HSC, B lymphoid and myeloid progenitors that confer an enhanced repopulating ability. *Lnk*-deficient mice have also revealed an important role for Lnk in B-cell lymphopoiesis, megakaryopoiesis and erythropoiesis, as a result of the absence of negative regulation of SCF, TPO and EPO signalling pathways. One important feature of the *Lnk*-/- mice phenotype is its resemblance to human myeloproliferative neoplasms (MPN): hypersensitivity to cytokines, increased number of haematopoietic progenitors, high platelet counts, splenomegaly together with fibrosis and extramedullary hematopoiesis (Velazquez et al., 2002; Campbell & Green, 2008). This has suggested an important role for Lnk in the development of these diseases. Indeed, loss of Lnk cooperates with oncogenes, such as JAK2 and BCR-ABL, to induce MPN in mice. These animals exhibit a disproportionate expansion of myeloid progenitors and immature precursors *in vitro* and *in vivo* (Bersenev et al., 2010). Moreover, aged *Lnk*-/- mice seem to spontaneously develop a Chronic Myeloid Leukemia (CML)-like MPN, suggesting a role for Lnk in myeloid expansion *in vivo*. However, this myeloid cell hyperproliferation fails to trigger blast crises, reflecting the need of *Lnk*-deficiency for additional oncogenic events to promote blast transformation. *Lnk*-deficient mice also exhibited an increase in endothelial progenitor cells (EPC) numbers that display an enhance capacity for colony formation. Different molecular, physiological and morphological approaches have shown that *Lnk* deficiency promotes vasculogenesis/angiogenesis and osteogenesis through the mobilization and recruitment of HSCs/EPCs via activation of the SCF/Kit signalling pathway in the ischemic and perifracture zone, respectively, thereby establishing an optimal environment for neovascularisation, bone healing and remodelling (Kwon et al., 2009, Matsumoto, et al., 2010). Taken together, these findings strongly suggest that Lnk regulates bone marrow EPC kinetics during vascular and bone regeneration.

4.3 *Cbl*-deficient mice

Mice deficient for *c-Cbl* and *Cbl-b* have been invaluable in demonstrating the important roles played by these proteins in fine-tuning signalling thresholds in immune cells. Despite close structural similarities, loss of c-Cbl and Cbl-b proteins evokes prominent phenotypic differences (Table 5). *c-Cbl*-null mice have an enlarged thymus, expanded hematopoietic progenitor pools with increased repopulating capacity, splenomegaly with extramedullary hematopoiesis, as well as changes in energy metabolism, and reduced fertility of male mice (Murphy et al., 1998; Naramura et al., 1998; Molero et al., 2004; El Chami et al., 2005, Rathinam et al., 2008). However, the most marked alteration in *c-Cbl* and *Cbl-b*-deficient animals is being associated with thymocyte and peripheral T-cell activation, respectively. *c-Cbl*-/- mice exhibit strong effects on thymocytes, with increase cell numbers in the thymus of the young adult and enhanced signal strength following TCR engagement. Moreover, perturbed thymocyte signalling does not depend on the TKB domain of c-Cbl, as a TKB knock-in did not rescue the phenotype (Thien et al., 2003). In contrast, *Cbl-b* ablation results in an impaired immunological tolerance induction and animals succumb to spontaneous and/or induced autoimmune diseases with widespread inflammatory organ (pancreas, lung) and tissue (adipose) damage (Bachmaier et al., 2000, 2007; Hirasaka et al., 2007). Importantly, *Cbl-b*-null mice are able to reject multiple types of tumours spontaneously (Chiang et al., 2007; Loeser et al., 2007).

The redundant and overlapping functions of Cbl family proteins are more evident from the striking phenotypes of *Cbl, Cbl-b* double-deficient mice. Deletion of both proteins in the germline leads to early embryonic lethality (Naramura et al., 2002). In contrast, T-cell specific double knock-out mice are viable, however, their T-cells develop independent of MHC-restricted thymic selection and these mice eventually succumb to autoimmune-like vasculitis early in adult life (Huang et al., 2006; Naramura et al., 2002). Similarly, B-cell specific *Cbl, Cbl-b* double deficiency leads to a failure to acquire tolerance to self antigens and the animals developed Systemic Lupus Erythematosus (SLE)-like autoimmune diseases (Kitaura et al., 2007). At the molecular level, cells from these double knock-out mice display delayed down-modulation of cell surface antigen receptors and prolonged activation of downstream signalling pathways.

Loss of *c-Cbl*, but not of *Cbl-b*, led to a significant expansion of HSC and haematopoietic progenitors. Strikingly, ablation of both proteins enhanced this phenotype and eventually all mice succumbed to aggressive myeloproliferative disease-like leukemia with peripheral organ involvement within two to three months after birth (Naramura et al., 2010). Moreover, blastic transformation of chronic myelogeneous leukemia in a *bcr/abl*-transgenic model is accelerated in the *c-Cbl* null background (Sanada et al., 2009). Combined, these observations support that c-Cbl can act as a tumor suppressor and that complete loss of Cbl functions is required to promote myeloid malignancy. In contrast to the tumor suppressor function of the wild-type c-Cbl, c-Cbl mutants isolated from human and murine neoplasms, as well as v-Cbl, show clear transforming capacity in terms of anchorage-independent growth in soft agar *in vitro* and tumour generation in nude mice *in vivo* (Sanada et al., 2009; Thien et al., 2001). Bone marrow cells transduced with c-Cbl mutants in the linker (70Z) or in the RING finger domain (R420Q) generate generalized mastocytosis, a myeloproliferative disease, and myeloid leukemia in lethally irradiated mice with long latency but high penetrance (Bandi et al., 2009). The transforming activity of these mutant forms of c-Cbl seems to be mediated by alteration of the E3 ubiquitin ligase activity. Most c-Cbl mutations in myeloid neoplasms are missense changes at highly conserved amino acid positions within the linker and RING finger domains, or involve splice-site sequences, leading to amino acid deletions within them. Supporting these findings, the generation of knock-in mutants carrying single point mutations in the TKB, linker or RING domains of c-Cbl protein has further validated the importance of these domains in Cbl-mediated tumorigenesis. Interestingly, mice with an equivalent RING finger domain mutation in *Cbl-b* do not show comparable changes in the haematopoietic compartment, indicating that Cbl-b is not capable of inhibiting c-Cbl functions (Rathinam et al., 2010). Taken together, mouse models with Cbl family ablation or point mutations have convincingly established the role of these proteins as important E3 ubiquitin ligases for the homeostasis of the haematopoietic and immune systems and as tumour suppressors.

4.4 *SOCS*-deficient mice

Since the discovery of SOCS proteins, much attention has been drawn to their physiological roles and their involvement in human diseases. Many of their common inhibitory activities on cytokine signalling demonstrated *in vitro*, do not seem to be essential *in vivo* as genetic ablation of CIS, SOCS1, SOCS2 and SOCS3 genes has demonstrated remarkable cytokine specificity for different SOCS molecules (Table 5).

SOCS1-deficient mice are growth retarded and died within 3 weeks of birth with a syndrome characterized by severe lymphopenia, activation of peripheral T cells, fatty degeneration and necrosis of the liver and multi-organ failure with rampant inflammation due to macrophage infiltration of major organs (Alexander et al., 1999; Marine et al., 1999a, Starr et al., 1998). The neonatal phenotypes appear primarily as the result of deregulated IFNγ signalling, because *SOCS1*[-/-] mice that are also deficient for IFNγ, do not die neonatally. Moreover, constitutive STAT1 activation and IFNγ-inducible genes were observed in *SOCS1* deficient mice, indicating that IFNγ signalling is regulated by SOCS1 and that its deregulation contributes to the lethal phenotype. However, the *SOCS1, IFNγ* double deficient mice ultimately died 6 months after birth with inflammation and polycystic kidneys, which suggests that SOCS1 regulation is not exclusive to IFNγ (Metcalf et al., 2002). The lethality in *SOCS1*[-/-] mice is also significantly delayed in the *RAG2*[-/-], *STAT1*[-/-], *STAT6*[-/-] and *STAT4*[-/-] backgrounds, thus implicating SOCS1 as a critical regulator of IFNγ, IL-4 and IL-12 signalling pathways (Alexander and Hilton, 2004).

In recent years, it has become clear that some of the SOCS members play critical roles in regulating T-cell differentiation, maturation and function by controlling different signalling events, as shown by the phenotypes displayed by *SOCS1* and *SOCS3* deficient mice. In this sense, T-cell specific conditional deletion of *SOCS1* showed that it is not sufficient to induce the lethal multi-organ disease; however it does cause T-cell specific abnormalities that include increased numbers of CD8[+] T cells and increased sensitivity to cytokines with common γ-chain receptors. SOCS1 also plays an important role in the regulation of Tregs. Higher number of Tregs is observed in the thymus and spleen of T-cell-specific *SOCS1*-deficient mice (Horino et al., 2008). This is probably due to higher IL-2 responses, because IL-2 enhances Tregs proliferation. Moreover, Lu and colleagues have recently showed that SOCS1-specific ablation in Tregs induced the development of spontaneous dermatitis, splenomegaly and lymphoadenopathy in these mice (Lu et al., 2009). These results point out SOCS1 as an important controller of Tregs.

Analysis of mice bearing the deletion of the SOCS box of *SOCS1* demonstrated the *in vivo* importance of the SOCS box for inhibition of IFNγ signalling by SOCS1. SOCS box deleted-deficient mice also die prematurely and suffer from reduced body weight. Inflammatory lesions are observed in skeletal and heart muscle, cornea, pancreas and dermis.

SOCS2 is thought to play a major role in the regulation of GH signalling. Indeed, mice deficient for *SOCS2* develop gigantism with enlargement of visceral organs and 3 months after birth weight 30-40% more than control mice, elevated mRNA levels of insulin-like growth factor (IGF-1) and enhanced responses to exogenous GH (Metcalf et al., 2000; Greenhalgh et al., 2005). Interestingly, over-expression of SOCS2 increases GH signalling and *SOCS2* transgenic mice develop mild gigantism (Favre et al., 1999). These results suggest a more complex role of SOCS2 in regulating GH signalling. To date, there are no evidences on the role of SOCS2 in the regulation of immune responses.

Deletion of *SOCS3* leads to embryonic lethality with embryos dying between 12 and 16 days of gestation (Marine et al., 1999b). Lethality was initially thought to result from excessive erythropoiesis due to enhanced EPO signalling. However, further studies showed that lethality was in fact due to placental insufficiency with poor development of embryonic vessels, spongiotrophoblasts, as well as increase in trophoblast giant cell differentiation (Roberts et al., 2001). Tetraploid aggregation assays resulting in SOCS3-deficient foetal components with SOCS3 sufficient placental tissues, generated live birth SOCS3-/- mice. These mice were smaller than littermates, exhibited cardiac hyperthrophy and finally succumbed by 25 days. Importantly, SOCS3 lethality could be rescued if mice were also deficient for Leukemia-Inhibitory factor (LIF) or its receptor (LIFR), indicating that SOCS3 is required for modulating LIF signalling in giant trophoblast cell differentiation (Takahashi et al., 2003, Robb et al., 2005).

SOCS3 has also been shown to play an important role in Th1 and Th2 cell differentiation. Indeed, blocking SOCS3 either by a dominant-negative mutant or in heterozygous SOCS3 mice diminishes the differentiation of Th2 cells, resulting in the skewing of T-cells towards the Th1 phenotype and reduced allergic responses (Seki et al., 2003; Kubo et al., 2006). Furthermore, over-expression of SOCS3 in T-cells provokes exacerbating Th2 cell-mediated eye-allergy, with inhibition of SOCS3 ameliorating the severity of the disease.

The receptors to which SOCS3 binds mostly activate STAT3, therefore, SOCS3 has been considered as a negative regulator of inflammation and an inhibitor relatively specific to STAT3. Indeed, mice with a conditional deletion of SOCS3 in haematopoietic and endothelial cells die as young adults due to severe inflammatory lesions in the peritoneal and pleural cavities (Croker et al., 2004, Robb et al., 2005). If G-CSF is administered to these mice, mimicking emergency granulopoiesis during infection, they exhibit massive neutrophil infiltration and destruction of liver, lung, muscle and spinal tissue, resulting from increased intensity and duration of G-CSF-induced STAT3 activation. These results thus indicate SOCS3 as a negative regulator of G-CSF and STAT3 in myeloid cells. Mice with SOCS3-deficient haematopoiesis display also high susceptibility to inflammatory joint disease in an IL-1-induced inflammatory model (Wong et al., 2006). Adenoviral gene transfer of SOCS3 or dominant negative STAT3 indeed reduced the proliferation of RA synovial fibroblasts and the severity of the disease in a mouse model that is also dependent on Th17 cells (Shouda et al., 2001). The generation of these same cells is enhanced in T-cell specific SOCS3-deficient mice and abrogation of SOCS3 binding site in gp130 knock-in mutant mice results in Th17-like arthritis (Taleb et al., 2009; Ogura et al., 2008). Together, these results show that the absence of SOCS3 has dramatic pro-inflammatory effects by promoting Th17 development and Th17-mediated disease.

Mice lacking CIS did not display any specific phenotype (Marine et al., 1999a). However, CIS-over-expressing transgenic mice recreate a phenotype quite similar to STAT5-deficient mice with defects in growth and lactation, GH and prolactin signalling, as well as in natural killer, natural killer T-cell and T-cell development (Matsumoto et al., 1999). These results support its role in JAK/STAT5 pathway.

The role of SOCS4 in vivo or in immune responses is to date unknown. However, in vivo studies on SOCS5 reveal its possible role in adaptive immunity, notably in Th1 and Th2 cell differentiation. SOCS5 transgenic mice show attenuation of IL-4-mediated STAT6 signalling, as well as reduced Th2 cell development and production of Th2-type-cytokines (Seki et al., 2002). Interestingly, SOCS5 over-expression augmented eosinophilic airway inflammation and septic peritonitis in mice (Ohshima et al., 2007; Watanabe et al., 2006). In contrast, SOCS5-deficent mice appear to have normal T-cell development and differentiation to both Th1 and Th2 cells (Brender et al., 2004). These contradictory phenotypes might be explained with the high homology between SOCS4 and SOCS5 denoting a redundant role of these proteins *in vivo*.

SOCS6-deficient mice do not display overt abnormalities, but just mild growth retardation, suggesting its role in cell growth (Krebs et al., 2002). However, SOCS6 over-expression results in inhibited insulin signalling and improvement in glucose tolerance, similarly to *p85*-deficient mice (Li et al., 2004). *SOCS7* ablation *in vivo* has mainly delineated its essential role in insulin signalling. *SOCS7*-deficient mice shows multiple defects at an early age with half of the homozygous progeny displaying severe hydrocephalus and growth retardation concomitant with hypoglycaemia and enhanced glucose metabolism that resulted in perinatal lethality (Banks et al., 2005; Krebs et al., 2004). On the other hand, SOCS7 seems to have a role in the regulation of allergic inflammatory disease. *SOCS7*-deficient mice have a propensity toward spontaneous development of cutaneous disease with infiltration of degranulated mast cells (Knisz et al., 2009). Thus, these studies suggest a role for SOCS7 in modulating the development of allergic diseases.

5. Inhibitory adaptors in human haematological diseases

As described in the previous section, animal models for the Dok, Lnk, Cbl and SOCS families have been invaluable in demonstrating the important roles played by these adaptor proteins in fine-tuning signalling thresholds in haematopoietic and immune cells. Some of these *in vivo* models recapitulate exactly or almost, essential features of different haematological and immune diseases, allowing us to identify new molecular players and mechanisms implicated in the initiation and progression of these malignancies.

Dok proteins

Studies on *Dok-1* and *Dok-2*-deficient mice demonstrated that these adaptors are essential to suppress the blastic transformation of the Bcr-Abl–induced CML-like disease. However, it is of note that in case of patients with CML, blast crisis mostly results in myeloid or B cell leukemia/lymphoma, usually not in the T cell variety. That Bcr-Abl mice carrying a p53 mutation also developed T cell lymphoma suggests involvement of genetic background (Honda et al., 2000). Moreover, as double *Dok-1/2* knockout mice developed myeloproliferative disease in the absence of Bcr-Abl, Dok-1 and Dok-2 may oppose a wide range of myeloid leukemogenesis in humans. Consistently, undetectable or marginal levels of their expression was observed in about half of the leukemic cell lines established from patients with myeloid leukaemia, regardless of whether it is CML or not (Yasuda et al., 2004). Further investigation of the tumour suppressive function of Dok-1 and Dok-2 in human malignancies, especially myeloid leukaemia including CML and CMMoL, might lead to an understanding of the molecular mechanisms of such diseases and contribute to designing effective therapies against them (Table 5).

Histiocytic sarcoma (HS) is a malignant proliferation of cells showing morphological and immunophenotypic features of mature histiocytes, which represent tissue-resident macrophages. Until recently, HS, which was also known as malignant histiocytosis, was often confused with anaplastic large B-cell lymphoma or with other malignant lymphomas

(Weiss et al., 2009). As the molecular etiology of this disease is unknown, there remains a need for realistic animal models. Mouse models that have been reported for HS frequently show multiple lesions including lymphomas and severe renal failure. The syndrome elicited in mice lacking all the three proteins, Dok-1, Dok-2, and Dok-3, more specifically resembles the disease found in humans and hence may serve as a useful model for the study of HS. Although elucidation of the mechanisms by which the ablation of Dok proteins specifically causes HS and how the tumour gains its aggressive phenotype awaits further studies, such studies will help unveil the hidden etiology of this rare aggressive human malignancy.

Lnk proteins

Lnk-deficient mice display a phenotype reminiscent of BCR-ABL negative (Ph-) MPNs, notably Essential Thrombocythemia (ET) and Primary Myelofibrosis (PMF) that has suggested a role for Lnk in the development of these diseases (Table 5). All MPNs are clonal disorders of HSC characterized by excessive proliferation of haematopoietic cells due to hypersensibility to normal cytokine regulation and absence of negative feed back regulation. The recent discovery of the Val617Phe acquired mutation of the *JAK2* gene (*JAK2*-V617F) represents the first reliable molecular marker of Ph- MPN (Campbell & Green, 2008). The pathogenic role of JAK2-V617F constitutive active kinase and more recently of mutated Mpl (*MPL*W-515L) most likely will go through abnormal activation of signalling molecules, among which Lnk likely plays an important negative regulatory role through its binding to JAK2-V617F and MPL-W515L forms. Indeed, recent work has demonstrated a modulation of Lnk level in megakaryocyte/platelets and CD34+ cells from MPNs patients (Baran-Marszak et al., 2010). Recently, the first *LNK* mutations in JAK2-V617F-negative MPN patients (ET and PMF) were identified (Oh et al., 2010). Both mutations are on exon 2, one (E208Q) is a missense mutation in the PH domain (ET patient), while the second mutation lead to a premature stop codon resulting in the absence of the protein (PMF patient). The prevalence of such mutations is rare (5% or less). However, other *LNK* mutations have been identified in leukemic transformation of MNP at a higher frequency [13%] (Pardani et al., 2010). Moreover, *LNK* exon 2 mutations were also found in pure erythrocytosis (Lasho et al., 2010). In this case, one mutation (A215V) was previously described in PMF blast crisis and another (E208X) results in absence of the protein. This finding suggests that the *LNK* mutations induce an MPN phenotype that may depend on different parameters, such as the presence of other mutations (Lasho et al., 2011).

Genome-wide association studies (GWAS) have recently revealed that different diseases share susceptibility variants. The *LNK/SH2B3* gene maps on chromosome 12q24 and a non-synonymous single nucleotide polymorphisms (SNP) in this gene has been reported in exon 2 resulting in a missense mutation at position 262 leading to a R262W amino acid substitution in the PH domain. Surprisingly, this nsSNP has recently been associated with inflammatory disorders, such as celiac disease (Hunt et al., 2008; Zhernakova et al., 2010), type 1 diabetes (Lavrikova et al., 2010), asthma (Gudbjartsson et al., 2009) multiple sclerosis (Alcina et al., 2010), and also to eight clinically relevant haematological parameters (Soranzo et al., 2009; Ganesh et al., 2009) in different populations. Furthermore, the *LNK* R262W variant has also been associated to cardiovascular diseases such as myocardial infarction, coronary heart disease and hypertension (Gudbjartsson et al., 2009; Ikram et al., 2010). All these data suggests that Lnk nsSNP could be a risk variant for these diseases contributing to their pathogenesis, and in consequence, providing a useful diagnostic marker.

Cbl proteins

Animal models have demonstrated the enhanced biological responses in the haematopoietic and immune system of Cbl family members when they are either genetically ablated or point mutated. It is in this context that the recent identification of mutations in CBL in patients with myeloid malignancies provides an important milestone (Table 5). Two groups simultaneously identified CBL mutations in Acute Myeloid Leukaemia (AML) patient samples (Sargin et al., 2007; Caligiuri et al., 2007). CBL mutations are most frequently observed in a distinct group of myeloid disorders named myelodysplastic syndromes/myeloproliferative neoplasms (MDS/MPN) that include: the Chronic Myelomonocytic Leukaemia (CMML), atypical Chronic Myeloid Leukaemia (aCML) and Juvenile Myelomonocytic Leukaemia (JMML). They originate from immature haematopoietic progenitors and are characterized by the production of dysplastic blood cells and myeloproliferative features. In most adult cases, mutations seem to be somatic, but germline mutations were reported in some JMML cases in children (Loh et al., 2009; Niemeyer et al., 2010; Martinelli et al., 2010). Genetic alterations in these haematological malignancies are strongly associated with hyperactivation of the Ras/MAPK signalling pathway due to activating mutations in signalling molecules involved in this pathway accounting for approximately 75%cases of JMML (Schubbert, et al., 2007). Strikingly, *CBL* mutations are found in 5% of aCML and up to 15% of JMML and CMML (Grand et al., 2009; Loh et al., 2009; Muramatsu et al., 2010; Shiba et al., 2010; Dunbar et al., 2008; Sanada et al., 2009). Most *CBL* mutations associated with myeloid malignancies are clustered around the linker and the RING finger domains and *in vitro* studies with these mutants have shown their lack of E3 ubiquitin ligase activity (Sargin et al., 2007; Grand et al., 2009; Sanada et al., 2009). Complete loss of *CBL*, deletions or mutations outside the linker/RING finger domains are rare, as well as mutations in *CBLB*. These findings suggest that expression of mutant Cbl proteins act as dominant negative inhibitor of wild-type Cbl or even of lost Cbl expression. A remarkable genetic feature of *c-CBL* mutations in these myeloid neoplasms is that mutations are homozygous in most cases, as a result of duplication of the mutated parental copy of 11q (where the *CBL* gene resides) and loss of the remaining wild-type allele, a genetic process called "acquired uniparental disomy" (aUPD) (Grand et al., 2009). This feature underlies the gain-of-function nature, rather than a loss-of-function, of the CBL mutations and may represent a defining oncogenic event. Indeed, mutations involving *RUNX1, JAK2, FLT3* and *TP53* have been shown to coexist with CBL mutations in myeloid neoplasms (Sanada et al., 2009; Perez et al., 2010; Tefferi, 2010; Makishima et al., 2011) suggesting that additional oncogenic events may contribute to the mutant Cbl-driven leukemogenic process.

SOCS proteins

There is now emerging evidence that SOCS expression is differentially regulated during Th cell differentiation and in Th-driven inflammatory diseases (Table 5). In Th1 inflammatory diseases (rheumatoid arthritis, ulcerative colitis, Crohn disease, contact and atopic dermatitis), SOCS1 expression is observed in lymphocytes and macrophages, as well as keratinocytes and stromal cells that are capable of antigen presentation, but granulocytes are negative (Egan et al., 2003; Federici et al., 2002). Importantly, SOCS3 expression levels seem to correlate with the severity of this type of inflammatory diseases (Seki et al., 2003; Shouda et al., 2001; Suzuki et al., 2001). The same is true for Th2-driven asthma that promotes lymphocyte, basophile and mast cell infiltration, where SOCS3 expression in Th2 lymphocytes is elevated. Furthermore, the association of the function of SOCS molecules in the allergic response has been supported by human studies analyzing the association of polymorphisms in *SOCS* genes with allergic disease in people. Interestingly, an association of a promoter polymorphism leads to a promoter with modified activity *in vitro*, suggesting that changes in *SOCS1* expression can have considerable effects on disease manifestations in patients (Harada et al., 2007). SOCS1 expression has been found decreased in some human cancers including hepatocellular carcinoma and myeloproliferative neoplasms and this is frequently associated with hyper-methylation of one or more *SOCS* genes (Yoshikawa et al., 2001; Watanabe et al., 2004; Quentmeier et al., 2008; Chaligné et al., 2009). In some cases, this methylation has been correlated to the degree of malignancy (Okochi et al., 2003; Yoshida et al., 2004). These observations strongly suggest that SOCS proteins may be tumour suppressors. Loss of SOCS expression may then contribute or favour tumour progression in synergy with other oncogenes. SOCS expression has also been implicated in the resistance to interferon in haematopoietic malignancies, such as leukaemia, lymphomas and multiple myeloma (Sakamoto et al., 2000, Sakai et al., 2002). Persistent expression of SOCS1 and/or SOCS3 has been detected in cutaneous T-cell lymphoma (CTCL), chronic myeloid leukaemia (CML), and some acute leukaemia (Brender et al., 2001b; Cho-Vega et al., 2004; Roman-Gomez et al., 2004). In these circumstances, elevated expression of SOCS coincides with constitutive activation of JAK/STAT pathways. Moreover, in certain myeloproliferative neoplasm, SOCS3 has been found hyper-phosphorylated, which enhances the half-life of the protein but interferes with its regulatory function (Hookham et al., 2007; Elliott et al., 2009; Suessmuth et al., 2009). These data suggests that perturbed SOCS expression may contribute to the malignant phenotype and favour disease progression, rather than being an early event in the oncogenic process.

6. Therapeutic application of inhibitory adaptors

Given the central role played by inhibitory adaptors in the regulation of different aspects of haematopoietic and immune cell function, they are predicted to serve as excellent new targets in the development of anti-oncogenic, anti-inflammatory and immunosuppressor reagents. The advantage of these adaptors as targets is their restricted expression in cells of the haematopoietic and immune system, at least of some of the members in the different families discussed here. The disadvantage for some of them (Dok, Lnk) is their lack of enzymatic activity for drug targeting. However, this can be surpassed by utilizing strategies based in the direct inhibition or blockade of their specific protein-protein interactions for targeting a particular signalling pathway. This approach relies on the current information available on the molecular structure of the adaptor functional domains and the identification of specific sequences or residues involved in the adaptor/partner interaction. In some pathological contexts, the association of the inhibitory adaptor with mutated or oncogenic forms of its targets is modified from that engaged with its normal counterpart (Baran-Marszak et al., 2010). These findings open the possibility to use the binding sequence in the adaptor to exclusively inhibit the oncogenic protein and signalling pathway, while sparing the normal cell signalling cascades. Indeed, successful development of small molecule inhibitors of protein-protein interaction has begun to emerge, validating it as a practical approach (Azmi & Mohammad, 2009). The use of dominant negative forms of these inhibitory proteins has also proved to be advantageous, notably for adaptors that have shown dual functions, as positive and negative regulators, as they allow modulate specifically their function depending on the cell type and biological response to be addressed. In the case of Lnk, its loss or inhibition causes the abnormal expansion and enhanced ability for engraftment of HSC (Takizawa et al., 2006); this feature can be used for bone marrow transplantation where the scarce number of these cells is always the limiting factor for the use of this therapy.

On the other hand, adaptors with catalytic activity, like the Cbl and SOCS proteins, have the double advantage of being used as adaptors and as E3 ligase. In the case of Cbl, it is clear that its ligase activity is central to the regulation of many oncogenic proteins, so drugs that could enhance this activity may provide new therapeutic strategies for limiting their constitutive signalling. A potential strategy is the screening for molecules that could mimic the activation of its E3 activity while retaining its targets binding. This can be use in basophile and mast cells of allergic patients as a therapy to treat allergy diseases. In the case of SOCS, a strategy based in the delivery of the SOCS3 protein using a recombinant cell penetrating moiety has proved to increase the concentration and activity of SOCS3 in the cells and suppressed the effects of acute inflammation (Jo et al., 2005). Moreover, therapeutic trials using SOCS antisense oligonucleotide, small hairpin RNA and peptide mimetics are currently investigated in animal models (Yoshimura et al., 2007). Importantly, a better understanding of the spectrum of signalling alterations provoked by mutant forms of the inhibitory adaptors identified in human pathologies is likely to reveal therapeutic strategies for patients with these mutations. In this context, the association of single nucleotide polymorphisms (SNP) in the genes of some of these adaptors (*LNK, SOCS*) with different inflammatory, myeloproliferative and vascular diseases suggests the implication of these molecules as risk factor and their potential use as biomarkers in these diseases. Lastly, future challenges in the study of inhibitory adaptors lie also in the development of performing techniques that will allow accurate monitoring of their signalling complexes at the molecular level. Indeed, precise regulation of protein interactions is of medical relevance, as modifications in the composition or localization of crucial components of these signalling networks can lead to the development of human diseases.

7. Conclusions

Over the past decade, it has become clear the pivotal role that cytokines play in the development and pathology of human diseases, including those of the haematopoietic and immune system. They perform their actions by regulating essential biological functions, such as cell proliferation, differentiation, cell morphology and migration. It is therefore not surprising that cytokine signal transduction pathways are tightly regulated. To achieve this, they have set up a variety of mechanisms and the rate at which the signal is turned off will be due to the net effect of all of these regulatory pathways. Although initially identified and best understood as mediators of positive signalling, adaptors have also shown an equally critical role in the negative control of signalling events. Inhibitory adaptors have been demonstrated important for maintaining homeostasis by preventing inappropriate cellular activation (Lnk, Cbl), by localizing enzymatically active regulatory molecules to specific subcellular compartments (Dok), and/or by terminating signalling cascades once they are initiated through targeting activated mediators to degradative pathways (Cbl, SOCS). In doing so, these molecules act upon three key signalling intermediates (the receptor,

JAK/other kinases, and STATs/downstream effectors) to completely switch off the signal. In contrast to SOCS and Lnk, which are induced in response to cytokines, Cbl and Dok (with the exception of Dok-2 in some cases) are constitutively present in the cell and may therefore function as more acute, early response regulators. The timing and specificity of each of these mechanisms, as well as how the inhibitors interact and cooperate with each other, is still an area for future investigation. Furthermore, the fact that the expression of these adaptors is itself regulated, points out further the complexity of the regulatory system. While gene-targeting studies have highlighted critical roles for the inhibitory adaptors in immune function, haematological malignancy and inflammation, the complexity of the mouse models, particularly with regard to multi-gene families, suggests that these studies should be carefully interpreted, and certainly more work is required before we can predict the consequences of using these molecules or their agonists/antagonists in a clinical setting. Thus, one of the challenges for the future is sorting out the roles of negative regulators of cytokine signalling in all the existing pathways activated in response to cytokines. This knowledge is likely to yield both new and confirmatory findings, with the anticipation of a better understanding of how these adaptors orchestrate the functional activity and fate of many partners to produce the desired intensity of a signalling response. Although a great deal of research remains to be done to clarify the roles of these inhibitors and their mutant forms in human diseases such as cancer and inflammation, it can be foreseen that it will lead to the development of strategies based on the up- or down-regulation of their properties for therapeutic purposes.

8. Acknowledgments

I thank the members of my laboratory and of the U978 Inserm for sharing their data and support. This work was supported by grants from the Institut National de la Santé et la Recherche Médicale (Inserm) and the Association pour la Recherche contre le Cancer (ARC, contrat no. SFI20101201732).

9. References

Abramson, J., Rozenblum, G., & Pecht, I. (2003). Dok protein family members are involved in signaling mediated by the type 1 Fcepsilon receptor. *Eur J Immunol.*, Vol.33, pp. 85–91

Alcina, A., Vandenbroeck, K., Otaegui, D., Saiz, A., Gonzalez, J.R., Fernandez, O., Cavanillas, M.L., Cénit, M.C., Arroyo, R., Alloza, I., García-Barcina, M., Antigüedad, A., Leyva, L., Izquierdo, G., Lucas, M., Fedetz, M., Pinto-Medel, M.J., Olascoaga, J, Blanco, Y., Comabella, M., Montalban, X., Urcelay, E., & Matesanz, F. (2010). The autoimmune disease-associated KIF5A, CD226 and SH2B3 gene variants confer susceptibility for multiple sclerosis. *Genes and Immun.*, Vol.11, pp. 439-445

Alexander, W.S., Starr, R., Fenner, J.E., Scott, C.L., Handman, E., Sprigg, N.S., Corbin, J.E., Cornisa, A.L., Darwiche, R., Owczarek, C.M., Kay, T.W., Incola, N.A., Hertzog, P.J., Metcalf, D., & Milton, D.J. (1999). SOCS1 is a critical inhibitor of interferon □ signalling and prevents the potentially fatal neonatal actions of this cytokine. *Cell,* Vol.9, pp. 597–608

Alexander WS, & Hilton DJ. (2004). The role of suppressors of cytokine signaling (SOCS) proteins in regulation of the immune response. *Annu Rev Immunol*, Vol.22, pp. 503–29

Azmi, A.S., & Mohammad, R.M. (2009). Non-peptidic small molecule inhibitors against Bcl-2 for cancer therapy. *J. Cell. Physiol.*, Vol.218, pp. 13-21

Babon, J.J., McManus, E., Yao, S., DeSouza, D.P., Mielke, L.A., Sprigg, N.S., Wilson, T.A., Hilton, D.J., Nicola, N.A., Baca, M., Nicholson, S.E., & Norton, R.S. (2006). The structure of SOCS3 reveals the basis of the extended SH2 domain function and identifies an unstructured insertion that regulates stability. *Mol. Cell.*, Vol.22, No.2, pp. 205-216

Bachmaier, K., Krawczyk, C., Kozieradzki, I., Kong, Y.-Y., Sasaki, T., Oliveira-dos-Santos, A., Mariathasan, S., Bouchard, D., Wakeham, A., Itie, A., Le, J., Ohashi, P.S., Sarosi, I., Nishina, H., Lipkowitz, S., & Penninger, J.M. (2000). Negative regulation of lymphocyte activation and autoimmunity by the molecular adaptor Cbl-b. *Nature*, Vol.403, pp. 211–216

Bachmaier, K., Toya, S., Gao, X., Triantafillou, T., Garrean, S., Park, G.Y., Frey, R.S., Vogel, S., Minshall, R., Christman, J.W., Tiruppathi, C., & Malik, A.B. (2007). E3 ubiquitin ligase Cbl-b regulates the acute inflammatory response underlying lung injury. *Nat. Med.*, Vol.13, pp. 920-926

Bandi, S.R., Brandts, C., Rensinghoff, M., Grundler, R., Tickenbrock, L., Kohler, G., Duyster, J., Berdel, W.E., Muller-Tidow, C., Serve, H., & Sargin, B. (2009). E3 ligase-defective Cbl mutants lead to a generalized mastocytosis and myeloproliferative disease. *Blood*, Vol.114, pp. 4197–208

Banks, A.S., Li, J., McKeag, L., Hribal, M.L., Kashiwada, M., Accili, D., & Rothman, P.B. (2005). Deletion of SOCS7 leads to enhanced insulin action and enlarged islets of Langerhans. *J Clin Invest.*, Vol.115, No.9, pp. 2462-2471

Baran-Marszak, F., Magdoud, H., Desterke, C., Alvarado, A., Roger, C., Harel, S., Mazoyer, E., Cassinat, B., Chevret, S., Tonetti, C., Giraudier, S., Fenaux, P., Cymbalista, F., Varin-Blank, N., LeBousse-Kerdilès, M.C., Kiladjian, J.J., & Velazquez, L. (2010). Expression level and differential JAK2-V617F-binding of the adaptor protein Lnk regulates JAK2-mediated signals in myeloproliferative neoplasms. *Blood*, Vol.116, No.26, pp. 5961-5971

Bartkiewicz, M., Houghton, A., & Baron, R. (1999). Leucine zipper-mediated homodimerization of the adaptor protein c-Cbl. A role in c-Cbl's tyrosine phosphorylation and its association with epidermal growth factor receptor. *J. Biol. Chem.*, Vol.274, No.43, pp. 30887–30895

Bersenev, A., Wu, C., Balcerek, J., & Tong, W. (2008). Lnk controls mouse hematopoietic stem cell self-renewal and quiescence through direct interactions with JAK2. *J. Clin. Invest.*, Vol.118, No.8, pp. 2832-2844

Bersenev, A., Wu, C., Balcerek, J., Jing, J., Kundu, M., Blobel, G.A., Chikwave, K.R., & Tong, W. (2010). Lnk constraints myeloproliferative diseases in mice. *J. Clin. Invest.*, Vol.120, No. 6, pp. 2058-2069

Bjorbaek, C., Buchholz, R.M., Davis, S.M., Bates, S.H., Pierroz, D.D., Gu, H., Neel, B.G., Myers, M.G. Jr, & Flier, J.S. (2001). Divergent roles of SHP-2 in ERK activation by leptin receptors. *J Biol Chem.*, Vol.276, pp. 4747–4755

Blake, T.J., Shapiro, M., Morse, H.C. III., & Langdon, W.Y. (1991). The sequences of the human and mouse *c-cbl* proto-oncogenes show *v-cbl* was generated by a large truncation encompassing a proline-rich domain and a leucine zipper-like motif. *Oncogene*, Vol.6, pp. 653-657

Boulay, I., Némorin, J.G., & Duplay, P. (2005). Phosphotyrosine binding-mediated oligomerization of downstream of tyrosine kinase (Dok)-1 and Dok-2 is involved in CD2-induced Dok phosphorylation. *J Immunol*, Vol.175, pp. 4483-4489

Boyle, K., Egan, P., Rakar, S., Wilson, T.A., Wicks, I.P., Metcalf, D., Hilton, D.J., Nicola, N.A., Alexander, W.S., Roberts, A.W., & Robb, L. (2007). The SOCS box of suppressor of cytokine signaling-3 contributes to the control of G-CSF responsiveness in vivo. *Blood*, Vol.110, pp. 1466-1474

Brender, C., Nielsen, M., Kaltoft, K., Mikkelsen, G., Zhang, Q., Wasik, M., Billestrup, N., & Odum, N. (2001b). STAT3-mediated constitutive expression of SOCS-3 in cutaneous T-cell lymphoma. *Blood.*, Vol.97, No.4, pp. 1056-1062.

Brender, C., Columbus, R., Metcal, D., Handman, E., Starr, R., Huntington, N., Tarlinton, D., Ødum, N., Nicholson, S.E., Nicola, N.A., Hilton, D.J., & Alexander, W.S. (2004). SOCS5 is expressed in primary B and T lymphoid cells but is dispensable for lymphocyte production and function. *Mol Cell Biol.*, Vol.24, No.13, pp. 6094-6103

Buza-Vidas, N., Antonchuk, J., Qian, H., Mansson, R., Luc, S., Zandi, S., Anderson, K., Takaki, S., Nygren, J.M., Jensen, C.T., & Jacobsen, S.E.W. (2006). Cytokines regulate postnatal hematopoietic stem cell expansion: opposing roles of thrombopoietin and LNK. *Genes & Dev.*, Vol.20, pp. 2018-2023

Cacalano, N.A., Sanden, D., & Johnston, J.A. (2001). Tyrosine-phosphorylated SOCS-3 inhibits STAT activation but binds to p120 RasGap and activates Ras. *Nat. Cell Biol.*, Vol.3, pp. 460-465

Caligiuri, M.A., Briesewitz, R., Yu, J., Wang, L., Wei, M., Arnoczky, K.J., Marburger, T.B., Wen, J., Perroti, D., Bloomfield, C.D., & Whitman, S.P. (2007). Novel c-CBL and CBL-b ubiquitin ligase mutations in human acute myeloid leukemia. *Blood*, Vol.110, pp. 1022-1024

Campbell, P.J., & Green, A.R. (2008). The myeloproliferative disorders. N Engl J Med., Vol. 355, pp. 2452-2466.

Carpino, N., Wisniewski, D., Strife, A., Marshak, D., Kobayashi, R., Stillman, B., & Clarkson, B. (1997). p62[dok]: a constitutively tyrosine-phosphorylated, GAP-associated protein in chronic myelogenous leukemia progenitor cells. *Cell*, Vol.88, pp. 197-204

Chaligné, R., Tonetti, C., Besancenot, R., Marty, C., Kiladjian, J.J., Socié, G., Bordessoule, D., Vainchenker, W., & Giraudier, S. (2009). SOCS3 inhibits TPO-stimulated, but not spontaneous, megakaryocytic growth in primary myelofibrosis. *Leukemia.*, Vol.23, No.6, pp. 1186-1190

Chan, M.P., Ilangumaran, S., La Rose, J., Chakrabartty, A., & Rottapel, R. (2003). Autoinhibition of the Kit receptor tyrosine kinase by the cytosolic juxtamembrane region. *Mol. Cell. Biol.*, Vol.23, pp. 3067-3078

Chiang, Y.J., Jang, I.K., Hodes, R., & Gu, H. (2007). Ablation of Cbl-b provides protection against transplanted and spontaneous tumors. *J. Clin. Invest.*, Vol.117, pp.1029-1036

Cho-Vega, J.H., Rassidakis, G.Z., Amin, H.M., Tsioli, P., Spurgers, K., Remache, Y.K., Vega, F., Goy, A.H., Gilles, F., & Medeiros, L.J. (2004). Suppressor of cytokine signaling 3 expression in anaplastic large cell lymphoma. *Leukemia.*, Vol.18, No.11, pp. 1872-1878

Croker, B.A., Metcalf, D., Robb, L., Wei, W., Mifsud, S., DiRago, L., Cluse, L.A., Sutherland, K.D., Hartley, L., Williams, E., Zhang, J.G., Hilton, D.J., Nicola, N.A., Alexander,

W.S., & Roberts, A.W. (2004). SOCS3 is a critical physiological negative regulator of G-CSF signaling and emergency granulopoiesis. *Immunity*, Vol.20, pp. 153-165

Crowder R.J., Enomoto, H., Yang, M., Johnson, E.M. Jr, & Milbrandt, J. (2004). Dok-6, a Novel p62 Dok family member, promotes Ret-mediated neurite outgrowth. *J Biol Chem*, Vol. 279, pp. 42072–42081

Davies, G.C., Ettenberg, S.A., Coats, A.O., Mussante, M., Ravichandran, S., Collins, J., Nau, M.M., & Lipkowitz, S. (2004). Cbl-b interacts with ubiquitinated proteins; differential functions of the UBA domains of c-Cbl and Cbl-b. *Oncogene*, Vol.23, No.42, pp. 7104–7115

De Sepulveda, P., Ilangumaran, S., & Rottapel, R. (2000). Suppressor of cytokine signaling-1 inhibits VAV function through protein degradation. *J Biol Chem*, Vol.275, pp. 14005–14008

Dhe-Paganon, S., Werner, E.D., Nishi, M., Hansen, L., Chi, Y.I., & Shoelson, S.E. (2004). A phenylalanine zipper mediates APS dimerization. *Nat. Struct. Mol. Biol.*, Vol. 11, No.10, pp. 968-974

Diakonova, M., Gunter, D.R., Herrington, J., & Carter-Su, C. (2002). SH2-B□ is a Rac-binding protein that regulates cell motility. *J. Biol. Chem.*, Vol.277, No.12, pp. 10669-10677

Di Cristofano, A., Carpino, N., Dunant, N., Friedland, G., Kobayashi, R., Strife, A., Wisniewski, D., Clarkson, B., Pandolfi, P.P., & Resh, M.D. (1998). Molecular cloning and characterization of p56[dok-2] defines a new family of RasGAP-binding proteins. *J. Biol. Chem.*, Vol.273, pp. 4827–4830

Dunbar, A.J., Gondek, L.P., O'Keefe, C.L., Makishima, H., Rataul, M.S., Szpurka, H., Sekeres, M.A., Wang, X.F., McDevitt, M.A., & Maciejewski, J.P. (2008). 250K single nucleotide polymorphism array karyotyping identifies acquired uniparental disomy and homozygous mutations, including novel missense substitutions of c-Cbl, in myeloid malignancies. *Cancer Res*, Vol.68, pp. 10349–10357

Egan, P.J., Lawlor, K.E., Alexander, W.S., & Wicks, I.P. (2003). Suppressor of cytokine signaling-1 regulates acute inflammatory arthritis and T cell activation. *J Clin Invest.*, Vol.111, No.6, pp. 915-924

El Chami N, Ikhlef F, Kaszas K, Yakoub S, Tabone E, Siddeek B, Cunha S, Beaudoin C, Morel L, Benahmed M, Régnier DC. (2005). Androgen-dependent apoptosis in male germ cells is regulated through the proto-oncoprotein Cbl. *J Cell Biol.*, Vol.171, No.4, pp.651-61

Elliott, J., Suessmuth, Y., Scott, L.M., Nahlik, K., McMullin, M.F., Constantinescu, S.N., Green, A.R., & Johnston, J.A. (2009). SOCS3 tyrosine phosphorylation as a potential bio-marker for myeloproliferative neoplasms associated with mutant JAK2 kinases. *Haematologica.*, Vol.94, No.4, pp. 576-80

Ema, H., Sudo, K., Seita, J., Matsubara, A., Morita, Y., Osawa, M., Takatsu, K., Takaki, S., & Nakauchi, H. (2005). Quantification of self-renewal capacity in single hematopoietic stem cells from normal and Lnk-deficient mice. *Develop. Cell*, Vol.8, pp. 907-914

Endo, T.A., Masuhara, M., Yokochi, M., Suzuki, R., Sakamoto, H., Mitsui, K., Matsumoto, A., Tanimura, S., Ohtsubo, M., Misawa, H., Miyazaki, T., Leonor, N., Taniguchi, T., Fujita, T., Kanakura, Y., Komiya, S., & Yoshimura, A. (1997). A new protein containing an SH2 domain that inhibits JAK kinases. *Nature*, Vol.387, pp. 921–924

Favre, H., Benhamou, A., Finidori, J., Kelly, P.A., & Edery, M. (1999). Dual effects of suppressor of cytokine signaling (SOCS-2) on growth hormone signal transduction. *FEBS Lett*, Vol.453, 63–66.

Favre, C., Gerard, A., Clauzier, E., Pontarotti, P., Olive, D., & Nunes, J.A. (2003). DOK4 and DOK5: new Dok-related genes expressed in human T cells. *Genes Immun.*, Vol.4, pp. 40–45

Federici M, Giustizieri ML, Scarponi C, Girolomoni G, & Albanesi C. (2002). Impaired IFN-gamma-dependent inflammatory responses in human keratinocytes overexpressing the suppressor of cytokine signaling 1. *J Immunol*, Vol.169, No.1, pp. 434-442

Fitau, J., Boulday, G., Coulon, F., Quillard, T. & Charreau, B. (2006). The adaptor molecule Lnk negatively regulates TNFalpha-dependent VCAM-1 expression in endothelial cells through inhibition of the ERK1 and 2 pathways. *J. Biol. Chem.*, Vol.281, No.29, pp. 20148-59

Frantsve, J., Schwaller, J., Sternberg, D.W., Kutok, J., & Gilliland, D.G. (2001). Socs-1 inhibits TEL-JAK2-mediated transformation of hematopoietic cells through inhibition of JAK2 kinase activity and induction of proteasome- mediated degradation. *Mol Cell Biol*, Vol.21, pp. 3547–3557

Garcia, A., Prabhakar, S., Hughan, S., Anderson, T.W., Brock, C.J., Pearce, A.C., Dwek, R.A., Watson, S.P., Heberstreit, H.F., & Zitzmann, N.A. (2004). Differential proteome analysis of TRAP-activated platelets: involvement of DOK-2 and phosphorylation of RGS proteins. *Blood*, Vol.103, pp. 2088-2095

Ganesh, S.K., Zakai, N.A., Van Rooij, F.J.A., Soranzo, N., Smith, A.V., Nalls, M.A., Chen, M.H., Kottgen, A., Glazer, N.L., Dehghan, A., Kuhnel, B., Aspelund, T., Yang, Q., Tanaka, T., Jaffe, A., Bis, J.C., Verwoert, G.C., Teumer, A., Fox, C.S., Guralnik, J.M., Ehret, G.B., Rice, K., Felix, J.F., Rendon, A., Eiriksdottir, G., Levy, D., Patel, K.V., Boerwinkle, E., Rotter, J.I., Hofman, A., Sambrook, J.G., Hernandez, D.G., Zheng, G., Bandinelli, S., Singleton, A.B., Coresh, J., Lumley, T., Uitterlinden, A.G., Vangils, J.M., Launer, L.J., Cupples, L.A., Oostra, B.A., Zwaginga, J.J., Ouwehand, W.H., Thein, S.L., Meisinger, C., Deloukas, P., Nauck, M., Spector, T.D., Gieger, C., Gudnason, V., van Duijn, C.M., Psaty, B.M., Ferrucci, L., Chakravarti, A., Greinacher, A., O'Donnell, C.J., Witteman, J.C., Furth, S., Cushman, M., Harris, T.B., & Lin, J.P. (2009). Multiple loci influence erythrocyte phenotypes in the CHARGE Consortium. *Nat. Genet.*, Vol.41, No.11, pp. 1191-1198

Geest, C.R. & Coffer, P. J. (2009). MAPK signaling pathways in the regulation of hematopoiesis. *J. Leuk. Biol.*, Vol.86, pp. 237-250

Gery, S., Gueller, S., Chumakova, K., Kawamata, N., Liu, L., & Koeffler, H.P. (2007). Adaptor protein Lnk negatively regulates the mutant MPL, MPLW515L associated with myeloproliferative disorders. *Blood*, Vol.110, No.9, pp. 3360-3364

Gery, S., Qi, C., Gueller, S., Hongtao, X., Tefferi, A., & Koeffler, H.P. (2009a). Lnk inhibits myeloproliferative disorder-associated JAK2 mutant, JAK2V617F. *J Leuk Biol.*, Vol.85, pp. 957-965

Gery, S., Gueller, S., Nowak, V., Sohn, J., Hofman, W.K., & Koeffler, H.P. (2009b). Expression of the adaptor protein Lnk in leukemia cells. *Exp Hematol.*, Vol.37, pp. 585-592

Grand, F.H., Hidalgo-Curtis, C.E., Ernst, T., Zoi, K., Zoi, C., McGuire, C., Kreil, S., Jones, A., Score, J., Metzgeroth, G., Oscier, D., Hall, A., Brandts, C., Serve, H., Reiter, A., Chase, A.J., & Cross, N.C.P. (2009). Frequent CBL mutations associated with 11q acquired uniparental disomy in myeloproliferative neoplasms. *Blood*, Vol.113, pp. 6182–6192

Greenhalgh, C.J., Metcalf, D., Thaus, A.L., Corbin, J.E., Uren, R., Morgan, P.O., Fabri, L.J., Zhang, J.G., Martin, H.M., Willson, T.A., Billestrup, N., Nicola, N.A., Baca, M.,

Alexander, W.S., & Hilton, D.J. (2002). Biological evidence that SOCS-2 can act either as an enhancer or suppressor of growth hormone signaling. *J Biol Chem*, Vol.277, pp. 40181–4

Grogan, T.M., Pileri, S.A., Chan, J.K.C., Helgadottir, A., Sulem, P., Jonsdottir, G.M., Thorleifsson, G., Helgadottir, H, Steinthorsdottir, V., Stefansson, H., Williams, C., Hui, J., Beilby, J., Warrington, N.M., James, A., Palmer, L.J., Koppelman, G.H., Heinzmann, A., Krueger, M., Boezen, H.M., Wheatley, A., Altmuller, J., Shin, H.D., Uh, S.T., Cheong, H.S., Jonsdottir, B., Gislason, D., Park, C.S., Rasmussen, L.M., Porsbjerg, C., Hansen, J.W., Backer, V., Werge, T., Janson, C., Jönsson, U.B., Ng, M.C., Chan, J., So, W.Y., Ma, R., Shah, S.H., Granger, C.B., Quyyumi, A.A., Levey, A.I., Vaccarino, V., Reilly, M.P., Rader, D.J., Williams, M.J., van Rij, A.M., Jones, G.T., Trabetti, E., Malerba, G., Pignatti, P.F., Boner, A., Pescollderungg, L., Girelli, D., Olivieri, O., Martinelli, N., Ludviksson, B.R., Ludviksdottir, D., Eyjolfsson, G.I., Arnar, D., Thorgeirsson, G., Deichmann, K., Thompson, P.J., Wjst, M., Hall, I.P., Postma, D.S., Gislason, T., Gulcher, J., Kong, A., Jonsdottir, I., Thorsteinsdottir, U., & Stefansson, K. Histiocytic sarcoma. In: Swerdlow SH, Campo E, Harris NL, et al. (eds). WHO Classification of Tumours of Haematopoietic and Lymphoid Tissues. 4th edn. International Agency for Research on Cancer: Lyon, 2008, pp 356–357

Gronski, M.A., Boulter, J.M., Moskophidis, D., Nguyen, L.T., Holmberg, K., Elford, A.R., Deenick, E.K., Kim, H.O., Penninger, J.M., Odermatt, B., Gallimore, A., Gascoigne, N.R., & Ohashi, P.S. (2004). TCR affinity and negative regulation limit autoimmunity. *Nat Med*, Vol.10, No.11, pp.1234–1239

Gudbjartsson, D. F., Bjornsdottir, U. S., Halapi, E., et al. (2009). Sequence variants affecting eosinophil numbers associate with asthma and myocardial infarction. *Nat. Genet.*, Vol.41, No.3, pp. 342-347

Gueller, S., Goodrigde, H.S., Niebuhr, B., Xing, H., Koren-Michowitz, M., Serve, H., Underhill, H.D., Brandts, C.H., & Koeffler, H.P. (2010). Adaptor protein Lnk inhibits c-fms-mediated macrophage function. *J. Leuk. Biol.*, Vol.88, pp. 699-706

Gueller, S., Hehn, S., Nowak, V., Gery, S., Serve, H., Brandts, C.H., & Koeffler, H.P. (2011). Adaptor protein Lnk binds to PDGF receptor and inhibits PDGF-dependent signaling. *Exp. Hematol.*, Vol.39, No.5, pp.591-600

Gueller, S., Gery, S., Nowak, V., Liu, L., Serve, H., & Koeffler, H.P. (2008). Adaptor protein Lnk associates with Y568 in c-Kit. *Biochem. J.*, Vol.415, pp. 241-245

Gueller, S., Hehn, S., Nowak, V., Gery, S., Serve, H., Brandts, C.H., & Koeffler, H.P. (2011). Adaptor protein Lnk binds to PDGF receptor and inhibits PDGF-dependent signaling. *Exp. Hematol.*, doi: 10.1016/j.exphem.2011.02.001

Gueller, S., Goodridge, H.S., Niebuhr, B., Xing, H., Koren-Michowitz, M., Serve, H., Underhill, D.M., Brandts, C.H., & Koeffler, H.P. (2010). Adaptor protein Lnk inhibits c-Fms-mediated macrophage function. *J. Leukoc. Biol.*, Vol.88, pp. 699-706

Guittard, G., Gérard, A., Dupuis-Coronas, S., Tronchère, H., Mortier, E., Favre, C., Olive, D., Zimmermann, P., Payrastre, B., & Nunès, J. (2009). Dok-1 and Dok-2 adaptor molecules are regulated by phosphatidylinositol 5-phosphate production in T cells. *J Immunol*, Vol.182, pp. 3974–3978

Gugasyan, R., Quilici, C., Grail, S.T.T.I., Verhagen, A.M., Roberts, A., Kitamura, T., Dunn, A.R., & Lock, P. (2002). Dok-related protein negatively regulates T cell development via its RasGTPase-activating protein and Nck docking sites. *J. Cell. Biol.*, Vol.158, pp. 115-125

Haan, S., Ferguson, P., Sommer, U., Hiremath, M., McVicar, D.W., Heinrich, P.C., Johnston, J.A., & Cacalano, N.A. (2003). Tyrosine phosphorylation disrupts elongin interaction and accelerates SOCS3 degradation. *J Biol Chem.*, Vol.278, No.34, pp.31972-31979

Harada M, Nakashima K, Hirota T, Shimizu M, Doi S, Fujita K, Shirakawa T, Enomoto T, Yoshikawa M, Moriyama H, Matsumoto K, Saito H, Suzuki Y, Nakamura Y, & Tamari M. (2007). Functional polymorphism in the suppressor of cytokine signaling 1 gene associated with adult asthma. *Am J Respir Cell Mol Biol.*, Vol.36, No.4, 491-496

He, X., Li, Y., Schembri-King, J., Jakes, S., & Hayashi, J. (2000). Identification of actin binding protein, ABP-280, as a binding partner of human Lnk adaptor protein. *Mol. Immunol.*, Vol.37, pp. 603-612

Hiragun, T., Peng, Z., & Beaven, M.A. (2005). Dexamethasone up-regulates the inhibitory adaptor protein Dok-1 and suppresses downstream activation of the mitogen-activated protein kinase pathway in antigen-stimulated RBL-2H3 mast cells. *Mol Pharmacol*, Vol.67, pp. 598–603

Hirasaka, K., Kohno, S., Goto, J., Furochi, H., Mawatari, K., Harada, N., Hosaka, T., Nakaya, Y., Ishidoh, K., Obata, T., Ebina, Y., Gu, H., Takeda, S., Kishi, K., & Nikawa, T. (2007). Deficiency of Cbl-b gene enhances infiltration and activation of macrophages in adipose tissue and causes peripheral insulin resistance in mice. *Diabetes*, Vol.56, pp. 2511-2522

Hilton, D.J., Richardson, R.T., Alexander, W.S., Viney, E.M., Willson, T.A., & Sprigg, N.S. (1998). Twenty proteins containing a C-terminal SOCS box form five structural classes. *Proc Natl Acad Sci USA*, Vol.95, pp.114–9

Honda, H., Ushijima, T., Wakazono, K., Oda, H., Tanaka, Y., Aizawa, S., Ishikawa, T., Yazaki, Y., & Hirai, H. (2000). Acquired loss of p53 induces blastic transformation in p210(bcr/abl)-expressing hematopoietic cells: a transgenic study for blast crisis of human CML. *Blood*, Vol.95, No.4, pp. 1144-1150

Honma M, Higuchi, O., Shirakata, M., Yasuda, T., Shibuya, H., Iemura, S., Natsume, T., & Yamanashi, Y. (2006). Dok-3 sequesters Grb2 and inhibits the Ras–Erk pathway downstream of protein-tyrosine kinases. *Genes Cells,* Vol.11, pp. 143–151

Hookham, M.B., Elliott, J., Suessmuth, Y., Staerk, J., Ward, A.C., Vainchenker, W., Percy, M.J., McMullin, M.F., Constantinescu, S.N., & Johnston, J.A. (2007). The myeloproliferative disorder-associated JAK2 V617F mutant escapes negative regulation by suppressor of cytokine signaling 3. *Blood*, Vol.109, No.11, pp. 4924-4929

Horino, J., Fujimoto, M., Terabe, F., serada, S., Takahashi, T., Soma, Y., Tanaka, K., Chinen, T., Yoshimura, A., Nomura, S., Kawase, I., Hayashi, N., Kishimoto, T., & Naka, T. (2008). Suppressor of cytokine signaling-1 ameliorates dextran sulfate sodium-induced colitis in mice. *Int. Immunol.*, Vol.20, pp. 753-762

Hu, J., & Hubbard, S.R. (2006). Structural basis for phosphotyrosine recognition by the Src Homology-2 domains of the adapter proteins SH2-B and APS. *J. Mol. Biol.*, Vol.361, pp. 69-79

Hu, J., Liu, J., Ghirlando, R., Saltiel, A.R., & Hubbard, S.R. (2003). Structural basis for recruitment of the adaptor protein APS to the activated Insulin receptor. *Mol. Cell.*, Vol.12, pp. 1379-1389

Huang, X., Li, Y., Tanaka, K., Moore, G., & Hayashi, J. (1995). Cloning and characterization of Lnk, a signal transduction protein that links T-cell receptor activation signal to phospholipase C1, Grb2, and phosphatidylinositol 3-kinase. *Proc. Natl. Acad. Sci. USA.* Vol.92, pp. 11618–11622

Huang, F., Kitaura, Y., Jang, I., Naramura, M., Kole, H.H., Liu, L., Qin, H., Schlissel, M.S., & Gu, H. (2006). Establishment of the major compatibility complex-dependent development of CD4+ and CD8+ T cells by the Cbl family proteins. *Immunity,* Vol.25, pp. 571-581

Hughan, S.C., & Watson, S.P. (2007). Differential regulation of adapter proteins Dok2 and Dok1 in platelets, leading to an association of Dok2 with integrin ☐IIb☐3. *J. Thromb Haemost,* Vol.5, pp. 387-394

Hunt, K., Zhernakova, A., Turner, G., Heap, G.A., Franke, L., Bruinenberg, M., Romanos, J., Dinesen, L.C., Ryan, A.W., Panesar, D., Gwilliam, R., Takeuchi, F., McLaren, W.M., Holmes, G.K., Howdle, P.D., Walters, J.R., Sanders, D.S., Playford, R.J., Trynka, G., Mulder, C.J., Mearin, M.L., Verbeek, W.H., Trimble, V., Stevens, F.M., O'Morain, C., Kennedy, N.P., Kelleher, D., Pennington, D.J., Strachan, D.P., McArdle, W.L., Mein, C.A., Wapenaar, M.C., Deloukas, P., McGinnis, R., McManus, R., Wijmenga, C., & van Heel, D.A. (2008). Newly identified genetic risk variants for celiac disease related to the immune response. *Nat. Genet.,* Vol.40, No.4, pp. 395-402

Hunter, S., Burton, E. A., Wu, S. C. & Anderson, S. M. (1999). Fyn associates with Cbl and phosphorylates tyrosine 731 in Cbl, a binding site for phosphatidylinositol 3-kinase. *J. Biol. Chem.,* Vol.274, pp. 2097–2106

Ikram, M.K., Xueking, S., Jensen, R.A., Cotch, M.F., Hewitt, A.W., Ikram, M.A., Wang, J.J., Klein, R., Klein, B.E., Breteler, M.M., Cheung, N., Liew, G., Mitchell, P., Uitterlinden, A.G., Rivadeneira, F., Hofman, A., de Jong, P.T., van Duijn, C.M., Kao, L., Cheng, C.Y., Smith, A.V., Glazer, N.L., Lumley, T., McKnight, B., Psaty, B.M., Jonasson, F., Eiriksdottir, G., Aspelund, T.; Global BPgen Consortium, Harris, T.B., Launer, L.J., Taylor K.D., Li, X., Iyengar, S.K., Xi, Q, Sivakumaran, T.A., Mackey, D.A., Macgregor, S, Martin, ,N..G., Young, T.L., Bis, J.C., Wiggins, K.L., Heckbert, S.R., Hammond, C.J., Andrew, T, Fahy S, Attia, J., Holliday E.G, Scott, R.J., Islam, F.M., Rotter, J.I., McAuley, A.K., Boerwinkle, E, Tai, E.S., Gudnason, V., Siscovick, D. S, Vingerling, J.R., & Wong.TY (2010). Four novel loci (19q13, 6q24, 12q24, and 5q14) influence the microcirculation in vivo. *PLoS Genet.,* Vol.6, No.10, e1001184

Irandoust, M.I., Aarts, L.H., Roovers, O., Gits, J., Erkeland, S.J., & Touw, I.P. (2007). Suppressor of signaling 3 controls lysosomal routing of G-CSF receptor. *EMBO J.,* Vol.26, pp. 1782-1793

Iseki, M., Kubo, C., Kwon, S.M., Yamaguchi, A., Kataoka, Y., Yoshida, N., Takatsu, S., & Takaki, S. (2004). Increased numbers of B-1 cells and enhanced responses against TI-2 antigen in mice lacking APS and adaptor molecule containing PH and SH2 domains. *Mol. Cell. Biol.,* Vol.24, pp. 2243-2250

Iseki, M., Kubo-Akashi, C., Kwon, S.M., Yamaguchi, A., Takatsu, K., & Takaki, S. (2005). APS, an adaptor molecule containing PH and SH2 domains, has a negative regulatory role in B cell proliferation. *Biochem. Biophys. Research. Commun.,* Vol.330, pp. 1005-1013

Jo, D., Liu, D., Yao, S., Collins, R.D., & Hawiger, J. (2005). Intracellular protein therapy with SOCS3 inhibits inflammation and apoptosis. *Nat Med.,* Vol.11, No.8, pp. 892-898

Joazeiro, C. A. P., Wing, S. S., Huang, H.-K., Leverson, J. D., Hunter, T. & Liu, Y.-C. (1999) The tyrosine kinase negative regulator c-Cbl as a RING-type, E2-dependent ubiquitin-protein ligase. *Science*, Vol.286, pp. 309–312

Kamura, T., Sato, S., Haque, D., Liu, L., Kaelin, W.G. Jr., Conaway, R.C., & Conaway, J.W. (1998). The elongin BC complex interacts with the conserved SOCS-box motif present in members of the SOCS, ras, WD- 40 repeat, and ankyrin repeat families. *Genes Dev.*, Vol.12, pp. 3872–3881

Keane, M.M., Rivero-Lezcano, O., Mitchell, J.A., Robbins, K.C., & Lipkowitz, S. (1995). Cloning and characterization of cbl-b: a SH3 binding protein with homology to the c-cbl proto-oncogene. *Oncogene*, Vol.10, pp. 2367-2377

Keane, M.M., Ettenberg, S.A., Nau, M.M., Banerjee, P., Cuello, M., Penninger, J., & Lipkowitz, S. (1999). Cbl-3: a new mammalian cbl family protein. *Oncogene*, Vol.18, pp. 3365-3375

Kent, D.G., Dykstra, B.J., Cheyne, J., Ma, E., & Eaves, C.J. (2008). Steel factor coordinately regulates the molecular signature and biologic function of hematopoietic stem cells. *Blood.*, Vol.112, pp. 560-567

Khwaja, A. (2006). The role of Janus kinases in haemopoiesis and haematological malignancy. *British Journal of Haematology*, Vol.134, pp. 366–384

Kitaura, Y., Jang, I.K., Wang, Y., Han, Y.C., Inazu, T., Cadera, E.J., Schlissel, M., Hardy, R.R., & Gu, H. (2007). Control of the B cell-intrinsic tolerance programs by ubiquitin ligases Cbl and Cbl-b. *Immunity*, Vol.26, pp. 567-578

Kimura, A., Kinjyo, I., Matsumara, Y., Mori, H., Mashima, R., Harada, M., Chien, K.R., Yasukawa, H., & Yoshimura, A. (2004). SOCS3 is a physiological negative regulator for granulopoiesis and granulocyte colony-stimulating factor receptor signaling. *J. Biol. Chem.*, Vol.279, pp. 6905-6910

Kinjyo, I., Hanada, T., Inagaki-Ohara, Mori, K., H., Aki, D., Ohishi, M., Yoshida, H., Kubo, M., & Yoshimura, A. (2002). SOCS1/JAB is a negative regulator of LPS-induced macrophage activation. *Immunity*, Vol.17, pp. 583–591

Kishi, K., Mawatari, K., Sakai-Wakamatsu, K., Yuasa, T., Wang, M., Ogura-Sawa, M., Nakaya, Y., Hatakeyama, S., & Ebina, Y. (2007). APS-mediated ubiquitination of the insulin receptor enhances its internalization, but does not induce its degradation. *Endocrinology*, Vol.54, No.1, pp. 77-88

Knisz, J., Banks, A., McKeag, L., Metcalfe, D.D., Rothman, P.B., & Brown, J.M. (2009). Loss of SOCS7 in mice results in severe cutaneous disease and increased mast cell activation. *Clin Immunol.*, Vol.132, No.2, pp. 277-284

Krawczyk, C., Bachmaier, K., Sasaki, T., Jones, R.G., Snapper, S.B., Bouchard, D., Kozieradzki, I., Ohashi, P.S., Alt, F.W., & Penninger, J.M. (2000). Cbl-b is a negative regulator of receptor clustering and raft aggregation in T cells. *Immunity*, Vol.13, pp. 463–473

Krebs, D.L., Uren, R.T., Metcalf, D., Rakar, S., Zhang, J.G., Starr, R., De Souza, D.P., Hanzinikolas, K., Eyles, J., Connolly, L.M., Simpson, R.J., Nicola, N.A., Nicholson, S.E., Baca, M., Hilton, D.J., & Alexander, W.S. (2002). SOCS-6 binds to insulin receptor substrate 4, and mice lacking the SOCS-6 gene exhibit mild growth retardation. *Mol Cell Biol.*, Vol.22, No.13, pp. 4567-4578.

Krebs, D.L., Metcalf, D., Merson, T.D., Voss, A.K., Thomas, T., Zhang, J.G., Rakar, S., O'bryan, M.K., Willson, T.A., Viney, E.M., Mielke, L.A., Nicola, N.A., Hilton, D.J., &

Alexander, W.S. (2004). Development of hydrocephalus in mice lacking SOCS7. *Proc Natl Acad Sci* U S A., Vol.101, No.43, pp. 15446-15451

Kwon, S.M., Suzuki, T., Kawamoto, A., Ii, M., Eguchi, M., Akimaru, H., Wada, M., Matsumoto, T., Masuda, H., Nakagawa, Y., Nishimura, H., Kawai, K., Takaki, S. & Asahara, T. (2009). Pivotal role of Lnk adaptor protein in endothelial progenitor cell biology for vascular regeneration. *Circ Res.* Vol.104, pp. 969-977

Kubo, M., Ozaki, A., Tanaka, S., Okamoto, M., & Fukushima, A. (2006). Role of suppressor of cytokine signaling in ocular allergy. *Curr. Opin. Allergy Clin. Immunol.*, Vol.6, pp. 361-366

Kubo-Akashi, C., Seki, M., Kwon, S.M., Takizawa, H., Takatsu, K., & Takaki, S. (2004). Roles of a conserved family of adaptor proteins, Lnk, SH2-B, and APS, for mast cell development, growth, and functions: APS-deficiency causes augmented degranulation and reduced actin assembly. *Biochem. Biophys. Research. Commun.*, Vol.315, pp. 356-362

Kurzer., J.H., Argetsinger, L.S., Zhou, Y.J., Kouadio, J.L.K., O'Shea, J.J., & Carter-Su, C. (2004). Tyrosine 813 is a site of JAK2 autophosphorylation critical for activation of JAK2 by SH2-B□. *Mol. Cell. Biol.*, Vol.24, No.10, pp. 4557-4570

Kurzer, J.H., Saharinen, P., Silvennoinen, O., & Carter-Su, C. (2006). Binding of SH2-B family members within a potencial negative regulatory region maintains JAK2 in an active state. *Mol. Cell. Biol.*, Vol.26, No.17, pp. 6381-6394

Kyo, S., Sada, K., Qu, X., Maeno, K., Miah, S.M., Kawauchi-Kamata, K., & Yamamura, H. (2003). Negative regulation of Lyn protein-tyrosine kinase by c-Cbl ubiquitin protein ligase in Fc epsilon RI-mediated mast cell activation. *Genes Cells*, Vol.8, No.10, pp. 825-836

Langdon, W.Y., Hartley, J.W., Klinken, S.P., Ruscetti, S.K., & Morse, H.C. (1989). V-cbl, an oncogene from a dual-recombinant murine retrovirus that induces early B-lineage lymphomas. *Proc. Natl. Acad. Sci.* USA, Vol.86, pp. 1168-1172

Lasho, T.L., Pardanani, A., & Tefferi, A. (2010). *LNK* mutations in *JAK2* mutation-negative erythrocytosis. *N. Engl. J. Med.*, Vol.363, No.12, pp. 1189-1190

Lasho, T.L., Tefferi, A., Finke, C., & Pardanani, A. (2011). Clonal hierarchy and allelic mutation segregation in a myelofibrosis patient with two distinct LNK mutations. *Leukemia*, Vol. 25; No.6, pp. 1056-1058

Lavrikova, E. Y., Nikitin, A. G., Kuraeva, T.L. Peterkova, V.A., Tsitlidze, N.M., Chistiakov, D.A., & Nosikov, V.V. (2011). The carriage of the type I diabetes-associated R262W variant of human LNK correlates with increased proliferation of peripheral blood monocytes in diabetic patients. *Pediatric Diabetes*, Vol.12, No.2, pp. 127-32

Leevers, S.J., Vanhaesebroeck, B., & Waterfield, M.D. (1999). Signalling through phosphoinositide 3-kinases: the lipids take centre stage. *Curr. Opin. Cell Biol.*, Vol.11, pp. 219-225

Lemay, S., Davidson, D., Latour, S., & Veillette, A. (2000). Dok-3, a novel adaptor molecule involved in the negative regulation of immunoreceptor signaling. *Mol. Cell. Biol.*, Vol.20, pp. 2743-2754

Li, Y., He, X., Schembri-King, J., Jakes, S., & Hayashi, J. (2000). Cloning and characterization of human Lnk, an adaptor protein with pleckstrin homology and Src homology 2 domains that can inhibit T cell activation. *J. Immunol.*, Vol.164, pp. 5199-5206

Li, L., Grønning, L.M., Anderson, P.O., Li, S., Edvardsen, K., Johnston, J., Kioussis, D., Shepherd, P.R., & Wang, P. (2004). Insulin induces SOCS-6 expression and its binding to the p85 monomer of phosphoinositide 3-kinase, resulting in improvement in glucose metabolism. *J Biol Chem.*, Vol.279, No.33, pp. 34107-34114

Li, M., Li, Z., Morris, D.L., & Rui, L. (2007). Identification of SH2B2□ as an inhibitor for SH2B1- and SH2B2□-promoted Janus kinase-2 activation and insulin signaling. *Endocrinology, Vol.148, pp. 1615-1621*

Liu, J., DeYoung, S.M., Hwang, J.B., O'Leary, E.E., & Saltiel, A.R. (2003). The roles of Cbl-b and c-Cbl in insulin-stimulated glucose transport. *J. Biol. Chem.*, Vol.278, No.38, pp. 36754–36762

Loeser, S., Loser, K., Bijker, S.M., Rangachari, M., van der Burg, S.H., Wada, T., Beissert, S., Melief, C.J., & Penninger, J.M. (2007). Spontaneous tumor rejection by cbl-b-deficient CD8+ T cells. *J. Exp. Med.*, Vol.204, pp. 879-891

Loh, M.L., Sakai, D.S., Flotho, C., Kang, M., Fliegauf, M., Archambeault, S., Mullighan, C.G., Chen, L., Bergstraesser, E., Bueso-Ramos, C.E., Emanuel, P.D., Hasle, H., Issa, J.P., van den Heuvel-Eibrink, M.M., Locatelli, F., Starý, J., Trebo, M., Wlodarski, M., Zecca, M., Shannon, K.M., & Niemeyer, C.M. (2009). Mutations in CBL occur frequently in juvenile myelomonocytic leukemia. *Blood*, Vol.114, pp. 1859-1863

Lu, L.F., Thai, T.H., Calado, D.P., Chaudhry, A., Kubo, M., Tanaka, K., Loeb, G.B., Lee, H., Yoshimura, A., Rajewsky, K., & Rudensky, A.Y. (2009). Foxp3-dependent microRNA155 confers competitive fitness to regulatory T cells by targeting SOCS1 protein. *Immunity.*, Vol.30, No.1, pp. 80-91

Lupher, M.L., Jr. Songyang, Z., Shoelson, S.E., Cantley, L.C., & Band, H. (1997). The Cbl phosphotyrosine-binding domain selects a D(N/D)XpY motif and binds to the Tyr292 negative regulatory phosphorylation site of ZAP-70. *J Biol Chem*, Vol.272, No.52, pp. 33140–33144

Makishima, H., Jankowska, A.M., McDevitt, M.A., O'Keefe, C., Dujardin, S., Cazzolli, H., Przychodzen, B., Prince, C., Nicoll, J., Siddaiah, H., Shaik, M., Szpurka, H., His, E., Advani, A., Paquette, R., & Maciejewski, J.P. (2011). CBL, CBLB, TET2, ASXLi, and IDH1/2 mutations and additional chromosomal aberrations constitute molecular events in chronic myelogenous leukemia. *Blood*, Vol. 117, No.21, pp. e198-e206

Marine, J.C., Topham, D.J., McKay, C., Wang, D., Parganas, E., Stravopodis, D., Yoshimura, A., & Ihle, J.N. (1999a). SOCS1 deficiency causes a lymphocyte-dependent perinatal lethality. *Cell*, Vol.98, pp. 609–16

Marine, J.C., McKay, C., Wang, D., Topham, D.J., Parganas, E., Nakajima, H., Penderville, H., Yasukawa, H., Sasaki, A., Yoshimura, A., & Ihle, J.N. (1999b). SOCS3 is essential in the regulation of fetal liver erythropoiesis. *Cell*, Vol.98, pp. 617–627

Martinelli, S., de Luca, A., Stellacci, E., Rossi, C., Checquolo, S., Lepri, F., Caputo, C., Silvano, M., Buscherini, F., Consoli, F., ferrara, G., Digilio, M.C., Cavaliere, M.L., van Hagen, J.M., Zampino, G., van der Burgt, I., Ferrero, G.B., Mazzanti, L., Screpanti, I., Yntema, H.G., Nillesen, W.M., Savarirayan, R., Zenker, M., Dallapiccola, B., Gelb, B.D., & Tartaglia, M. (2010). Heterozygous germline mutations in the CBL tumor-suppressor gene cause a Noonan syndrome-like phenotype. *Am. J. Hum. Genet.*, Vol.87, pp. 250-257

Mashima, R., Honda, K., Yang, Y., Morita, Y., Inoue, A., Arimura, S., Nishina, H., Ema, H., Nakauchi, H., Seed, B., Oda, H., & Yamanashi, Y. (2010). Mice lacking Dok-1, Dok-2, and Dok-3 succumb to aggressive histiocytic sarcoma. *Lab Invest.* Vol.90, No.9, pp. 1357-1364

Matsumoto, A., Seki, Y., Kubo, M., Ohtsuka, S., Suzuki, A., Hayashi, I., Tsuji, K., Nakahata, T., Okabe, M., Yamada, S., & Yoshimura, A. (1999). Suppression of STAT5 functions in liver, mammary glands, and T cells cytokine-inducible SH2-containing protein 1 transgenic mice. *Mol. Cell. Biol.*, Vol.9, No.9, pp. 6396-6407

Matsumoto, T., Ii, M., Nishimura, H., Shoji, T., Mifune, Y., Kawamoto, A., Kuroda, R., Fukui, T., Kawakami, Y., Kuroda, T., Kwon, S.M., Iwasaki, H., Horii, M., Yokoyama, A., Oyamada, A., Lee, S.Y., Hayashi, S., Kurosaka, M., Takaki, S., & Asahara, T. (2010). Lnk-dependent axis of SCF-cKit signal for osteogenesis in bone fracture healing. *J. Exp. Med.*, Vol.207, pp. 2207-2223

Metcalf, D., Greenhalgh, C.J., Viney, E., Willson, T.A., Starr, R., Nicola, N.A., Hilton, D.J., & Alexander, W.S. (2000). Gigantism in mice lacking suppressor of cytokine signalling-2. *Nature*, Vol.405, pp. 1069-1073

Metcalf, D.S., Mifsud, L., Di Rago, N., Nicola, N. A., Hilton, D.J., & Alexander, W.S. (2002). Polycistic kidneys and chronic inflammatory lesions are the delayed consequences of loss of the suppressor of cytokine signaling-1 (SOCS-1). *Proc. Natl. Acad. Sci. U.S.A.*, Vol.99, pp. 943-948

Minami, A., Iseki, M., Kishi, K., Wang, M., Ogura, M., Furukawa, N., Hayashi, S., Yamada, M., Obata, T., Takeshita, Y., Nakaya, Y., Bando, Y., Izumi, K., Moodie, S.A., Kajiura, f., Matsumoto, M., Takatsu, K., Takaki, S., & Ebina, Y. (2003). Increased insulin sensitivity and hypoinsulinemia in APS knockout mice. *Diabetes*, Vol.52, pp. 2657-2665

Minamoto, S., Ikegame, K., Ueno, K., Narazaki, M., Naka, T., Yamamoto, H., Matsumoto, T., Saito, H., Hosoe, S., & Kishimoto, T. (1997). Cloning and functional análisis of new members of STAT induced STAT inhibitor (SSI) family: SSI-2 and SSI-3. *Biochem. Biophys. Res. Commun.*, Vol.237, No.1, pp. 79-83

Molero JC, Jensen TE, Withers PC, Couzens M, Herzog H, Thien CB, Langdon WY, Walder K, Murphy MA, Bowtell DD, James DE, Cooney GJ. (2004). c-Cbl-deficient mice have reduced adiposity, higher energy expenditure, and improved peripheral insulin action. *J Clin Invest.*, Vol.114, No.9, pp.1326-33

Molfetta, R., Belleudi, F., Peruzzi, G., Morrone, S., Leone, L., Dikic, I., Piccoli, M., Frati, L., Torrisi, M.R., Santoni, A., & Paolini, R. (2005). CIN85 regulates the ligand-dependent endocytosis of the IgE receptor: a new molecular mechanism to dampen mast cell function. *J Immunol*, Vol.175, pp. 4208-4216

Moodie, S.A., Alleman-Sposeto, J., & Gustafson, T.A. (1999). Identification of the APS protein as a novel insulin receptor substrate. *J. Biol. Chem.*, Vol.274, pp. 11186-11193

Muramatsu H, Makishima H, Jankowska AM, Yoshida, N., Xu, Y., Nishio, N., Hama, A., Yagasaki, H., Takahashi, Y., Kato, K., Manabe, A., Kojima, S., & Maciejewski, J.P. (2010). Mutations of E3 ubiquitin ligase Cbl family members but not TET2 mutations are pathogenic in juvenile myelomonocytic leukemia. *Blood*, Vol.15, pp. 1969-1975

Murphy, M. A., Schnall, R. G., Venter, D. J., Barnett, L., Bertoncello, I., Thien, C. B. F., Langdon, W. Y., & Bowtell, D. D. L. (1998). Tissue hyperplasia and enhanced T cell signalling via ZAP-70 in c-Cbl deficient mice. *Mol. Cell. Biol.*, Vol.18, pp. 4872-4882

Naka, T., Narazaki, M., Hirate, M., Matsumoto, T., Minamoto, S., Aono, A., Nishimoto, N., Kajita, T., Taga, T., Yoshizaki, K., Akira, S., & Kishimoto, T. (1997). Structure and function of a new STAT-induced STAT inhibitor. *Nature*, Vol.387, pp. 924-929

Nakagawa, R., Naka, T., Tsutsui, H., Fujimoto, M., Kimura, A., Abe, T., Seki, E., Sato, S., Takeuchi, O., Takeda, K., Akira, S., Yamanishi, K., Kawase, I., Nakanishi, K., & Kishimoto, T. (2002). SOCS-1 participates in negative regulation of LPS responses, *Immunity*, Vol.17, pp. 677–687

Naramura, M., Kole, H. K., Hu, R.-J., & Gu, H. (1998). Altered thymic positive selection and intracellular signals in Cbl-deficient mice. *Proc. Natl. Acad. Sci. U.S.A.*, Vol.95, pp. 15547–15552

Naramura, M., Jang, I.K., Kole, H., Huang, F., Haines, D., & Gu, H. (2002). c-Cbl and Cbl-b regulate T cell responsiveness by promoting ligand-induced TCR downmodulation. *Nat. Immunol.*, Vol.3, pp. 1192–1199

Naramura, M., Nandwani, N., Gu, H., Band, V., & Band, H. (2010). Rapidly fatal myeloproliferative disorders in mice with deletion of Casitas B-cell lymphoma (Cbl) and Cbl-b in hematopoietic stem cells. *Proc. Natl. Acad. Sci. U.S.A.*, Vol.107, N0. 37, pp. 16274-16279

Narazaki, M., Fujimoto, M., Matsumoto, T., Morita, Y., Saito, H., Kajita, T., Yoshizaki, K., Naka, T., & Kishimoto, T. (1998). Three distinct domains of SSI-1/SOCS-1/JAB protein are required for its suppression of interleukin 6 signaling. *Proc Natl Acad Sci USA*, Vol.95, pp. 13130–13134

Nelms, K., O'Neill, T.J., Li, S., Hubbard, S.R., Gustafson, T.A., & Paul, W.E. (1999). Alternative splicing, gene localization, and binding of SH2-B to the insulin receptor kinase domain. *Mamm Genome*, Vol.10, pp. 1160-1167

Némorin , J.G., & Duplay, P. (2000). Evidence that Lck-mediated phosphorylation of p56dok-2 and p62dok may play a role in CD2 signalling. *J. Biol. Chem.*, Vol.275, pp. 14590-14597

Nicholson, S.E., Willson, T.A., Farley, A., Starr, R., Zhang, J.G., Baca, M., Alexander, W.S., Metcalf, D., Hilton, D.J., & Nicola, N.A. (1999). Mutational analyses of the SOCS proteins suggest a dual domain requirement but distinct mechanisms for inhibition of LIF and IL-6 signal transduction. *EMBO J.*, Vol.18, pp. 375–385.

Nicholson, S.E., De Suoza, D., Fabri, L.J,, Corbin, J., Willson, T.A., Zhang, J.G., Silva, A., Asimakis, M., Farley, A., Nash, A.D., Metcalf, D., Hilton, D.J., Nicola, N.A., & Baca, M. (2000). Suppressor of cytokine signalling-3 preferentially binds to the SHP-2-binding site on the shared cytokine receptor subunit gp 130. *Proc Natl Acid Sci USA*, Vol.97, pp. 6493–6498

Niemeyer, C., Kang, M.W., Shin, D.H., Furlan, I., Erlacher, M., Bunin, N.J., Bunda, S., Finklestein, J.Z., Sakamoto, K.M., Gorr, T.A., Mehta, P., Schmid, I., Kropshofer, G., Corbacioglu, S., Lang, P.J., Klein, C., Schlegel, P.G., Heinzmann, A., Schneider, M., Starý, J., van den Heuvel-Eibrink, M.M., Hasle, H., Locatelli, F., Sakai, D., Archambeault, S., Chen, L., Russell, R.C., Sybingco, S.S., Ohh, M., Braun, B.S., Flotho, C., & Loh, M.L. (2010). Germline CBL mutations cause developmental abnormalities and predispose to juvenile myelomonocytic leukemia. *Nat. Genet.*, Vol.42, No.9, pp. 794-800

Niki, M., Di Cristofano, A., Zhao, M., Honda, H., Hirai, H., Van Aelst, L., Cordon-Cardo, C., & Pandolfi, P.P. (2004). Role of Dok-1 and Dok-2 in leukemia suppression. *J. Exp. Med.*, Vol.200, No.12, pp. 1689-1695

Ng, C.H., Xu, S., & Lam, K.P. (2007). Dok-3 plays a non redundant role in negative regulation of B-cell activation. *Blood*, Vol.110, pp. 259–266

Nobuhisa, I., Takizawa, M., Takaki, S., Inoue, H., Okita, K., Ueno, M., Takatsu, K., & Taga, T. (2003). Regulation of hematopoietic development in the Aorta-Gonad-Mesonephros region mediated by Lnk adaptor protein. *Mol. Cell. Biol.*, Vol.23, No.23, pp. 8486-8494

Ogura, H., Murakami, M., Okuyama, Y., Tsuruoka, M., Kitabayashi, C., Kanamoto, M., Nishihara, M., Iwakura, Y., & Hirano, T. (2008). Interleukin-17 promotes autoimmunity by triggering a positive-feedback loop via interleukin-6 induction. *Immunity*, Vol.29, pp. 628-636

Oh, S.T., Simonds, E.F., Jones, C., Hale, M.B., Goltsev, Y., Gibbs Jr, K.D., Merker, J.D., Zehnder, J.L., Nolan, G.P., & Gotlib, J. (2010). Novel mutations in the inhibitory adaptor protein LNK drive JAK-STAT signaling in patients with myeloproliferative neoplasms. *Blood*, 116, No.6, pp. 988-992

Ohshima, M., Yokoyama, A., Ohnishi, H., Hamada, H., Kohno, N., Higaki, J., & Naka, T. (2007). Overexpression of suppressor of cytokine signalling-5 augments eosinophilic airway inflammation in mice. *Clin Exp Allergy.*, Vol.37, No.5, pp. 735-742

Ohtsuka, S., Takaki, S., Iseki, M., Miyoshi, K., Nakagata, N., Kataoka, Y., Yoshida, N., Takatsu, K., & Yoshimura, A. (2002). SH2-B is required for both male and female reproduction. *Mol. Cell. Biol.*, Vol.22, pp. 3066-3077

Okochi O, Hibi K, Sakai M, Inoue S, Takeda S, Kaneko T, & Nakao A. (2003). Methylation-mediated silencing of SOCS-1 gene in hepatocellular carcinoma derived from cirrhosis. *Clin Cancer Res.*, Vol.9, No.14, pp. 5295-5298

Ortmann, R. A., Cheng, T., Visconti, R., Frucht, D. M. & O'Shea, J.J. (2000). Janus kinases and signal transducers and activators of transcription: their roles in cytokine signaling, development and immunoregulation. *Arthritis Res*, Vol.2, pp. 16-32

Osborne, M.A., Dalton, S., & Kochan, J.P. (1995). The yeast tribrid system: genetic detection of trans-phosphorylated ITAM-SH2-interactions. *Biotechnology*, Vol.13, pp. 1474-1478

Ott, V.L., Tamir, I., Niki, M., Pandolfi, P.P., & Cambier, J.C. (2002). Downstream of kinase, p62(dok), is a mediator of Fc gamma IIB inhibition of Fc epsilon RI signaling. *J Immunol.*, Vol.168, pp. 4430–4439

Paolini, R., Molfetta, R., Beitz, L.O., Zhang, J., Scharenberg, A.M., Piccoli, M., Frati, L., Siraganian, R., & Santoni, A. (2002). Activation of Syk tyrosine kinase is required for c-Cbl-mediated ubiquitination of Fcepsilon RI and Syk in RBL cells. *J Biol Chem*, Vol.277, No.40, pp. 36940–36947

Pardani, A., Lasho, T., Finke, C., Oh, S.T., Gotlib, J., & Tefferi, A. (2010). LNK mutation studies in blast-phase myeloproliferative neoplasms, and in chronic-phase disease with TET2, IDH, JAK2 or MPL mutations. *Leukemia*, Vol.24, No.10, pp. 1713-1718

Pawson, T. & Scott, J. D. (1996). Signaling Through Scaffold, Anchoring, and Adaptor Proteins. *Science*, Vol.278, pp. 2075-2080

Perez, B., Kosmider, O., Cassinat, B., Renneville, A., Lachenaud, J., Kaltenbach, S., Bertrand, Y., Chomienne, C., Fontenay, M., Preudhomme, C., & Cavé, H. (2010). Genetic typing of CBL, ASXL1, RUNX1, TET2, and JAK2 in juvenile myelomonocytic leukaemia reveals a genetic profile distinct from chronic myelomonocytic leukaemia. *Br. J. Haematol.*, Vol.151, pp. 460-468

Qu, X., Sada, K., Kyo, S., Maeno, K., Miah, S.M., & Yamamura, H. (2004). Negative regulation of FcepsilonRI-mediated mast cell activation by a ubiquitin-protein ligase Cbl-b. *Blood*, Vol.103, No.5, pp. 1779–1786

Quentmeier, H., Geffers, R., Jost, E., Macleod, R.A., Nagel, S., Röhrs, S., Romani, J., Scherr, M., & Zaborski, M., & Drexler, H.G. (2008). SOCS2: inhibitor of JAK2V617F-mediated signal transduction. *Leukemia.*, Vol.22, No.12, pp. 2169-2175

Ram, P.A., & Waxman, D.J. (1999). SOCS/CIS protein inhibition of growth hormone-stimulated STAT5 signaling by multiple mechanisms. *J Biol Chem.*, Vol.274, pp. 35553–35561

Rathinam, C., Thien, C.B.F., Langdon, W.Y., Gu, H., & Flavell, R.A. (2008). The E3 ubiquitin ligase c-Cbl restricts development and functions of hematopoietic stem cells. *Genes Dev.*, Vol.22, pp. 992-997

Rathinam, C., Thien, C.B.F., Flavell, R.A., & Langdon, W.Y. (2010). Myeloid leukemia development in c-Cbl RING finger mutant mice is dependent on FLT3 signaling. *Cancer Cell*, Vol.18, pp. 341-352

Reichsteiner, M., & Rogers, S.W. (1996). PEST sequences and regulation by proteolysis. *Trends Biochem. Sci.*, Vol.21, pp. 267-271

Ren, D., Li, M., Duan, C., & Rui, L. (2005). Identification of SH2-B as a key regulator of leptin sensitivity, energy balance, and body weight in mice. *Cell. Metab.*, Vol.2, pp. 95-104

Riedel, H., Wang, J., Hansen, H., & Yousaf, N. (1997). PSM, an insulin-dependent, pro-rich, PH, SH2 domain containing partner of the insulin receptor. *J. Biochem.*, Vol.122, pp. 1105-1113

Robb, L., Boyle, K., Rakar, S., Hartley, R., Lochland, J., & Roberts, A.W. (2005). Genetic reduction of embryonic leukemia-inhibitory factor production rescues placentation in SOCS3-null embryos but does not prevent inflammatory disease. *Proc Natl Acad Sci* USA, Vol.102, pp.16333-16338

Roberts, A.W., Robb, L., Rakar, S., Hartley, L., Cluse, L., Nicola, N.A., Metcalf, D., Hilton, D.H., & Alexander, W.S. (2001). Placental defects and embryonic lethality in mice lacking suppressor of cytokine signaling 3. *Proc Natl Acad Sci* USA, Vol.98, pp. 9324–9329

Roman-Gomez, J., Jimenez-Velasco, A., Castillejo, J.A., Cervantes, F., Barrios, M., Colomer, D., Heiniger, A., & Torres, A. (2004). The suppressor of cytokine signaling-1 is constitutively expressed in chronic myeloid leukemia and correlates with poor cytogenetic response to interferon-alpha. *Haematologica.*, Vol.89, No.1, pp. 42-48

Rudd, E.C. (2001). Lnk adaptor: novel negative regulator of B cell lymphopoiesis. *Science's STKE*: PE1.

Rui, L., Mathews, L.S., Hotta, K., Gustafson, T.A., & Carter-Su, C. (1997). Identification of SH2-B☐ as a substrate of the tyrosine kinase JAK2 involved in Growth hormone signaling. *Mol. Cell. Biol.*, Vol.17, No.11, pp- 6633-6644

Rui, L., Gunter, D.R., Herrington, J., & Carter-Su, C. (2000). Differential binding to and regulation of JAK2 by the SH2 domain and N-terminal region of SH2-B☐. *Mol. Cell. Biol.*, Vol.20, No.9, pp. 3168-3177

Rui, L., Yuan, M., Frantz, D., Shoelson, S., & White, M.F. (2002). SOCS-1 and SOCS-3 block insulin signaling by ubiquitin-mediated degradation of IRS1 and IRS2. *J Biol Chem*, Vol.277, pp. 42394–42398

Ryan, P., Davies, G.C., Nau, M.M., & Lipkowitz, S. (2006). Regulating the regulator: negative regulation of Cbl ubiquitin ligases. *Trends Biochem. Sci.*, Vol.31, No.2, pp. 79-88

Sakai, I., Takeuchi, K., Yamauchi, H., Narumi, H., & Fujita, S. (2002). Constitutive expression of SOCS3 confers resistance to IFN-alpha in chronic myelogenous leukemia cells. *Blood.*, Vol.100, No.8, pp.2926-31

Sakamoto, H., Kinjyo, I., & Yoshimura, A. (2000). The Janus kinase inhibitor, Jab/SOCS-1, is an interferon-gamma inducible gene and determines the sensitivity to interferons. *Leuk Lymphoma.*, Vol.38, No.1-2, pp.49-58

Sargin, B., Choudhary, C., Crosetto, N., Schmidt, M.H.H., Grundler, R., Rensinghoff, M., Thiessen, C., Tickenbrock, L., Schwäble, J., Brandts, C., August, B., Koschmieder, S., Bandi, S.R., Duyster, J., Berdel, W.E., Müller-Tidow, C., Dikic, I., & Serveet, H. (2007). Flt3-dependent transformation by inactivating c-Cbl mutations in AML. *Blood*, Vol.110, pp. 1004–12

Sanada, M., Suzuki, T., Shih, L.Y., Otsu, M., Kato, M., Yamazaki, S., Tamura, A., Honda, H., Sakata-Yamagimoto, M., Kumano, K., Oda, H., Yamagata, T., Takita, J., Gotoh, N., Nakazaki, K., Kawamanta, N., Onodera, M., Nobuyoshi, M., Hayashi, Y., Harada, H., Kurokawa, M., Chiba S., Mori, H., Ozawa, K., Omine, M., Hirai, H., Nakauchi, H., Koeffler, H. P. & Ogawa, S. (2009). Gain-of-function of mutated c-CBL tumour suppressor in myeloid neoplasms. *Nature*, Vol.460, pp. 904–908

Sasaki, A., Yasukawa, H., Susuki, A., Kamizono, S., Syoda, T., Kinyo, I, Sasaki, M., Johnston, J.A., & Yoshimura, A. (1999). Cytokine-inducible SH2 protein-3 (CIS3/SOCS3) inhibits Janus tyrosine kinase by binding through the N-terminal kinase inhibitory region as well as SH2 domain. *Genes Cells*, Vol.4, pp. 339-351

Sasaki, A., Yasukawa, H., Shouda, T., Kitamura, T., Dikic, I., & Yoshimura, A. (2000). CIS3/SOCS-3 suppresses erythropoietin (EPO) signaling by binding the EPO receptor and JAK2. *J Biol Chem.*, Vol.275, pp. 29338–29347

Sasaki, A., Inagaki-Ohara, K., Yoshida, T., Yamanaka, A., Sasaki, M., Yasukawa, H., Koromilas, A.E., & Yoshimura, A. (2003). The N-terminal truncated isoform of SOCS3 translated from an alternative initiation AUG codon under stress conditions is stable due to the lack of a major ubiquitination site, Lys-6. *J Biol Chem*, Vol.278, pp. 2432–2436

Schade, A.E., Wlodarski, M.W. & Maciejewski, J.P. (2006). Pathophysiology Defined by Altered Signal Transduction Pathways. The Role of JAK-STAT and PI3K Signaling in Leukemic Large Granular Lymphocytes. *Cell Cycle*, Vol.5, No.22, pp. 2571-2574

Schmitz, J.,Weissenbach, M., Haan, S., Heinrich, P.C., & Schaper, F. (2000). SOCS3 exerts its inhibitory functions on interleukin-6 signal transduction through the SHP2 recruitment site of gp130. *J Biol Chem.*, Vol.275, pp. 12848–12856

Schubbert, S., Shannon, K., & Bollag, G. (2007). Hyperactive Ras in developmental disorders and cancer. *Nat. Rev. Cancer.*, Vol.7, pp. 295-308

Seita, J., Ema, H., Ooehara, J., Ymazaki, S., Tadokoro, Y., Yamasaki, A., Eto, K., Takaki, S., Takatsu, S., & Nakauchi, H. (2007). Lnk negatively regulates self-renewal of hematopoietic stem cells by modifying thrombopoietin-mediated signal transduction. *Proc. Natl. Acad. Sci. USA.*, Vol.104, No.7, pp. 2349-2354

Seki, Y., Hayashi, K., Matsumoto, A., Seki, N., Tsukada, J., Ransom, J., Naka, T., Kishimoto, T., Yoshimura, A., & Kubo, M. (2002). Expression of the suppressor of cytokine signaling-5 (SOCS5) negatively regulates IL-4-dependent STAT6 activation and Th2 differentiation. *Proc Natl Acad Sci USA.*, Vol.99, No.20, pp. 13003-13008

Seki, Y., Inoue, H., Nagata, N., Hayashi, K., Fukuyama, S. Matsumoto, K., Komine, O. , Hamano, S., Himeno, K., Inagaki-Ohara, K., Cacalano, N., O'Garra, A., Oshida, T.,

Saito, H., Johnston, J.A., Yoshimura, A., & Kubo, M. (2003). SOCS-3 regulates onset and maintenance of T(H)2-mediated allergic responses, *Nat Med*, Vol.9, pp. 1047–1054

Senis, Y.A., Antrobus, R., Severin, S., Parguiña, A.F., Rosa, I., Zitzmann, N., Watson, S.P., & Garcia, A. (2009). Proteomic analysis of integrin ⬚IIb⬚3 outside-in signaling reveals Src-kinase-independent phosphorylation of Dok-1 and Dok-3 leading to SHIP-1 interactions. *J. Thromb Haemost*, Vol.7, pp. 1718-1726

Shao, Y., Yang, C., Elly, C., & Liu, Y.C. (2004). Differential regulation of the B cell receptor-mediated signaling by the E3 ubiquitin ligase Cbl. *J Biol Chem*, Vol.279, No.42, pp. 43646–43653

Shiba N, Kato M, Park, M.J., Sanada, M., Ito, E., Fukushima, K., Sako, M., Arakawa, H., Ogawa, S., & Hayashi, Y. (2010). CBL mutations in juvenile myelomonocytic leukemia, but not in pediatric myelodysplastic syndrome. *Leukemia*, Vol.24, No.4, pp. 1090-1092

Shinohara, H., Inoue, A., Toyama-Sorimachi, N., Nagai, Y., Yasuda, T., Suzuki, H., Horai, R., Iwakura, Y., Yamamoto, T., Karasuyama, H., Miyake, K., & Yamanashi, Y. (2005). Dok-1 and Dok-2 are negative regulators of lipopolysaccharide induced signaling. *J Exp Med*, Vol.201, pp. 333–339

Shouda, T., Yoshida, T., Hanada, T., Wakioka, T., Oishi, M., Miyoshi, K., Komiya, S., Kosai, K., Hanakawa, Y., Hashimoto, K., Nagata, K., & Yoshimura, A. (2001). Induction of the cytokine signal regulator SOCS3/CIS3 as a therapeutic strategy for treating inflammatory arthritis. *J. Cin. Invest.* 108, pp. 1781-1788

Simon, C., Dondi, E., Chaix, A., De Sepulveda, P., Kubiseski, T.J., Varin-Blank, N., & Velazquez L. (2008). Lnk adaptor protein down-regulates specific Kit-induced signaling pathways in primary mast cells. *Blood.*, Vol.112, pp. 4039-4047

Siewert, E., Muller-Esterl, W., Starr, R., Heinrich, P.C., & Schape, F. (1999). Different protein turnover of interleukin-6-type cytokine signaling components. *Eur J Biochem*, Vol.265, pp. 251–257

Sohn, H.W., Gu, H., & Pierce, S.K. (2003). Cbl-b negatively regulates B cell antigen receptor signaling in mature B cells through ubiquitination of the tyrosine kinase Syk. *J Exp Med*, Vol.197, No.11, pp. 1511–1524.

Songyang, Z., Yamanashi, Y., Liu, D., & Baltimore, D. (2001). Domain-dependent function of the ras-GAP-binding protein p62Dok in cell signaling. *J Biol Chem*, Vol.276, pp. 2459-2465

Soranzo, N., Spector, T. D., Mangino, M., Kühnel, B., Rendon, A., Teumer, A., Willenborg, C., Wright, B., Chen, L., Li, M., Salo, P., Voight, B.F., Burns, P., Laskowski, R.A,, Xue, Y., Menzel, S., Altshuler, D., Bradley, J.R., Bumpstead, S., Burnett, M.S., Devaney, J., Döring, A., Elosua, R., Epstein, S.E., Erber, W., Falchi, M., Garner, S.F., Ghori, M.J., Goodall, A.H., Gwilliam, R., Hakonarson, H.H., Hall, A.S., Hammond, N., Hengstenberg, C., Illig, T., König, I.R., Knouff, C.W., McPherson, R., Melander, O., Mooser, V., Nauck, M., Nieminen, M.S., O'Donnell, C.J., Peltonen, L., Potter, S.C., Prokisch, H., Rader, D.J., Rice, C.M., Roberts, R., Salomaa, V., Sambrook, J., Schreiber, S., Schunkert, H., Schwartz, S.M., Serbanovic-Canic, J., Sinisalo, J., Siscovick, D.S., Stark, K., Surakka, I., Stephens, J., Thompson, J.R., Völker, U., Völzke, H., Watkins, N.A., Wells, G.A., Wichmann, H.E., Van Heel, D.A., Tyler-Smith, C., Thein, S.L., Kathiresan, S., Perola, M., Reilly, M.P., Stewart, A.F., Erdmann, J., Samani, N.J., Meisinger, C., Greinacher, A., Deloukas, P., Ouwehand, W.H., Gieger, C. (2009). A genome-wide meta-analysis identifies 22 loci associated with eight haematological parameters in the HaemGen consortium. *Nat. Genet.*, Vol.41, No.11, pp. 1182-1190

Starr, R., Willson, T.A., Viney, E.M., Murra, L.J.L., Rayner, J.R., Jenkins, B.J., Gonda, T.J., Alexander, W.S., Metcalf, D., Nicola, N.A., & Hilton, D.J. (1997). A family of cytokine-inducible inhibitors of signalling. *Nature*, Vol.387, pp. 917–921

Starr, R., Metcalf, D., Elefanty, A.G., Brysha, M., Willson, T.A., Nicola, N.A., Hilton, D.J., & Alexander, W.S. (1998). Liver degeneration and lymphoid deficiencies in mice lacking suppressor of cytokine signaling-1. *Proc. Natl. Acad. Sci. USA*, Vol.95, No.24, pp. 14395-14399

Stork, B., Neumann, K., Goldbeck, I., Alers, S., Kähne, T., Naumann, M., Engelke, M., & Wienands, J. (2007). Subcellular localization of Grb2 by the adaptor protein Dok-3 restricts the intensity of Ca2+ signaling in B cells. *EMBO J*, Vol.26, pp. 1140–1149

Suessmuth, Y., Elliott, J., Percy, M.J., Inami, M., Attal, H., Harrison, C.N., Inokuchi, K., McMullin, M.F., & Johnston, J.A. (2009). A new polycythaemia vera-associated SOCS3 SH2 mutant (SOCS3F136L) cannot regulate erythropoietin responses. *Br J Haematol.*, Vol.147, No.4, pp. 450-458

Suzu S, Tanaka-Douzono, M., Nomaguchi, K., Yamada, M., Hayasawa, H., Kimura, F., & Motoyoshi, K. (2000). p56^{dok-2} as a cytokine-inducible inhibitor of cell proliferation and signal transduction. *EMBO J*, Vol.19, pp. 5114–5122

Suzuki A, Hanada T, Mitsuyama K, Yoshida T, Kamizono S, Hoshino T, Kubo M, Yamashita A, Okabe M, Takeda K, Akira S, Matsumoto S, Toyonaga A, Sata M, & Yoshimura A. (2001). CIS3/SOCS3/SSI3 plays a negative regulatory role in STAT3 activation and intestinal inflammation. *J Exp Med.*, Vol.193, No.4, pp. 471-481

Takaki, S., Watts, J.D., Forbush, K.A., Nguyen, N.T., Hayashi, J., Alberola-Ila, J., Aebersold, R., & Perlmutter, R.M. (1997). Characterization of Lnk. An adaptor protein expressed in lymphocytes. *J. Biol. Chem.*, Vol.272, pp. 14562–14570

Takaki, S., Sauer, K., Iritani, B.M., Chien, S., Ebihara, Y., Tsuji, K.I., Takatsu, K., & Perlmutter, R.M. (2000). Control of B cell production by the adaptor protein Lnk: definition of a conserved family of signal-modulating proteins. *Immunity.* Vol.13, pp. 599–609

Takaki, S., Morita, H., Tezuka, Y., & Takatsu, K. (2002). Enhanced hematopoiesis by hematopoietic progenitor cells lacking intracellular adaptor protein, Lnk. *J Exp Med.*, Vol.195, pp. 151-160

Takaki, S., Tezuka, Y., Sauer, K., Kubo, C., & Kwon, S.M., Armstead, E., Nakao, K., Katsuki, M., Perlmutter, R.M., & Takatsu, K. (2003). Impaired lymphopoiesis and altered B cell subpopulations in mice overexpressing Lnk adaptor protein. *J Immunol*, Vol.170, pp. 703-710

Takahashi, Y., Carpino, N., Cross, J.C., Torres, M., Parganas, E. & Ihle, J.N. (2003). SOCS3: an essential regulator of LIF receptor signaling in trophoblast giant cell differentiation, *EMBO J*, Vol.22, pp. 372–384

Takizawa, H., Kubo-Akashi, C., Nobuhisa, I., Kwon, S.M., Iseki, M., Taga, T., Takatsu, K., & Takaki, S. (2006). Enhanced engraftment of hematopoietic stem/progenitor cells by the transient inhibition of an adaptor protein, Lnk. *Blood*, Vol.107, No.7, pp. 2968-2975

Takizawa, H., Eto, K., Yoshikawa, A., Nakauchi, H., Takatsu, K., & Takaki, S. (2008). Growth and maturation of megakaryocytes is regulated by Lnk/SH2B3 adaptor protein through crosstalk between cytokine- and integrin-mediated signals. *Exp. Hematol.*, Vol.36, No.7, pp. 897-906

Takizawa, H., Nishimura, S., Takayama, N., Oda, A., Nishikii, H., Morita, Y., Kakimura, S., Yamazaki, S., Okamura, S., Tamura, N., Goto, S., Sawaguchi, A., Manabe, I., Takatsu, K., Nakauchi, H., Takaki, S., & Eto, K. (2010). Lnk regulates integrin aIIb☐3 outside-in signaling in mouse platelets, leading to stabilization of thrombus development in vivo. *J. Clin. Invest.*, Vol.120, No.1, pp. 179-190

Taleb, S., Romain, M., Ramkhelawon, B., Uyttenhove, C., Pasterkamp, G., Herbin, O., Esposito, B., Perez, N., Yasukawa, H., Van Snick, J., Yoshimura, A., Tedgui, A., & Mallat, Z. (2009). Loss of SOCS3 expression in T cells reveals a regulatory role for interleukin-17 in atherosclerosis. *J Exp Med*, Vol.206, pp. 2067-2077

Tamir, I., Stolpa, J.C., Helgason, C.D., Nakamura, K., Bruhns, P., Daeron, M., & Cambier, J. (2000). The RasGap-binding protein p62dok is a mediator of inhibitory Fc☐RIIB signals in B cells. *Immunity*, Vol.12, pp. 347-358

Tefferi, A. (2010). Novel mutations and their functional and clinical relevance in myeloproliferative neoplasms: JAK2, MPL, TET2, ASXL1, CBL, IDH and IKZF1. *Leukemia*, Vol.24, pp. 1128-1138

Thien, C.B., Bowtell, D.D., & Langdon, W.Y. (1999). Perturbed regulation of ZAP-70 and sustained tyrosine phosphorylation of LAT and SLP-76 in c-Cbl-deficient thymocytes. *J Immunol*, Vol.162, No.12, pp. 7133–7139.

Thien, C. B. F., Walker, F. & Langdon, W. Y. (2001) Ring finger mutations that abolish c-Cbl-directed polyubiquitination and downregulation of the EGF receptor are insufficient for cell transformation. *Mol. Cell*, Vol.7, pp. 355–365

Thien, C.B.F., & Langdon, W.Y. (2001). Cbl: many adaptations to regulate protein tyrosine kinases. *Nat. Rev. Mol. Cell. Biol.*, Vol. 2, pp. 294-305.

Thien, C.B.F., Scaife, R.M., Papadimitriou, J.M., Murphy, M.A., Bowtell, D.D.L. & Langdon, W.Y. (2003). A mouse with a loss-of-function mutation in the c-Cbl TKB domain shows perturbed thymocyte signaling without enhancing the activity of the ZAP-70 tyrosine kinase. *J. Exp. Med.*, Vol.197, pp. 503–513

Tong, W., & Lodish, F.H. (2004). Lnk inhibits Tpo-mpl signaling and Tpo-mediated megakaryocytopoiesis. *J Exp Med*, Vol.200, pp. 569-580

Tong, W., Zhang, J., & Lodish, F.H. (2005). Lnk inhibits erythropoiesis and Epo-dependent JAK2 activation and downstream signaling pathways. *Blood.*, Vol.105, pp. 4604-4612

Tsygankov, A. Y., Mahajan, S., Fincke, J. E. & Bolen, J. B. (1996). Specific association of tyrosine-phosphorylated c-Cbl with Fyn tyrosine kinase in T cells, *J. Biol. Chem.*, Vol.271, pp. 27130–27137

Velazquez, L., Cheng, A.M., Fleming, H.E., Furlonger, C., Vesely, S., Bernstein, A., Paige, C.J., & Pawson, T. (2002). Cytokine Signaling and Hematopoietic Homeostasis Are Disrupted in Lnk-deficient Mice. *J. Exp. Med.*, Vol.195, No. 12, pp. 1599-1611

Verdier, F., Chretien, S., Muller, O., Varlet, P., Yoshimura, A., Gisselbrecht, S., Lacombe, C., & Mayeux, P. (1998). Proteasomes regulate erythropoietin receptor and signal transducer and activator of transcription 5 (STAT5) activation. Possible involvement of the ubiquitinated Cis protein. *J Biol Chem*, Vol.273, pp. 28185–28190

Vuica, M., Desiderio, S., & Schneck, J.P. (1997). Differential effects of B cell receptor and B cell receptor-Fc☐RIIB1 engagement on Docking of Csk to GTPase-activating protein (GAP)-associated p62. *J. Exp. Med.*, Vol.186, pp. 259-267

Wakioka, T., Sasaki, A., Mitsui, K., Yokouchi, M., Inoue, A., Komiya, S., & Yoshimura, A. (1999). APS, an adaptor protein containing Pleckstrin homology (PH) and Src homology-2 (SH2) domains inhibits the JAK-STAT pathway in collaboration with c-Cbl. *Leukemia.*, Vol.13, pp. 760–767

Waiboci, L.W., Ahmed, C.M., Mujtaba, M.G., Flowers, L.O., Martin, J.P., Haider, M.I., & Johnson, H.M. (2007). Both the suppressor of cytokine 1 (SOCS-1) kinase-inhibitory region and SOCS-1 mimetic bind to JAK2 autophosphorylation site: implications for the development of a SOCS-1 antagonist. *J. Immunol.*, Vol.178, pp. 5058-5068

Wan, M., Li, Y., Xue, H., Li, Q., & Li, J. (2006). TNF-□ induces Lnk expression through PI3K-dependent signaling pathway in human umbilical vein endothelial cells. *J. Surg. Research.*, Vol.136, pp. 53-57

Watanabe, H., Kubo, M., Numata, K., Takagi, K., Mizuta, H., Okada, S., Ito, T., & Matsukawa, A. (2006). Overexpression of suppressor of cytokine signaling-5 in T cells augments innate immunity during septic peritonitis. *J Immunol.*, Vol.177, No.12, pp. 8650-8657

Weiss, L.M., & Chang, K.L. Pathology of Langerhans cell histiocytosis and other histiocytic proliferations. In: Greer JP, Foerster J, Rodgers GM, et al. (eds). Wintrobe's Clinical Hematology. 12th edn. Lippincott Williams & Wilkins: Philadelphia, 2009, pp 1582–1588

Werz, C., Köhler, K., Hafen, E., & Stocker, H. (2009). The Drosophila SH2B family adaptor Lnk acts in parallel to Chico in the Insulin signaling pathway. *PLos Genet.*, Vol.5, No.8, e1000596, doi: 10.1371/journal.pgen.1000596

White, G.E., Cotterill, A., Addley, M.R., Soilleux, E.J., & Greaves, D.R. (2001). Suppressor of cytokine signaling protein SOCS3 expression is increased at sites of acute and chronic inflammation. *J. Mol. Hist.*, Vol.42, pp. 137-151

Wollberg, P., Kennartsson, J., Gottridsson, E., Yoshimura, A., & Rönnstrand, L. (2003). The adapter protein APS associates with the multifunctional docking sites Tyr-568 and Tyr-936 in c-Kit. *Biochem. J.*, Vol.370, pp. 1033-1038

Wong, P.K., Egan, P.J., Croker, B.A., O'Donnell, K., Sims, N.A., Drake, S., Kiu, H., McManus, E.J., Alexander, W.S., Roberts, A.W., & Wicks, I.P. (2006). SOCS-3 negatively regulates innate and adaptive immune mechanisms in acute IL-1 dependent inflammatory arthritis. *J. Clin. Invest.*, Vol.116, pp. 1571-1581

Yabana, N., & Shibuya, M. (2002). Adaptor protein APS binds the NH2-terminal autoinhibitory domain of guanine exchange factor Vav3 and augments its activity. *Oncogene*, Vol.21, pp. 7720-7729

Yamanashi, Y., & Baltimore, D. (1997). Identification of the Abl- and rasGAP-associated 62 kDa protein as a docking protein, Dok. *Cell*, Vol.88, pp. 205–211

Yamanashi, Y., Tamura, T., Kanamori, T., Yamane, H., Nariuchi, H., Yamamoto, T., & Baltimore, D. (2000). Role of the rasGAP-associated docking protein p62dok in negative regulation of B cell receptor-mediated signaling. *Genes Dev*, Vol.14, pp. 11–16

Yasuda, T., Maeda, A., Kurosaki, M., Tezuka, T., Hironaka, K., Yamamoto, T., & Kurosaki, T. (2000). Cbl suppresses B cell receptor-mediated phospholipase C (PLC)-gamma2 activation by regulating B cell linker protein-PLC-gamma2 binding. *J Exp Med*, Vol.191, pp. 641–650

Yasuda, T., Tezuka, T., Maeda, A., Inazu, T., Yamanashi, Y., Gu, H., Kurosaki, T., & Yamamoto, T. (2002). Cbl-b positively regulates Btk-mediated activation of phospholipase C-gamma2 in B cells. *J Exp Med*, Vol.196, pp. 51–63

Yasuda, T., Shirakata, M., Iwama, A., Ishii, A., Ebihara, Y., Osawa, M., Honda, K., Shinohara, H., Sudo, K, Tsuji, K., Nakauchi, H., Iwakura, Y., Hirai, H., Oda, H., Yamamoto, T., &

Yamanashi, Y. (2004). Role of Dok-1 and Dok-2 in myeloid homeostasis and suppression of leukemia. *J. Exp. Med.*, Vol.200, No.12, pp. 1681-1687

Yasukawa, H., Misawa, H., Sakamoto, H., Masuhara, M., Sasaki, A., & Wakioka, T. (1999). The JAK-binding protein JAB inhibits Janus tyrosine kinase activity through binding in the activation loop. *EMBO J*, Vol.18, pp. 1309-20

Yokouchi, M., Suzuki, R., Masuhara, M., Komiya, S., Inoue, A., & Yoshimura, A. (1997). Cloning and characterization of APS, an adaptor molecule containing PH and SH2 domains that is tyrosine phosphorylated upon B-cell receptor stimulation. *Oncogene*, Vol.15, pp. 7-15

Yokouchi, M., Kondo, T., Sanjay, A., Houghton, A., Yoshimura, A., Komiya, S., Zhang, H. & Baron, R. (2001). Src-catalyzed phosphorylation of c-Cbl leads to the interdependent ubiquitination of both proteins. *J. Biol. Chem.*, Vol.276, pp. 35185-35193

Yoshida, T., Ogata, H., Kamio, M., Joo, A., Shiraishi, H., Tokunaga, Y., Sata, M., Nagai, H., & Yoshimura, A. (2004). SOCS1 is a suppressor of liver fibrosis and hepatitis-induced carcinogenesis. *J Exp Med.*, Vol.199, No.12, pp. 1701-1707

Yoshikawa, H., Matsubara, K., Qian, G.S., Jackson, P., Groopman, J.D., Manning, J.E., Harris, C.C., & Herman, J.G. (2001). SOCS-1, a negative regulator of the JAK/STAT pathway, is silenced by methylation in human hepatocellular carcinoma and shows growth-suppression activity. *Nat Genet.*, Vol.28, No.1, pp. 29-35

Yoshimura, A., Ohkubo, T., Kiguchi, T., Jenkins, N.A., Gilbert, D.J., Copeland, N.G.,Hara, T., & Miyajima, A. (1995). A novel cytokine-induced gene CIS encodes an SH2-containing protein that binds to tyrosine-phosphorylated interleukin 3 and erythropoietin receptors. *EMBO J.*, Vol.14, pp. 2816-26

Yoshimura, A., Naka, T., & Kubo, M. (2007). SOCS proteins, cytokine signalling and immune regulation. *Nat Rev Immunol.*, Vol.7, No.6, pp. 454-65

Zhang, J.G., Farley, A., Nicholson, S.E., Wilson, T.A., Zugaro, L.M., simpson, R.J., Moritz, R.L., Cary, D., Richardson, R., Hausmann, G., Kile, B.J., Kent, S.B., Alexander, W.S., Metcalf, D., Hilton, D.J., Nicola, N.A., & Baca, M. (1999). The conserved SOCS box motif in suppressors of cytokine signaling binds to elongins B and C and may couple bound proteins to proteasomal degradation. *Proc. Natl. Acad. Sci.* USA, Vol.96, No.5, pp. 2071-2076

Zhang, J.G., Metcalf, D., Rakar, S., Asimakis, M., Greenhalgh, C.J., Willson, T.A., Starr, R., Nicholson, S.E., Carter, W., Alexander, W.S., Hilton, D.J., Nicola, N.A. (2001). The SOCS box of suppressor of cytokine signaling-1 is important for inhibition of cytokine action in vivo. *Proc Natl Acad Sci* USA, Vol.98, pp.13261-13265

Zhang, J., Chiang, Y.J., Hodes, R.J., & Siraganian, R.P. (2004). Inactivation of c-Cbl or Cbl-b differentially affects signaling from the high affinity IgE receptor. *J Immunol*, Vol.173, No.3, pp. 1811-1818

Zheng, N., Wang, P., Jeffrey, P. D. & Pavletich, N. P. (2000) Structure of a c-Cbl-UbcH7 complex: RING domain function in ubiquitin-protein ligases. *Cell*, Vol.102, pp. 533-539

Zhernakova, A., Elbers, C.C., Ferwerda, B., Romanos, J., Trynka, G., Dubois, P.C., de Kovel, C.G., Franke, L., Oosting, M., Barisani, D., Bardella, M.T.; Finnish Celiac Disease Study Group, Joosten, L.A., Saavalainen, P., van Heel, D.A., Catassi, C., Netea, M.G., & Wijmenga, C. (2010). Evolutionary and functional analysis of Celiac risk loci reveals SH2B3 as a protective factor against bacterial infection. *Am. J. Hum. Genet.*, Vol.86, pp. 970-977

4

Nitric Oxide / Cyclic Nucleotide Regulation of Globin Genes in Erythropoiesis

Vladan P. Čokić[1], Bojana B. Beleslin-Čokić[2], Gordana Jovčić[1],
Raj K. Puri[3] and Alan N. Schechter[4]

[1]*Laboratory of Experimental Hematology, Institute for Medical Research, Belgrade,*
[2]*Clinic of Endocrinology, Diabetes and Diseases of Metabolism, School of Medicine,*
University Clinical Center, Belgrade,
[3]*Division of Cellular and Gene Therapies, Center for Biologics Evaluation and Research,*
Food and Drug Administration, Bethesda,
[4]*Molecular Medicine Branch, National Institute of Diabetes and Digestive and Kidney*
Diseases, National Institutes of Health, Bethesda,
[1,2]*Serbia*
[3,4]*USA*

1. Introduction

1.1. Hemoglobin synthesis

The human hematopoiesis initiates in the second to third embryonic weeks with formation of mesoderm-derived blood islands in the extraembryonic mesoderm of the developing secondary yolk sac (Migliaccio et al., 1986). Erythropoiesis involves proliferation and differentiation of committed erythroid progenitors to mature red blood cells (erythrocytes). Although globins represents <0.1% of proteins at the proerythroblast level, it reaches 95% of all proteins at the level of reticulocytes (Nienhuis & Benz, 1977). Physiologically, the expression of the globin genes is generally regulated in such a way that at any point in development the output of the beta (β)-globin-like chains equals the alpha (α)-globin chains (Lodish & Jacobsen, 1972). The α-globin gene cluster contains three genes and several pseudogenes arranged from the telomere toward the centromere in the following order: 5'-ξ2-$\psi\xi$1-$\psi\alpha$2-$\psi\alpha$1-α2-α1-θ1-3' (Higgs et al., 1998). The human β-globin locus consists of five functional β-like globin genes, that are arranged in the order of their expression during development (5'-ε-$^G\gamma$-$^G\gamma$-δ-β-3'), and an upstream regulatory element, the locus control region (LCR), that is physically composed of five DNase I-hypersensitive sites (HSs) (Grosveld et al., 1987). The most widely studied changes during red cell ontogeny are the shifts or "switches" in globin types. Embryonic erythroblasts are characterized by the synthesis of the unique hemoglobins Gower I ($\zeta_2\varepsilon_2$), Gower II ($\alpha_2\varepsilon_2$), and Hb Portland ($\zeta_2\gamma_2$). The zeta (ζ)- and epsilon (ε)-globin chains are embryonic α-like and β-like chains, respectively. Thus, a switch from ζ- to α- and ε- to gamma (γ)-globin gene production begins during the embryonic phase of erythropoiesis but is not complete until fetal erythropoiesis is well established. During the transition from yolk sac to fetal liver erythropoiesis (5–8 weeks), erythroid precursors within the fetal liver co-express embryonic (ζ- or ε-) and fetal (α- or γ-) globins both in vivo and in vitro (Peschle et al., 1984). The predominant type of hemoglobin synthesized during fetal liver erythropoiesis is fetal hemoglobin (HbF, $\alpha_2\gamma_2$). HbF is formed by γ-globin chain A or G according to the amino acid at the 136 position in the γ chain, i.e., alanine or glycine. The proportion of $^G\gamma$ to $^A\gamma$ is constant throughout fetal development: about 75% of $^G\gamma$ and 25% of $^A\gamma$. However, in adult red cells, the small amount of HbF is composed mainly of $^A\gamma$ (60% vs. 40% of $^G\gamma$) (Jensen et al., 1982). α- and β-globin chains combine as a tetramer of two α- and two β-globin polypeptides along with a heme moiety to form the adult hemoglobin molecule (HbA, $\alpha_2\beta_2$). HbA, detectable at the earliest stages of fetal liver erythropoiesis, is also synthesized as a minor component throughout this period, but HbA₂ ($\alpha_2\delta_2$), minor hemoglobin in the adult, is undetectable in these early stages. From about the 30th gestational week onward, β-globin synthesis steadily increases, so that by term 50%–55% of hemoglobin synthesized is HbA. By 4-5 weeks of postnatal age, 75% of the hemoglobin is HbA, this percentage increasing to 95% by 4 months as the fetal-to-adult hemoglobin switch is completed. HbF levels in circulating red cells are in a plateau for the first 2–3 weeks (as a result of the decline in total erythropoiesis that follows birth), but HbF gradually declines and normal levels (<1%) are achieved by 200 days after birth.

1.2 The GATA-1/2 and Krüppel-like factors role in hemoglobin switching

The regulation of globin gene switching is a very complex process requiring the coordination of different signaling pathways and molecular reactions. Many transcription factors controlling globin gene expression have been identified and characterized. These factors form a complex network of protein-protein and protein-DNA interactions with each other, globin gene promoters, LCR HSs, and other cis-acting intergenic regions (Stamatoyannopoulos, 2005). The GATA family of proteins (GATA1–6) comprises zinc finger transcription factors that both activate and repress target genes containing a consensus GATA binding motif (Orkin, 1992). Binding sites with this motif are present in many positions in the α- and β-globin loci, as well as many other erythroid-expressed genes. The founding member of this family, GATA1, was discovered as a β-globin locus-binding protein (Pruzina et al., 1991). GATA1 is essential for erythroid cell maturation in vivo (Pevny et al., 1989). In addition, GATA1 homodimerizes and interacts with other transcription factors, such as SP-1 and erythroid Krüppel-like factor (EKLF/KLF1), further contributing to the complex network of GATA factor interactions (Gregori et al., 1996). GATA2 is primarily expressed in primitive erythropoiesis, but later in development GATA1 expression predominates (Leonard et al., 1993). Downregulation of GATA2 is important for progression of erythroid cell differentiation (Persons et al., 1999). The protein Friend of GATA1 (FOG) is co-expressed with GATA1 during embryonic development in erythroid cells (Tsang et al., 1997). GATA1 binds a region upstream of both the HBG1- and HBG2-promoter, necessary for HbF silencing, in a FOG1 dependent manner leading to recruitment of the suppressive NuRD-complex (Harju-Baker et al., 2008). GATA-1, together with FOG-1, functions as an anchor in the formation of chromatin looping, and is required for physical interactions between the β LCR and β globin promoter (Vakoc et al., 2005).

The Krüppel-like factors are a family of C2H2 zinc finger DNA binding proteins that are important in controlling developmental programs. KLF1 gene is an erythroid cell-specific zinc finger transcription factor, containing a DNA-binding domain located at its C-terminus, composed of three 'Krüppel-like' C2H2 zinc finger motifs, and a proline-rich transactivation domain at its N-terminus (Miller & Bieker, 1993). KLF1 preferentially activates the β-globin gene promoter by binding with high affinity to the CACCC element (Bieker & Southwood, 1995). KLF1 is essential for adult β-globin gene transcription and binds to the βLCR and β-globin promoters, required for direct interactions between the βLCR and the β-globin gene in humans (Donze et al., 1995, Scheme 1). Patients with hereditary persistence of HbF, with elevated levels of HbF, have mutations in the gene encoding erythroid transcription factor KLF1 (Borg et al., 2010). Recent findings demonstrate that KLF1, and the co-activator BRG1, are designated by short-chain fatty acid derivatives to activate the fetal globin genes. The SWI/SNF complex chromatin-modifying core ATPase BRG1 is required for γ-globin induction by short-chain fatty acid derivatives, and is actively recruited to the γ-globin promoter in the KLF1-dependent manner (Perrine et al., 2009). KLF1-GATA1 fusion proteins activated δ-, γ-, and β-globin promoters, and significantly up-regulated delta (δ)- and γ-globin RNA transcript and protein expression in human erythroleukemic cells (Zhu et al., 2011). DRED (direct repeat erythroid-definitive) was identified as a repressor of the ε-globin gene, it appears to prevent binding of KLF1 to the ε-globin gene promoter and silences ε-globin expression during definitive erythropoiesis (Tanimoto et al., 2000). KLF2 also regulates the expression of the human embryonic ε-globin gene but not the adult β-globin gene (Basu et al., 2005). Another erythroid-specific transcription factor, called fetal Krüppel-like factor (KLF11), activates γ- and ε-globin genes in human erythroleukemic cells (Asano et al., 1999, Scheme 1). KLF11 also activates γ-globin transcription via the CACCC element in the promoter (Asano et al., 2000). The protein encoded by this gene is a zinc finger transcription factor that binds to SP1-like sequences in ε- and γ-globin gene promoters.

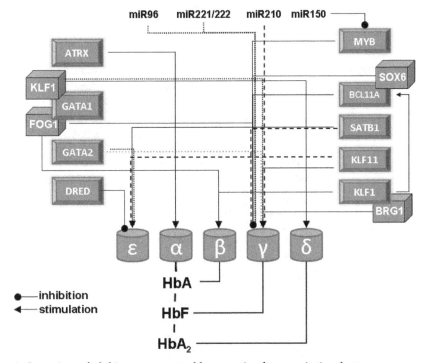

Sheme 1. Overview of globin genes control by examined transcription factors.

1.3 Other factors that participate in hemoglobin switching

A nuclear protein, special AT-rich binding protein 1 (SATB1), regulates genes through targeting chromatin remodeling and its overexpression increases ε-globin and decreases γ-globin gene expression (Wen et al., 2005, Scheme 1). Global changes to chromatin, including acetylation, phosphorylation, and methylation play roles in LCR activation. Histone acetylation occurs during chromatin remodeling and hyperacetylation is associated with transcriptional activation of a locus (Pazin & Kadonaga, 1997). Similar to acetylation, phosphorylation of histone H3 disrupts DNA-nucleosome interaction and increases transcription factor accessibility to DNA. SATB1 overexpression increased ε-globin and decreased γ-globin gene expression accompanied by histone hyperacetylation and hypomethylation in chromatin from the ε-globin promoter and HS2, and histone hypoacetylation and hypermethylation associated with the γ-globin promoter (Wen et al., 2005). Mitogen activated protein kinase (MAPK) pathways, as well as the stress activated p38 pathway, activate histone H3 phosphorylation (Cheung et al., 2000). Studies on p38 knockout mice established a role for the p38 stress pathway in the switch from primitive to definitive erythropoiesis (Tamura et al., 2000). Mutations in the transcription factor alpha thalassemia/mental retardation syndrome X-linked (ATRX), nearly always downregulate α-globin expression, provide potentially important insight into the trans-regulation of globin gene expression (Gibbons et al., 1995). Alpha hemoglobin stabilizing protein (AHSP) is an erythroid-specific protein that forms a stable complex with free alpha-hemoglobin (Kihm et al., 2002). It has been found that AHSP expression was highly dependent on the larger subunit of nuclear factor erythroid-derived 2 (NFE2) (Guo-wei et al., 2010). The transcription factor NFE2 activation of globin production was stimulated by cAMP-dependent protein kinase (PKA) in erythroid cells (Casteel et al., 1998).

BCL11A gene (encoding the transcription factor B-cell lymphoma/leukemia 11A) maintains silencing of γ-globin expression in adult erythroid cells and functions as a direct transcriptional regulator of the fetal to adult hemoglobin switch in humans. BCL11A protein levels vary in erythroid progenitors over the course of human ontogeny. BCL11A is expressed as short variant proteins in primitive erythroid progenitors that largely express γ-globin and as full-length forms at the adult stage with silenced γ-globin genes (Sankaran et al., 2008). In erythroid progenitors, BCL11A physically interacts with the NuRD chromatin remodelling complex, and the erythroid transcription factors, GATA1 and FOG1. In addition, KLF1, as a key activator of BCL11A, controls globin gene switching by directly activating β-globin and indirectly repressing γ-globin gene expression (Zhou et al., 2010). BCL11A binds the upstream LCR, ε-globin, and the intergenic regions between γ-globin and δ-globin genes. BCL11A and SOX6 co-occupy the human β-globin cluster along with GATA1, and cooperate in silencing γ-globin transcription in adult human erythroid progenitors (Xu et al., 2010, Scheme 1). SOX6 has also been suggested to enhance definitive erythropoiesis in mouse by stimulating erythroid cell survival, proliferation and terminal maturation (Dumitriu et al., 2006). A broad genome expression profile studies led to the identification of common genetic polymorphisms in the locus of the β-globin gene, a region between the HBS1-like gene HBS1L and the oncogene MYB, as well as within the gene BCL11A (Galarneau et al., 2010). HBS1L-MYB intergenic polymorphism on chromosome 6q23 is associated with elevated HbF levels. MYB and HBS1L expression was significantly reduced in erythroid cultures of individuals with high HbF levels, whereas overexpression of MYB in human erythroleukemic cells inhibited γ-globin expression supporting role of MYB in HbF regulation (Jiang et al., 2006). The human erythroid precursor cells from individuals with higher HbF and higher F cell levels have lower MYB expression associated with lower erythrocyte count but higher erythrocyte volume (Jiang et al., 2006).

MicroRNAs (miRNAs or miRs) are small, 19 to 25 nucleotide long, non-coding RNAs, which target mRNAs in a sequence-specific manner, inducing translational repression or decay. Increased miRNA-210 levels elevated γ-globin levels in hereditary persistence of HbF (Bianchi et al., 2009), while the let-7 family has been associated with hemoglobin switching (Noh et al., 2009). Recently, two miRNAs, miR-221 and miR-222, have been identified to regulate HbF expression in erythropoietic cells via the kit receptor (Gabbianelli et al., 2010). miRNA-150 repression of MYB in hematopoietic progenitor cells, of human bone marrow origin, supported MYB's importance in erythroid and megakaryocytic differentiation (Lu et al., 2008). It has been reported that miRNA-96, miRNA-146a, let-7a, miR-888 and miR-330a-3p are significantly more abundant in reticulocytes obtained from adults than from umbilical cord blood and therefore are potential inhibitors of γ-globin expression. The miR-96 has been identified as a direct inhibitor of γ-globin expression (Azzouzi et al., 2011, Scheme 1). These findings demonstrate that miRNAs contribute to HbF regulation by the post-transcriptional inhibition of γ-globin expression during adult erythropoiesis.

2. Microarray analysis of globin related genes during ontogenesis

2.1 Introduction

Several groups have examined the gene expression profile of human CD34+ hematopoietic progenitor cells from bone marrow (BM), peripheral blood (PB) and cord blood (CB) using microarray technology (He et al., 2005; Ng et al., 2004; Steidl et al., 2002). The modulation of gene expression during ontogeny, in fetal liver (FL)- and CB-derived CD34+CD38− hematopoietic progenitor cells, appears to overlap broadly with early response genes of growth factor stimulated adult (BM) hematopoietic progenitor cells (Oh et al., 2000). Recent studies have begun to define a general gene expression profiling for human erythroid cells from different origins - adult BM and PB (Goh et al., 2007; Gubin et al., 1999; Fujishima et al., 2004). In general, it has been hypothesized that globin gene switching may be mediated by proteins expressed during different stages of ontogeny.

Following the same intention, we have performed serial gene expression profiling in human differentiating erythroid cells by oligonucleotide microarrays. The several expressed genes (GATA1, ALAS2, EPOR, globins, etc.) linked to known erythroid differentiation confirms the validity of our approach in establishing the appropriate in vitro cell culture conditions. To study the mechanism of globin gene switching, we have performed gene expression profiling of erythroid progenitor cells derived from hematopoietic tissues during ontogeny, using a large Gene Array to gain insight into the associated molecular pathways. Gene expression patterns of CD71+ erythroid progenitor cells, differentiated from human FL, CB, BM, PB and granulocyte colony-stimulating factor (G-CSF) mobilized PB (mPB), were compared to establish the expression patterns of representative genes.

2.2 Material and methods

2.2.1 Liquid erythroid cell cultures

CD34+ hematopoietic progenitor cells were purified by positive immunomagnetic selection using the MACS cell isolation system (Miltenyi Biotec, Auburn, CA). Fresh BM, PB and G-CSF stimulated mPB CD34+ cells were collected (AllCells LLC, Berkeley, CA) and proceeded with selection. CB CD34+ cells (AllCells LLC) and FL CD34+ cells (Cambrex Bio Science, Inc., Walkersville, MD) were collected and frozen. For analysis, CD34+ cells were resuspended in medium with erythropoietin (EPO), as already described (Cokic et al., 2003). After 6 days of EPO treatment, 5×10^5 cells were washed and incubated for 20 minutes in the presence of the monoclonal antibody anti-CD71 Tricolor for cell staining (Beckman-Coulter, Miami, FL). Cells were then washed, fixed and acquired on an LSRII flow cytometer (BD Biosciences, San Jose, CA). Data were analyzed with Flowjo software (Tree Star, San Carlos, CA). After 6 days of erythropoietin treatment and incubation at 37°C (5% CO_2, 95% humidity), we used the RNeasy protocol for isolation of total RNA from erythroid progenitor cells (Qiagen, Valencia, CA) according to the manufacturer's instructions. Concentration and integrity of total RNA was assessed using an 8453 UV/Visible Spectrophotometer (Hewlett-Packard GmbH, Waldbronn, Germany) and Agilent 2100 Bioanalyzer Software (Agilent Technologies, Waldbronn, Germany).

2.2.2 Microarray studies

In microarray studies, the numbers of total genes overexpressed in erythroid cells of CB, BM and PB origin were determined from three independent samples as biological repeats. FL and mPB-derived samples were analyzed in independent duplicate samples at day 6 of erythroid liquid culture. High quality oligonucleotide glass arrays were produced containing a total of 16,659 seventy-mer oligonucleotides (Operon Inc. Valencia, CA). The array includes probes for 2121 hypothetical proteins and 18-expressed sequence tags (ESTs) and spans approximately 50% of the human genome (Operon Inc.). The arrays were produced in house by spotting oligonucleotides on poly-L-lysine coated glass slides by Gene Machines robotics (Omnigrid, San Carlos, CA).

Total human universal RNA (HuURNA) isolated from a collection of adult human tissues to represent a broad range of expressed genes from both male and female donors (BD Biosciences, Palo Alto, CA) served as a universal reference control in the competitive hybridization. Labeled cDNA probes were produced as described (Risinger et al., 2003). cDNA was purified by the MinElute column (Qiagen). Binding buffer PB was added to the coupled cDNA, and the mixture applied to the MinElute column and centrifuged. After discharging the flow-through, washing buffer PE was added to the column, and centrifuged. Then the columns were placed into a fresh eppendorf tube and elution buffer added to the membrane, incubated and centrifuged and probe collected. The probe was dried in speed-vac. Finally, 5 µl of 2X coupling buffer and 5 µl Cy3 and Cy5 dye (GE Healthcare Bio-Sciences Corp., Piscataway, NJ) were mixed into the control (HuURNA) and experimental cDNAs (huES cell-derived) respectively and incubated at room temperature in dark for 90 minutes. After incubation, the volume was raised to 60 µl by DEPC water and then cDNA was purified by the MinElute column and eluted with 13 µl elution buffer by centrifugation. For hybridization, 36 µl hybridization mixture was pre-heated at 100°C for 2 minutes and cooled for 1 minute. Total volume of probe was added on the array and covered with cover slip. Slides are placed in hybridization chamber and 20µl water was added to the slide, and incubated overnight at 65°C. Slides were then washed for 2 minutes each in 2X SSC, 1X SSC and 0.1X SSC and spin-dried. Microarray slides were scanned in both Cy3 (532nm) and Cy5 (635nm) channels using Axon GenePix 4000B scanner (Axon Instruments, Inc., Foster City, CA) with a 10-micron resolution. Scanned microarray images were exported as TIFF files to GenePix Pro 3.0 software for image analysis. The average of the total Cy3 and Cy5 signal gave a ratio that was used to normalize the signals. Each microarray experiment was globally normalized to make the median value of the log2-ratio equal to zero. The Loess normalization process corrects for dye bias, photo multiplier tube voltage imbalance, and variations between channels in the amounts of the labeled cDNA probes hybridized. The data files representing the differentially expressed genes were then created. For advanced data analysis, gpr and jpeg files were imported into microarray database, and normalized by software tools provided by NIH Center for Information Technology (http://nciarray.nci.nih.gov/). Spots with confidence interval of 99 (≥ 2 fold) with at least 150-fluorescence intensity for both channel and 30 µm spot size were considered as good quality spots for analysis. Paired t test was used in microarray analysis.

2.3 Results

2.3.1 Predominantly elevated genes expression in ontogenic tissues

In the presence of EPO and other cytokines, CD34+ cells were differentiated in vitro into erythroid progenitor cells. Besides flow cytometry for analysis of *in vitro* erythroid differentiation, we already reported measurement of hemoglobin content by benzidine staining and high-performance liquid chromatography in erythroid progenitor cells during their *in vitro* differentiation in same culture conditions (Cokic et al., 2003, 2008). The transferrin receptor (CD71) is present on early erythroid cells but is lost as reticulocytes differentiate into mature erythrocytes (Cokic et al., 2003). At day 6 of erythroid cell culture, the erythroid progenitor cells were sorted as 100% CD71+, a well-known early marker of erythroid differentiation. In microarray studies, the quantities of tissue specific overexpressed genes were determined from two to four independent samples (biological repeats). During microarray analysis genes are upregulated or downregulated versus HuURNA, what we used as a control alongside each sample. We observed largely upregulated genes in all tissues (Table 1).

Besides common highly expressed genes in erythroid progenitor cells: CD71, Rh-associated glycoprotein (RHAG), SERPINE1 mRNA binding protein 1 (SERBP1); the highly expressed genes in erythroid cells of FL origin are ribonuclease, RNase A family 2 and 3 (RNASE2/3) and serpin peptidase inhibitor, clade B (SERPINB1, Table 1).

The highly expressed genes in erythroid cells of CB origin are hemoglobin gamma A (HBG1), NFE2 and eosinophil peroxidase (EPX). The greatly expressed genes in erythroid cells of BM origin are latexin (LXN), coproporphyrinogen oxidase (CPOX) and carbonic anhydrase II (CA2). The highly expressed genes in erythroid cells of mPB origin are KLF1, aminolevulinate, delta-, synthase 2 (ALAS2) and THO complex 2 (THOC2). The genes with reduced expressed in erythroid cells of PB origin are proteoglycan 2 (PRG2), Charcot-Leyden crystal protein (CLC), EPX and v-myb myeloblastosis viral oncogene homolog

Gene Name	Description	Fold induction vs. HuURNA (±SD)				
		FL	CB	BM	mPB	PB
HBG1	hemoglobin, gamma A	4.2±0.7	4.5±0.9	4.1±1	4.3±0.2	4.7±0.6
CLC	Charcot-Leyden crystal protein	4.3±0.4	4.3±0.7	4.6±0.6	4.8±0.4	2.9±0.6
PRG2	proteoglycan 2, bone marrow	5±0.3	4.2±0.9	4.7±0.5	4.1±0.7	2.9±0.4
RNASE2	ribonuclease, RNase A family, 2	**4.3±0.7**	3.7±0.9	3.1±0.6	3.5±0.7	1.4±0.8
HBD	hemoglobin, delta	2±1.3	3.5±0.3	4.3±0.4	4.2±0.4	3.2±0.5
EPX	eosinophil peroxidase	**4±0.2**	**3.4±0.8**	2.9±0.7	2.6±1.1	0.9±0.5
SRGN	serglycin	4.3±1	2.8±1	4.4±1.3	4.6±0.4	2.1±0.5
TFRC	transferrin receptor (p90, CD71)	3.1±1	3.3±1.2	4.4±0.3	4.3±0.03	3±0.9
HBE1	hemoglobin, epsilon 1	3±1.2	2.6±1.5	**4.4±1.7**	**4.6±0.01**	3.4±1.3
RHAG	Rh-associated glycoprotein	2.7±1.3	3.2±1.2	2.1±0.9	3.1±0.7	2.1±0.5
MPO	myeloperoxidase	3.8±0.2	3.2±0.6	3.4±0.1		
MYB	v-myb myeloblastosis viral oncogene homolog	3±0.3	3.1±0.7	2.6±0.4	3.5±0.4	1.7±1
RNASE3	ribonuclease, RNase A family, 3	**3.6±1.2**	2.7±1.5	2±1	3.1±0.7	0.6±0.2
LXN	latexin	1.5±0.4	1.9±0.7	**4.7±1**	**4.1±0.5**	2.7±0.2
CD36	CD36 molecule (thrombospondin rec)	1.6±1.1	2.6±0.5	**4±1**	3.2±0.5	2.1±0.8
CPOX	coproporphyrinogen oxidase	2±0.8	2.7±0.6	**3.5±0.7**	2.9±0.4	1.8±0.6
CA2	carbonic anhydrase II	0.15	1±0.3	**3.3±0.6**	1.8±0.2	1.7±0.5
CYTL1	cytokine-like 1	1.4±0.8	1.7±0.4	2.8±0.4	**3.7±0.3**	2.4±0.3
KLF1	Kruppel-like factor 1 (erythroid)	1±0.4	1.7±0.5	2.5±0.9	**3.6±0.3**	2.3±0.2
ALAS2	aminolevulinate, delta-, synthase 2	1.5±0.4	1.4±0.3	2.5±0.9	**3.5±0.7**	2.7±0.3
CPA3	carboxypeptidase A3 (mast cell)	1	0.9±0.3	1.9±0.7	**3.2±0.4**	1.2±0.5
THOC2	THO complex 2	0.6±0.4	0.9±0.5	1.4±0.7	**3.1±0.2**	1.6±0.5
GATA1	globin transcription factor 1	0.9	2.1±0.4	2.7±0.6	2.5±0.3	2.3±0.3
NFE2	nuclear factor (erythroid-derived 2)	1.4±0.4	1.9±0.5	2.6		1.6±0.5
SERPINB1	serpin peptidase inhibitor, clade B	**2.5±0.2**	1.8±0.3	1.7±0.4	0.9±0.3	0.7±0.3
SERBP1	SERPINE1 mRNA binding protein 1	2.1±0.4	2.4±0.5	1.9±0.7	1.9±0.5	1.6±0.6

Table 1. Largely up-regulated genes vs. HuURNA among different tissues: FL, CB, BM, mPB, PB. Bolded black values represent increased genes expression, whereas bolded gray values represent decreased genes expression in comparison to other tissues.

(MYB). Presence of certain gene in the least two samples (66% filtering), in one group of tissues, reduced largely the total gene expression in all tissues. Using the range of microarray analysis and filtering reduction, the erythroid cells of FL tissue origin expressed 1772 genes, CB-derived erythroid cells expressed 3846 genes, BM derived erythroid cells expressed 1827 genes, mPB derived erythroid cells expressed 4008 genes, and PB derived erythroid cells expressed 1320 genes. The observed gene expression is more than doubled in CB and mPB tissues in comparison to other tissues.

2.3.2 A comparison in genes expression of erythroid cells during subsequent stages of development

Using Venn diagrams we compared total gene expression, determined by microarray analysis, among all examined ontogenic tissues. By 66% filtering, we analyzed only genes

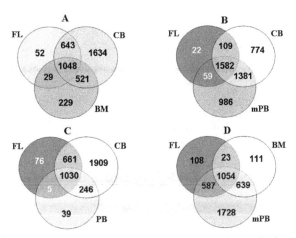

Fig. 1. **Venn diagram of genes expression in erythroid progenitor cells between FL and other developmental tissues.** A: Comparison among FL, CB and BM tissues; B: Comparison among FL, CB and mPB tissues; C: Comparison among FL, CB and PB tissues; D: Comparison among FL, BM and mPB tissues.

present in at least two donor samples per tissue. We compared gene expression of FL-derived erythroid cell with other ontogenic derived tissues in Figure 1. Shared genes expression was more prominent between CB and FL/mPB derived erythroid cells, than between FL and BM/PB tissues (Figure 1A-C). Moreover, the FL- and CB-derived erythroid cells have the more common genes with mPB-derived erythroid cells than with BM and PB tissues (Figures 1D, 2C). The genes related to FL tissue shared the similar expression with BM- and PB-derived cells (Figure 2A). In addition, the genes expression in mPB-derived erythroid cells contains the majority of genes expressed in FL, BM and PB tissues (Figure 2B,

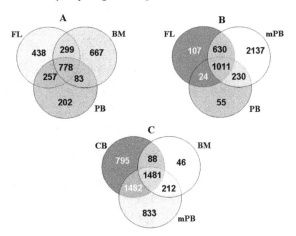

Fig. 2. **Venn diagram of genes expression in erythroid progenitor cells among ontogenic tissues.** A: Comparison among FL, BM and PB tissues; B: Comparison among FL, mPB and PB tissues; C: Comparison among CB, BM and mPB tissues.

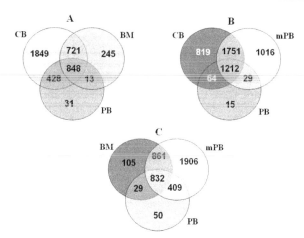

Fig. 3. **Venn diagram of genes expression in erythroid progenitor cells between PB and other ontogenic tissues.** A: Comparison among CB, BM and PB tissues; B: Comparison among CB, mPB and PB tissues; C: Comparison among BM, mPB and PB tissues.

3C), but not in CB tissue (Figures 2C, 3B). Also, mPB-derived erythroid cells shared more genes with BM tissue than with PB tissue (Figure 3C). The genes expression in CB-derived erythroid cells overwhelmed the gene expression in BM tissues and almost completely in PB tissue (Figure 3A).

Comparison in genes expression between FL- and CB-derived erythroid cells revealed couple statistically significant genes (p<0.01, Table 2): POLE3 and BRP44. Negative values in Tables represent downregulated genes expression in ontogenic tissues in contrast to HuURNA, whereas positive values represent upregulated genes.

Gene	Description	p value	FL Mean±SD	CB Mean±SD	Tissue presence
POLE3	polymerase epsilon 3	0.0022	0.4±0.22	0.8±0.4	FL, CB, mPB, PB
SNRPD3	small nuclear ribonucleoprotein D3	0.0036	0.8±0.02	1.6±0.4	FL, CB, mPB
ZFP36	zinc finger protein 36	0.0072	-1.6±0.07	-2.3±0.6	FL, CB, mPB
BRP44	brain protein 44	0.0063	-0.14±0.09	0.5±0.1	All tissues

Table 2. Comparison of statistically significant (p<0.01) genes between FL and CB tissues.

Brain protein 44 (BRP44) gene expressions was highly significantly increased in CB-derived erythroid cells vs. FL-derived cells (Table 2), but was reduced in comparison to PB-derived cells (Table 8). BRP44 gene was stable expression in all examined ontogenic tissues, whereas POLE 3 gene expression was absent in BM tissue (Table 2). Comparison in genes expression between FL- and BM-derived erythroid cells exposed more statistically significant genes (Table 3): SBNO2, WDR1 and CTAG2 present in all tissues.

WD repeat domain 1 (WDR1) gene expressions was significantly increased in BM- vs. PB-derived erythroid cells (Table 10), but was reduced in comparison to FL-derived cells (Table

3). Evaluation in genes expression between FL- and mPB-derived erythroid cells exposed also statistically significant genes (Table 4): ME2 present just in FL and mPB tissues, highly upregulated EEF1B2 expressed in all tissues. IFI30 was downregulated in mPB-derived erythroid cells, but was upregulated in FL-derived cells (Table 4).

Gene	Description	p value	FL Mean±SD	BM Mean±SD	Tissue presence
SPRR2B	small proline-rich protein 2B	0.0001	-0.8±0.03	-0.9±0.5	FL, CB, BM,mPB
SRI	sorcin	0.0014	0.9±0.04	1.1±0.2	All tissues
KPNA2	karyopherin alpha 2	0.002	0.5±0.005	1 ±0.2	All tissues
SDHC	succinate dehydrogenase complex, subunit C	0.0021	0.1±0.05	0.2±0.2	All tissues
NCOA4	nuclear receptor coactivator 4	0.0048	2±0.3	1.8±0.4	All tissues
SBNO2	strawberry notch homolog 2	0.005	-1.5±0.02	-1.1±0.6	All tissues
TTC3	tetratricopeptide repeat domain 3	0.0057	0.3±0.08	0.6±0.1	FL, CB, BM,mPB
PTTG1	pituitary tumor-transforming1	0.0078	0.7±0.05	1±0.2	All tissues
WDR1	WD repeat domain 1	0.0079	0.5±0.002	0.3±0.1	All tissues
MINK1	Misshapen-like kinase 1	0.0089	-1.2±0.1	-0.9±0.5	All tissues
CTAG2	cancer/testis antigen 2	0.0094	-0.1±0.25	-0.2±0.54	All tissues

Table 3. Comparison of statistically significant (p<0.01) genes between FL and BM tissues.

Gene	Description	p value	FL Mean±SD	mPB Mean±SD	Tissue presence
ME2	malic enzyme 2, NAD(+)-dependent, mitochondrial	0.0068	1.19±0.15	0.9±0.14	FL, mPB
INSIG1	insulin induced gene 1	0.0073	-0.08±0.4	-0.01±0.4	FL, mPB
EEF1B2	eukaryotic translation elongation factor 1 beta 2	0.0009	1.77±0.12	2.3±0.12	All tissues
ZNF224	zinc finger protein 224	0.0015	-0.2±0.06	0.9±0.06	FL, CB, BM, mPB
CSDE1	cold shock domain containing E1, RNA-binding	0.004	0.56±0.08	0.6± 0.02	All tissues
IFI30	Interferon, gamma-inducible protein 30	0.0059	0.06±0.05	-2±0.07	FL, CB, BM, mPB
PSMD11	proteasome 26S, non-ATPase,11	0.0091	0.67±0.17	0.18±0.16	All tissues
PGAM1	phosphoglycerate mutase 1	0.0093	0.87±0.15	0.06±0.16	FL, CB, mPB, PB
PTPRC	protein tyrosine phosphatase, receptor type, C	0.0093	1.42±0.75	1.5±0.75	FL, CB, BM, mPB

Table 4. Comparison of statistically significant (p<0.01) genes between FL and mPB tissues.

Comparison between FL- and PB-derived erythroid cells revealed just two significant genes: TOP1 and CAT (Table 5). TOP1 and CAT genes have higher levels in FL tissue than in PB.

Gene	Description	p value	FL Mean±SD	PB Mean±SD	Tissue presence
TOP1	topoisomerase I	0.0017	1.3±0.34	0.9±0.7	All tissues
CAT	catalase	0.0042	1.8±0.18	1.3±0.26	FL, CB, mPB, PB

Table 5. Comparison of statistically significant (p<0.01) genes between FL and PB tissues.

Evaluation in genes expression between CB- and BM-derived erythroid cells exposed several genes: WAPAL, GRB2, GOLIM4, etc. (Table 6). CTDSP1 has the elevated expression in CB tissue, while TPST2 has the higher expression in BM tissue (Table 6).

Gene	Description	p value	CB Mean±SD	BM Mean±SD	Tissue presence
SCAMP2	secretory carrier membrane protein 2	0.0022	0.4±0.22	0.8±0.4	CB, BM, PB
ABCF2	ATP-binding cassette, sub-family F	0.0075	-0.2±0.17	0.22±0.08	CB, BM, PB
ZNF16	zinc finger protein 16	0.0093	0.2±0.2	0.6±0.18	CB, BM, PB
GRIPAP1	GRIP1 associated protein 1	0.0014	-0.6±0.45	-0.06±0.45	All tissues
WAPAL	wings apart-like homolog	0.0023	1.3±0.1	1.7±0.1	All tissues
TPST2	tyrosylprotein sulfotransferase 2	0.0029	0.8±0.26	1.6±0.21	All tissues
TPSB2	tryptase beta 2	0.0035	-0.7±0.43	1±0.33	All tissues
CCNB2	cyclin B2	0.0037	1.3±0.21	1.7±0.19	All tissues
RPS13	ribosomal protein S13	0.0041	1.9±0.23	1.5±0.21	All tissues
GRB2	growth factor receptor-bound protein 2	0.0067	-0.06±0.4	0.4±0.38	All tissues
GSK3A	glycogen synthase kinase 3α	0.0071	-1±0.04	-0.8±0.06	All tissues
CTDSP1	carboxy-terminal domain, A polypeptide small phosphatas 1	0.0077	0.4±0.23	-0.05±0.01	All tissues
ZNF43	zinc finger protein 43	0.0086	0.9±0.11	1.2±0.09	All tissues
GOLIM4	golgi integral membrane protein 4	0.0094	0.4±0.04	0.85±0.07	All tissues

Table 6. Comparison of statistically significant (p<0.01) genes between CB and BM tissues.

Zinc finger protein 43 (ZNF43) has also significantly increased gene expressions in BM-derived erythroid cells compared to CB- and PB-derived erythroid cells (Tables 6, 10). Golgi integral membrane protein 4 (GOLIM4) gene has also significantly increased expressions in BM-derived erythroid cells compared to CB- and mPB-derived erythroid cells (Tables 6, 9). Assessment in genes expression between CB- and mPB-derived erythroid cells uncovered several genes: ARF4, PHIP, ACIN1, etc. (Table 7). ARF4 has highly upregulated gene expression in CB-derived cells compared to mPB tissue.

Measurement in genes expression profile between CB and PB tissues revealed the downregulated genes PPFIA4 and WIPI2, as well as upregulated genes FBL and BRP44 (Table 8). WIPI2 was less downregulated in PB tissue than in CB tissue.

Determination of statistical significance between BM and mPB tissues showed the prevalent quantity of genes: MYCL2, ADIPOR2 and POP7 present in CB, BM and mPB tissues; NFATC3, YY1, GCA present in all tissues except PB; YWHAZ, TACC3, UBE2D3 present in BM, mPB and PB tissues (Table 9).

Gene	Description	P value	CB Mean±SD	mPB Mean±SD	Tissue presence
GRN	granulin	0.0007	-1.1±0.35	-1.5±0.16	All tissues
PHIP	pleckstrin homology domain interacting protein	0.0009	0.5±0.38	1.4±0.29	All tissues
ARF4	ADP-ribosylation factor 4	0.0037	0.4±0.3	0.04±0.15	FL, CB, BM, mPB
UBE2V1	ubiquitin-conjugating enzyme E2 variant 1	0.0044	0.7±0.06	0.4±0.04	All tissues
ACIN1	apoptotic chromatin condensation inducer 1	0.0058	0.6±0.11	0.3±0.05	All tissues
XRCC6	X-ray repair complementing defective repair in Chinese hamster cells 6	0.0067	1.2±0.13	0.8±0.11	All tissues
F2R	coagulation factor II (thrombin) receptor	0.0072	-0.2±0.22	-0.9±0.21	FL, CB, BM, mPB
SNRPA	small nuclear ribonucleo-protein polypeptide A	0.008	1.6±0.37	1.1±0.02	FL, CB, mPB
LGALS1	lectin, galactoside-binding, soluble, 1	0.0093	-1.3±0.48	-0.5±0.57	FL, CB, mPB

Table 7. Comparison of statistically significant (p<0.01) genes between CB and mPB tissues.

Gene	Description	p value	CB Mean±SD	PB Mean±SD	Tissue presence
PPFIA4	protein tyrosine phos-phatase, f polypeptide, interacting protein α 4	0.0016	-1.3±0.37	-0.06±0.44	All tissues
WIPI2	WD repeat domain, phosphoinositide interacting 2	0.0043	-0.3±0.08	-0.02±0.14	All tissues
FBL	fibrillarin	0.0056	1.5±0.29	0.9±0.36	All tissues
BRP44	brain protein 44	0.0059	0.5±0.13	1±0.14	All tissues

Table 8. Comparison of statistically significant (p<0.01) genes between CB and PB tissues.

Gene	Description	p value	BM Mean±SD	mPB Mean±SD	Tissue presence
MYCL2	v-myc avian myelocytomatosis viral oncogene homolog 2	0.0006	-0.7±0.26	-1.4±0.26	CB, BM, mPB
SKAP2	src kinase associated phosphoprotein 2	0.0012	-1.1±0.3	-1.6±0.31	CB, BM, mPB
MPHOSPH9	Mphase phosphoprotein mpp9	0.0012	-0.7±0.18	-1.3±0.19	CB, BM, mPB
SLC25A39	solute carrier family 25, member 39	0.0013	1.5±0.13	0.9±0.07	CB, BM, mPB

Gene	Description	p value	BM Mean±SD	mPB Mean±SD	Tissue presence
UBE2NL	ubiquitin-conjugating enzyme E2N-like	0.0015	0.9±0.17	0.6±0.17	CB, BM, mPB
POP7	Processing of precursor 7, ribonuclease P/MRP subunit	0.0027	-0.4±0.21	0.28±0.12	CB, BM, mPB
ANKH	ankylosis, progressive homolog	0.0031	-0.5±0.22	-1.2±0.21	CB, BM, mPB
ADIPOR2	adiponectin receptor 2	0.0045	0.6±0.32	0.6±0.01	CB, BM, mPB
ZBTB43	zinc finger and BTB domain containing 43	0.0041	-0.9±0.22	-1.4±0.21	CB, BM, mPB
RBM8A	RNA binding motif protein 8A	0.0048	-0.9±0.45	-0.3±0.13	CB, BM, mPB
ZYG11B	zyg-11 homolog B	0.0062	-0.2±0.28	-0.9±0.23	CB, BM, mPB
APBB2	amyloid beta precursor protein-binding, family B, member 2	0.0074	-0.8±0.16	-1.1±0.17	CB, BM, mPB
CEP97	centrosomal protein 97kDa	0.0082	-0.6±0.09	-1.4±0.1	CB, BM, mPB
KLRD1	killer cell lectin-like receptor subfamily D	0.0011	-0.4±0.16	-1.3±0.16	FL, CB, BM, mPB
TOMM34	translocase of outer mitochondrial membrane 34	0.0035	-0.5±0.21	-0.6±0.15	FL, CB, BM, mPB
NFATC3	nuclear factor of activated T-cells, cytoplasmic, calcineurin-dependent 3	0.0045	1.3±0.19	0.9±0.23	FL, CB, BM, mPB
YY1	YY1 transcription factor	0.0047	1.4±0.18	0.8±0.22	FL, CB, BM, mPB
SSB	Sjogren syndrome antigen B	0.0050	2.7±0.72	2.3±0.003	FL, CB, BM, mPB
UBC	ubiquitin C	0.0069	-1±0.53	-1.3±0.08	FL, CB, BM, mPB
UBA1	ubiquitin-like modifier activating enzyme 1	0.0083	-0.4±0.6	-0.6±0.17	FL, CB, BM, mPB
LRRC59	leucine rich repeat containing59	0.0086	1.9±0.25	1.5±0.03	FL, CB, BM, mPB
GCA	grancalcin, EF-hand calcium binding protein	0.0098	1.2±0.21	0.4±0.17	FL, CB, BM, mPB
TACC3	transforming, acidic coiled-coil containing protein 3	0.0011	0.02±0.01	-0.3±0.03	BM, mPB, PB
LMNB1	lamin B1	0.0014	1±0.1	-0.1±0.04	BM, mPB, PB
SREBF2	sterol regulatory element binding	0.0019	-0.6±0.05	-2.1±0.18	BM, mPB, PB
UBE2D3	ubiquitin-conjugating enzyme E2D 3	0.0032	1.02±0.06	0.5±0.001	BM, mPB, PB
YWHAZ	tyrosine 3-mono oxygenase/tryptophan 5-monooxygenase activation protein, zeta polypeptide	0.0042	1.4±0.08	0.7±0.04	BM, mPB, PB

Gene	Description	p value	BM Mean±SD	mPB Mean±SD	Tissue presence
GOLIM4	golgi integral membrane protein 4	0.0044	0.8±0.02	0.29±0.05	BM, mPB, PB
GLE1	GLE1 RNA export mediator homolog	0.0049	-0.4±0.02	0.29±0.12	BM, mPB, PB
CORO1C	coronin actin binding protein 1C	0.0049	1.4±0.1	0.6±0.08	BM, mPB, PB
ARHGDIB	Rho GDPdissociation inhibitorβ	0.0075	1.4±0.02	1.2±0.03	BM, mPB, PB
TMEM187	transmembrane protein 187	0.0082	-0.4±0.08	-0.9±0.03	BM, mPB, PB
TIMM23	translocase of inner mitochon-drial membrane 23 homolog	0.0088	0.9±0.1	0.3±0.05	BM, mPB, PB
PSMB5	proteasome subunit, β type, 5	0.0092	0.3±0.02	0.02±0.02	BM, mPB, PB

Table 9. Comparison of statistically significant (p<0.01) genes between BM and mPB tissues.

YY1 transcription factor has significantly increased gene expressions in BM-derived erythroid cells compared to PB- and mPB-derived erythroid cells (Tables 9, 10). Measurement of statistical significance between BM and PB tissues revealed the following significant genes: NUCKS1 and KDM3B prevalent in BM tissue, ATF5 and ATP5L prevalent in BM tissue (Table 10).

Gene	Description	p value	BM Mean±SD	PB Mean±SD	Tissue presence
NUCKS1	nuclear casein kinase and cyclin-dependent kinase substrate 1	0.0092	1.1±0.62	0.7±0.12	CB, BM,PB
KDM3B	lysine (K)-specific demethylase 3B	0.0002	0.8±0.01	0.15±0.03	BM, mPB, PB
WDR1	WD repeat domain 1	0.0018	0.3±0.1	-0.2±0.03	BM, mPB, PB
YY1	YY1 transcription factor	0.0018	1.4±0.2	0.25±0.14	BM, mPB, PB
FEN1	flap structure-specific endonuclease 1	0.004	2.7±0.1	1.13±0.2	BM, mPB, PB
ATF5	activating transcription factor 5	0.0057	-0.8±0.1	-0.2±0.14	BM, mPB, PB
ZNF43	zinc finger protein 43	0.0058	1.2±0.08	0.5±0.15	BM, mPB, PB
ATP5L	ATP synthase, H+ transporting, mitochondrial F0 complex, subunit G	0.0071	0.3±0.08	0.78±0.09	BM, mPB, PB
HLA-C	MHC class I human leukocyte antigen	0.0046	-2.7±0.7	-2.1±0.88	CB,BM,PB

Table 10. Comparison in statistically significant (p<0.01) gene between BM and PB tissues.

Flap structure-specific endonuclease 1 (FEN1) gene has significantly decreased expressions in PB-derived erythroid cells compared to BM- and mPB-derived erythroid cells (Tables 10, 11). Similarity in genes expression between mPB and PB tissues was limited on four significant genes: TXNIP, EIF3E, FEN1 and FECH (Table 11). TXNIP was present and downregulated just in mPB and PB tissues, whereas EIF3E and FEN1 was highly upregulated in all tissues and predominantly in mPB-derived erythroid cells. FECH has more prominent expression in PB- than in mPB-derived cells.

Gene	Description	p value	mPB Mean±SD	PB Mean±SD	Tissue presence
TXNIP	Brain-expressed HHCPA78 homolog VDUP1	0.0063	-1.3±0.05	-0.14±0.18	mPB, PB
EIF3E	eukaryotic translation initiation factor 3, subunit E	0.0003	2.5±0.14	1.2±0.24	All tissues
FEN1	flap structure-specific endonuclease 1	0.0028	2±0.21	1.13±0.21	All tissues
FECH	ferrochelatase	0.0074	1.6±0.7	2.5±0.59	FL, CB, mPB, PB

Table 11. Comparison in statistically significant ($p < 0.01$) gene between mPB and PB tissues.

2.3.3 Signaling pathways related to globin genes expression

It has been already reported that γ globin genes expression is regulated by nitric oxide (NO) and p38 MAPK signaling pathways (Cokic et al., 2003; Ramakrishnan & Pace, 2011). We examined the genes related to those pathways in erythroid progenitor cells during ontogeny in succeeding tissues (Figure 4). Protein kinase, cAMP-dependent, regulatory, type II, beta (PRKAR2B) has the highest expression in NO signaling pathways linked genes throughout the ontogeny reaching the top in PB-derived erythroid cells. Calmodulin 2 (CALM2) gene demonstrates decline in expression during ontogeny, as well as protein phosphatase 3 beta isoform (PPP3CB, Figure 4A). Downregulation in gene expression during ontogeny was shown for protein kinase, cAMP-dependent, regulatory, type I, alpha (PRKAR1A) and calmodulin 3 (CALM3). Regarding p38 MAPK signaling pathway, transforming growth factor, beta 1 (TGFB1) gene expression was predominant in FL- and BM-derived erythroid cells, while heat shock 27kDa protein 1 (HSPB1) was decreased in BM-derived erythroid cells (Figure 4B). Linked to p38 MAPK, v-myc myelocytomatosis viral oncogene homolog (MYC) has the most upregulated gene expression throughout the ontogeny (Figure 4B).

2.3.4 Discussion

To recognize sets of genes that reveal the essential mechanisms in hematopoiesis, as potential novel therapeutic targets, several groups have performed individual gene expression profiling in erythroid cells from certain tissues during ontogenesis. We extended those studies, of gene expression pattern of ontogenic tissues, to compare gene expression from fetal to adult hematopoiesis as a more reflective and comprehensive overview of erythropoiesis. Gene expression in normal human erythroid progenitor cells has been described and generally static expression analysis was performed on cultured human erythroid progenitor CD71+ cells derived from CD34+ cells in the presence of EPO and cocktail of cytokines. We presented the number of total genes overexpressed in evaluated tissues, the most dominant in CB and mPB tissues. Also, the highly expressed genes are SERPINE1, PRG2, CLC, HBG1, NFE2 and EPX. General genes expression was more present between CB and FL/mPB derived erythroid cells, than between FL and adult tissues.

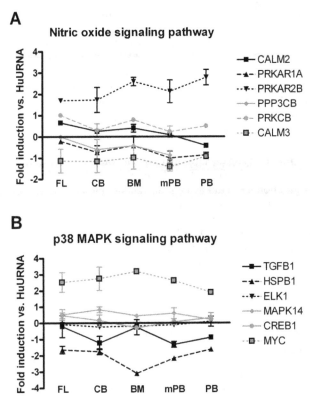

Fig. 4. **Gene expression in signaling pathways related to globins stimulation determined by microarray analysis.** A: Induction of Nitric oxide signaling pathway related genes in erythroid progenitor cells during human ontogeny. B: Induction of p38 MAPK signaling pathway related genes in erythroid progenitor cells during human ontogeny.

Comparison between certain tissues revealed the statistically significant genes: TOP1, CAT, IFI30 in FL tissue, ARF4, CTDSP1 in CB tissue, WDR1, ATF5, YWHAZ in BM tissue, EIF3E and FEN1 in mPB tissue, FECH in PB tissue. PRKAR2B has the highest expression in NO signaling pathways, while MYC has the most upregulated gene expression in p38 MAPK signaling pathway in erythroid progenitor cells throughout ontogeny.

3. Nitric oxide interaction with signaling pathways related to erythropoiesis

It has been found that proliferation of erythropoietic cells is more related to activation of JAK-STAT and MAPK p42/44 signaling pathways, whereas the survival of erythropoietic cells correlated better with activation of PI-3K-AKT, JAK-STAT and MAPK p42/44 pathways (Ratajczak et al., 2001). During erythroid maturation, the p38 MAPK regulates γ-globin transcription through its downstream effector cAMP response element binding protein 1 (CREB1) which binds the Gγ-globin 3′,5′-cyclic adenosine monophosphate (cAMP) response element (Ramakrishnan & Pace, 2011). NO is a diffusible free radical that plays a role as a chemical messenger involved in vasodilator, neurotransmitter, and anti-platelet aggregation. NO is produced and released from three different isoforms of NO synthase (NOS) that convert the l-arginine and molecular oxygen to citrulline and NO in cells: endothelial (eNOS), inducible (iNOS), and neuronal (nNOS) (Cokic & Schechter, 2008). NO readily diffuses across cell membranes into neighboring cells, or may produce effects distant from its site of production transported by vehicles such as low-molecular weight S-nitrosotiols, S-nitrosylated proteins including hemoglobin and albumin, and nitrosyl-metal complexes which liberate NO spontaneously or after cleavage by ectoenzymes (Bogdan, 2001). A significance of NO in erythroid differentiation has been founded on demonstration that NO donors inhibit growth of erythroid primary cells and colony cultures (Maciejewski et al., 1995). Besides observation that NO inhibited erythroid differentiation induced by butyric acid, antitumour drugs aclarubicin and doxorubicin, but not by hemin (Chénais et al., 1999), additional study demonstrated inhibitory effect of NO in the hemin-induced erythroid differentiation (Kucukkaya et al., 2006). NO decreased colony-forming unit-erythrocytes (CFU-E) and CFU-granulocyte macrophage (CFU-GM) formation derived from human bone marrow mononuclear cells. Moreover, NO increased CFU-GM and decreased CFU-E formation derived from CD34+ hematopoietic progenitor cells (Shami & Weinberg, 1996). Although NO increased intracellular levels of guanosine 3',5'-cyclic monophosphate (cGMP) in bone marrow cells, addition of a membrane permeable cGMP analogue did not reproduce previously mentioned effects of NO in bone marrow derived colonies (Shami & Weinberg, 1996). We have previously shown that HbF stimulation is dependent on NO/cGMP signaling pathway in erythroid progenitor cells (Cokic et al., 2003). NO-releasing agents and cGMP analogues inhibit murine erythroleukemia cell differentiation and suppress erythroid-specific gene expression such as beta-globin and delta-aminolevulinate synthetase (Suhasini et al., 1995). Serum nitrate and nitrite (NOx) concentrations correlated inversely with hemoglobin levels (Choi et al., 2002).

EPO increased the level of phosphorylated eNOS and stimulated NO production and cGMP activity during hypoxia (Beleslin-Cokic et al., 2004; Su et al., 2006). Phospho-eNOS and eNOS were significantly induced by hypoxia (Beleslin-Čokić et al., 2011). NO participates in stability control of hypoxia inducible factor (HIF)-1α and induces HIF-1α accumulation and HIF-1-DNA binding (Kovacević-Filipović et al., 2007). Hypoxia and EPO increased erythropoietin receptor (EPOR) gene expression and protein level (Beleslin-Čokić et al., 2011). The physiologically low oxygenation of bone marrow is a regulator of hematopoiesis maintenance, and physiological levels of O_2 should be considered as an important environmental factor that significantly influences cytokine activity (Brüne & Zhou, 2007; Krstic et al., 2009a). The proportion of γ–globin mRNA (the $\gamma/(\gamma+\beta)$ mRNA ratio) increased with reduced oxygen, reaching a maximum value at 5% O_2 of 1.5 to 4-fold higher than at 20% O_2, and then decreased as the O_2 dropped to 2%. In parallel, the proportion of HbF (the HbF/(HbF+HbA) ratio) also peaked at 5% O_2. Reported increase in the HbF was generally lower than that of the γ-globin mRNA, suggesting that although globin mRNA accumulation is primarily under transcriptional regulation, additional post-transcriptional processing such as globin chain stability contribute to the amount of produced hemoglobins (Rogers et al., 2008).

4. Nitric oxide influence on hematopoietic microenvironment in bone marrow

Various growth factors, cytokines, and chemokines are secreted by human hematopoietic progenitor cells, myeloblasts, erythroblasts, and megakaryoblasts to regulate normal hematopoiesis in an autocrine/paracrine manner. Furthermore, each stromal cell in the bone marrow may provide the preferable microenvironment for a rapid expansion of the lineage-restricted progenitor cells (Kameoka et al., 1995; Majka et al., 2001). We showed that the human endothelial cells and macrophages contain NOS activity, representing the potential pool for NO production. The erythroid progenitor cell co-cultures with either macrophages or endothelial cells, stimulated by NO-inducers, demonstrated more elevated levels of γ-globin gene expression than in the erythroid cells only (Čokić et al., 2009). This observation suggests that NO could come out of the bone marrow stromal cells and diffuse into the erythroid progenitor cells largely participating in γ-globin gene induction, linked to stromal cells augmented capability for NO production. This supplemented NO production, in the hematopoietic microenvironment, has the potential to enhance HbF synthesis in erythroid progenitor cells, which still have low hemoglobin levels and presumably low scavenging activity. Accumulating evidence emphasized the involvement and important role of NO in the regulation of hematopoiesis (Krstić et al., 2009, 2010). Spleen is also an active hematopoietic organ where response of hematopoietic cells to cytokines depends on the tissue microenvironment (Jovčić et al., 2007). Improper signaling inside bone marrow stromal cells can lead to their failure and inconsistent microenvironmental niche for hematopoietic stem cells. It has been recently shown that basal NO/cGMP/cGMP-dependent protein kinase (PKG) activity is necessary for preserving bone marrow stromal cell survival and promoting cell proliferation and migration (Wong & Fiscus, 2011). Co-culture studies of human macrophages, as well as human bone marrow endothelial cell line, with erythroid progenitor cells resulted in induction of γ-globin mRNA expression in the presence of cytostatic hydroxyurea. NOS-dependent stimulation of NO by lipopolysaccharide and interferon-γ has been observed in human macrophages. In addition, lipopolysaccharide and interferon-γ together increased γ-globin gene expression in human macrophage/erythroid cell co-cultures (Čokić et al., 2009). These observations are in accord to the intimate contact between erythroid and stromal cells, effects and associations in physiological hematopoietic microenvironment. The endothelial cells as well as macrophages, normal components of bone marrow stroma, play an active role in the modulation of human hematopoietic stem cell growth (Ascensao et al., 1984; Davis et al., 1005; Hanspal & Hanspal, 2004). The murine endothelial cell lines also stimulate the proliferation and differentiation of erythroid precursors, where close cell contact is necessary for erythropoiesis (Ohneda & Bautch, 1997). Mice deficient in eNOS, expressed by bone marrow stromal cells, demonstrated a defect in progenitor cell mobilization (Aicher et al., 2003). Hemoglobin synthesis of erythroleukemia cells line was increased after co-culture with endothelial cells and monolayers of bone-marrow-derived macrophages, as well as with cell-free culture media conditioned by blood-monocyte-derived macrophages (Zuhrie et al., 1988). NO has also an important role in bone marrow angiogenesis, together with vascular endothelial growth factor (VEGF), with implications in patients with leukemic malignancies (Antic et al., 2010, 2011). NO-cGMP pathway stimulates the proliferation and osteoblastic differentiation of primary mouse bone marrow-derived mesenchymal stem cells and osteoblasts (Hikiji et al., 1997). NO donors, as well as proteasome inhibitors, inhibited cytokine induced intercellular adhesion molecule 1 (ICAM-1) and vascular cell adhesion molecule 1 (VCAM-1) expression (Cobb et al., 1996; De Caterina et al., 1995). The proteasome inhibition also significantly enhanced endothelial-dependent vasorelaxation of rat aortic rings (Stangl et al., 2004), as well as NO production in endothelial cells (Cokic et al., 2007).

5. Cyclic nucleotides induction of globin genes expression

5.1 NO/cGMP stimulation of γ-globin gene expression

We demonstrated that NO increases γ-globin gene expression in erythroid cells during differentiation. Inhibition of soluble guanylate cyclase (sGC) prevents NO-induced increase in γ-globin gene expression (Cokic et al., 2003). In addition, we have shown that the well known γ-globin gene inducer hydroxyurea stimulated HbF by the NO-dependent activation of sGC in human erythroid progenitor cells (Cokic et al., 2003). It has been shown that both sGC activators and cGMP induce γ-globin gene expression in human erythroleukemic cell line and primary erythroblasts (Ikuta et al., 2001). Therefore, intracellular pathway including sGC and PKG induced expression of the γ-globin gene (Ikuta et al., 2001). Moreover, it has been reported that hydroxyurea increased NOx levels and NOS-dependent γ-globin transcription in erythroleukemic and primary erythroid cells. This γ-globin gene activation demonstrated cGMP-dependence (Lou et al., 2009). We found that during human erythroid differentiation in vitro, eNOS mRNA and protein levels were initially high but then declined steadily, as did the production of NO derivatives, in contrast with steady elevation of hemoglobin levels, a potent scavenger of NO (Cokic et al., 2008). According to our previous results, hydroxyurea dose- and time-dependently induced rapid but transient activation of eNOS in endothelial cells (Cokic et al., 2006). Hydroxyurea stimulated NO production in endothelial cells, both as short and long term effects (Cokic et al., 2006, 2007). Chronic hydroxyurea therapy significantly increased NO, cGMP, and HbF levels in patients with sickle cell anemia (Nahavandi et al., 2002). cGMP levels were found to be significantly higher in red blood cells (RBCs) of sickle cell patients than in RBCs of normal individuals, and were further increased in RBCs of sickle cell patients on hydroxyurea therapy (Conran et al., 2004). NOS activity was also higher in RBCs of sickle cell disease patients on hydroxyurea therapy than in untreated patients (Iyamu et al., 2005). It is in accordance with results that l-arginine alone does not increase serum NOx production in steady-state patients, however it does when given together with hydroxyurea (Morris et al., 2003). Neither l-arginine alone nor l-arginine in combination with NOS inhibitor effected hydroxyurea-mediated induction of HbF synthesis in erythroid progenitors (Haynes et al., 2004). L-arginine did not change the suppression of burst forming unit-erythroid (BFU-E) colony growth and stimulation of HbF synthesis by hydroxyurea in erythroid progenitors (Baliga et al., 2010). Inhibition of NOS attenuated the hydroxyurea and l-arginine effects on BFU-E colony growth and HbF synthesis (Baliga et al., 2010), but did not decrease NOx production in RBCs during incubation with hydroxyurea (Nahavandi et al., 2006).

5.2 Nitric oxide synthase levels in red blood cells

It has been demonstrated that human RBCs contain iNOS and eNOS as well as calmodulin, suggesting that RBCs may synthesize its own NO (Jubelin & Gierman, 1996). This notion was supported by the observation that RBCs have an active eNOS protein (Chen & Mehta, 1998). Addition of l-arginine to RBCs stimulated NO production (measured as plasma nitrite) in a dose-dependent manner (Nahavandi et al., 2006), whereas it did not significantly change NOx levels (Chen & Mehta, 1998). However, it was later reported that RBCs possess iNOS and eNOS, but the proteins are without catalytic activity (Kang et al., 2000). Recent studies, revealed eNOS protein activity in the cytosol and in the internal side of membrane RBCs, serving essential regulatory functions for RBCs deformability and platelet aggregation (Kleinbongard et al., 2006). In vitro NOx production by RBCs (normal and sickle) is increased by treatment with hydroxyurea, but it's not decreased by NOS inhibition (Nahavandi et al., 2006). In difference to this result, we showed that hydroxyurea increased NO production via induction of eNOS activity in endothelial cells (Cokic et al., 2006). Thus, hydroxyurea may increase the plasma concentration of NO by combining endothelial cell NOS activity and interaction with oxy/deoxy hemoglobin in RBCs. We found previously that hydroxyurea increased cAMP and cGMP levels in human endothelial cells (Cokic et al., 2006), as well as NO levels via activation of eNOS and proteasome inhibition (Cokic et al., 2007). Previous reports indicated that cAMP elevation activated the L-arginine/NO system and induced vasorelaxation in rabbit femoral artery in vivo and human umbilical vein in vitro (Xu et al., 2000). It is known that agents that increase cAMP stimulate eNOS activity in human umbilical vein endothelial cells (Ferro et al., 1999). A recent report revealed that a rapid increase in endothelial NO production by bradykinin is mediated exclusively by PKA signaling pathway (Bae et al., 2003). PKA signaling acts by increasing phosphorylation of Ser1177 and dephosphorylation of Thr495 to activate eNOS (Michell et al., 2001). Shear stress stimulates phosphorylation of bovine eNOS at the corresponding serine in a PKA-dependent, but PKB/Akt-independent, manner, whereas NO production is regulated by the mechanisms dependent on both PKA and PKB/Akt (Boo et al., 2002).

5.3 A role of cAMP-dependent pathway in γ-globin gene induction

During erythroid differentiation adenylate cyclase and cAMP phosphodiesterase activity, as well as cellular cAMP concentrations, decline in a synchronized manner (Setchenska et al., 1981). The cAMP-dependent pathway plays a negative role in a γ-globin gene expression in K562 erythroleukemic cell line, in contrast to a cGMP positive role (Inoue et al., 2004). It has been also found that, upon activation of the cAMP pathway, expression of the γ-globin gene is induced in adult erythroblasts (Kuroyanagi et al., 2006). The subsequent study found that the cAMP-dependent pathway efficiently induced γ-globin expression in adult erythroblasts of beta-thalassaemia (Bailey et al., 2007). In patients with beta-thalassaemia intermedia, cAMP levels were elevated in both RBCs and nucleated erythroblasts but no consistent elevation was found with cGMP levels. The transcription factor cAMP response element binding protein (CREB) was phosphorylated in nucleated erythroblasts and its phosphorylation levels correlated with γ-globin gene expression of the patients (Bailey et al., 2007). According to previous study, guanylate cyclase inhibition minimally reduced HbF induction, whereas adenylate cyclase inhibition markedly decreased HbF induction by hydroxyurea in CD34+-derived erythroid cells. Activation of the adenylate cyclase modestly induced HbF production, while hydroxyurea failed to significantly stimulate adenylate cyclase activity on days 7 to 10 of erythroid cells liquid culture (Keefer et al., 2006). However, in our cultures we found that in early erythroid progenitor cell cultures (day 4), hydroxyurea stimulated cAMP production (Cokic et al., 2008). It has been also postulated that cJun activates the Gγ-globin promoter via an upstream cAMP response element in a way equivalent to CREB1 (Kodeboyina et al., 2010).

5.4 Cyclic nucleotides interaction with phosphodiesterases

It has been shown that nitrite increased blood flow in the human circulation as well as vasodilatation of rat aortic rings. Formation of both NO gas and NO-modified hemoglobin resulted from the nitrite reductase activity of deoxyhemoglobin and deoxygenated erythrocytes levels (Cosby et al., 2003). Studies of nitrite activation of sGC demonstrated that nitrite alone activated sGC in solution (Jeffers et al., 2005). In our performed in vitro studies nitrite failed to induce cGMP, in purified form of sGC in solution, what confirmed a major role of NO molecule in hydroxyurea interaction with sGC (Cokic et al., 2008). It has been also demonstrated that eNOS is rapidly activated and phosphorylated on both Ser1177 and Thr495 in the presence of cGMP-dependent protein kinase II and the catalytic subunit of PKA in endothelial cells. These processes are more prominent in the presence of Ca^{2+}/calmodulin (Butt et al., 2000). The transient rises of cGMP levels induced by bradykinin and endothelin-1, which caused release of Ca^{2+} from internal stores, were similarly enhanced by activation of adenylate cyclase and increased cAMP levels. The cAMP seems to enhance NO formation, which depends on Ca^{2+} release from internal stores (Reiser, 1992). An elevated cGMP level attenuated the store-operated Ca^{2+} entry in vascular endothelial cells (Kwan et al., 2000). The cGMP-mediated $[Ca^{2+}]i$-reducing mechanisms may operate as a negative reaction to protect endothelial cells from the damaging effect of excessive $[Ca^{2+}]i$. The main targets of cGMP are phosphodiesterases (PDEs), resulting in interference with the cAMP-signaling pathway (Vaandrager & de Jonge, 1996). cAMP hydrolyzing PDE isozymes in endothelial cells are represented by PDE2 and PDE4 as cGMP-stimulated and cGMP-insensitive PDE, respectively. In endothelial cells, PDE4 inhibition may up-regulate basal production of NO, being supported by PDE2 inhibition (Lugnier et al., 1999). cGMP-inhibited PDE3 was expressed in K562 erythroleukemic cells at a high level (Inoue et al., 2004), while PDE3/4 inhibitor treatment reduced asymmetrical dimethylarginine, an endogenous NOS inhibitor, and elevated NO/cGMP levels (Pullamsetti et al., 2011). In addition, PDE9A gene expression is increased in CD34+-derived erythroid cells and K562 erythroleukemic cells. Inhibition of PDE9A enzyme significantly increased production of the γ-globin gene in K562 cells (Almeida et al., 2008).

6. Nitric oxide-related therapy in hemoglobinopathies

NO inhibits HbS polymer formation and has anti-sickling properties. NO may disrupt HbS polymers by abolishing the excess positive charge of HbS, resulting in increased oxygen affinity in patients with sickle cell disease (Ikuta et al., 2011). In sickle cell disease, HbS polymerization and intravascular sickling lead to reperfusion injury, hemolysis, decreased NO bioavailability and oxidative stress. Increased expression of HbF decreased intravascular sickling, accompanied by decreased hemolysis, oxidative stress and increased NO metabolites (NOx) levels (Dasgupta et al., 2010). Nitrite can react similarly with adult oxy- and deoxy-hemoglobin (HbA), resulting in oxidative denitrosylation of nitrosyl-hemoglobin and rapid dissociation of NO. RBCs containing oxy-HbF (F-cells) had accelerated oxidative denitrosylation. So, induction of HbF present in sickle cell disease may enhance vasodilatation in addition to direct inhibition of polymerization of deoxy sickle hemoglobin (Salhany, 2008). The role of NO in erythrocyte function, sickle cell anemia, malaria, and damage to banked blood has been already reviewed, as well as the use of NO targeted therapies for erythrocyte disease (Maley et al., 2010). Pain from vaso-occlusive crisis is the major cause of hospitalization in patients with sickle cell disease, where beneficial therapeutic effects of inhaled NO have been demonstrated (Head et al., 2010). Decreased exhaled nitric oxide levels (FE_{NO}) have been described in patients with sickle cell disease, together with deficiency in plasma arginine. Additional study shows that sickle cell disease patients, with and without a history of acute chest syndrome, have similar FE_{NO} at baseline when compared with healthy controls (Sullivan et al., 2010).

The protecting effects of exogenous NO on murine cerebral malaria are associated with decreased brain vascular expression of inflammatory markers, ICAM-1 and P-selectin, resulting in attenuated endothelial damage and facilitating blood flow (Zanini et al., 2011). Previous reports demonstrated reduced NO levels in severe malaria related to impaired production of NO, reduced mononuclear cell iNOS expression and NOS substrate arginine (Anstey et al., 1996; Lopansri et al., 2003). Responsible factors for low NO levels in malaria include scavenging of NO by free hemoglobin and superoxide anion, and reduced levels of nitrate, a NO precursor molecule (Lopansri et al., 2003). Endothelial activation plays a central role in the pathogenesis of severe malaria with angiopoietin-2 as a key regulator. NO is a major inhibitor of angiopoietin-2 release from endothelium and has been shown to decrease endothelial inflammation and reduce the adhesion of parasitized RBCs. Low-flow inhaled NO is an attractive new candidate for the adjunctive treatment of severe malaria (Hawkes et al., 2011). Exhaled NO was also lower in severe malaria in comparison to moderately severe falciparum malaria and controls. Intravenous administration of l-arginine increased exhaled NO in moderately severe malaria (Yeo et al., 2007).

7. Conclusion: Nitric oxide and soluble guanylate cyclase

Besides direct stimulation of sGC in erythroid cells, NO is produced by stromal cells of bone marrow hematopoietic microenvironment. NOS enzymes in stromal cells are activated via PKA, supported by intracellular Ca^{2+} elevation. NO has been released into the intercellular space and then passed through the plasma membrane of erythroid cells, where it binds directly to ferrous-deoxy heme of sGC, activating the enzyme. Activation of NO-sGC increases conversion of GTP to cGMP, resulting in elevation of cGMP and subsequent activation of cGMP-dependent protein kinases (PKG) and cGMP-hydrolyzing PDEs. Activation of sGC and PKG increases expression of the γ-globin gene in erythroid cells. NO reduces cAMP levels in erythroid cells, whereas cAMP appears to enhance NO formation. The NO-mediated cAMP-reducing mechanisms may operate as a negative feedback in control of cAMP levels. In addition, cGMP enhances cAMP level and cAMP-signalling pathway by competing for the PDEs active site that has modest cyclic nucleotides selectivity (e.g., PDE3 isozymes). By this way, cGMP inhibits the activity of cAMP-specific PDE3, which results in the increase in intracellular cAMP levels and thereby leads to the activation of PKA. Activation of the cAMP-dependent pathway also induces expression of the γ-globin gene in erythroblasts. The phosphorylation levels of CREB correlated with elevated γ-globin gene expression. Moreover, inhibition of PDE9A enzyme significantly increases production of the γ-globin gene. Therefore, it appears that activation of the linked cGMP- and cAMP-signalling pathways regulates γ-globin expression.

Presented results contribute to the understanding of the significance of NO participation in γ-globin induction. These results should support future studies, with the emphasis focused on the hematopoietic microenvironment, in search of therapy of sickle cell disease. In addition to the possibility of NOS presence and activity in mature RBCs, our data show strong eNOS protein levels and function in more primitive human erythroid progenitor and precursor cells, where control of gene expression occurs. While mechanisms involved in globin gene expression have been recognized at different levels within the regulatory hierarchy, relations between molecular pathways are only emerging. Our presented microarray results demonstrated the broad gene expression profile and related pathways linked to stimulation of globin genes during ontogeny. The presented genes and signaling pathways, involved in the mechanism of globin genes activation, might be targets for therapeutic agents that upregulate γ-globin gene expression and HbF levels in hemoglobinopathies. This ontogenic overview linked to specific genes and transcriptional programs in normal erythropoiesis may contribute to further understanding of erythroid progenitor cell development.

8. Acknowledgments

This research was supported by the Intramural Research Program of the NIH and NIDDK and by grant from the Serbian Ministry of Education and Science (175053).

9. References

Aicher, A., Heeschen, C., Mildner-Rihm, C., Urbich, C., Ihling, C., Technau-Ihling, K., Zeiher, A.M., & Dimmeler, S. (2003). Essential role of endothelial nitric oxide synthase for mobilization of stem and progenitor cells. *Nature medicine*, Vol. 9, No. 11, (Nov 2003), pp.1370-1376, ISSN 1078-8956

Almeida, C.B., Traina, F., Lanaro, C., Canalli, A.A., Saad, S.T., Costa, F.F., & Conran, N. (2008). High expression of the cGMP-specific phosphodiesterase, PDE9A, in sickle cell disease (SCD) and the effects of its inhibition in erythroid cells and SCD neutrophils. *British journal of haematology*, Vol. 142, No. 5, (Sep 2008), pp. 836-844, ISSN 1365-2141

Anstey, N.M., Weinberg, J.B., Hassanali, M.Y., Mwaikambo, E.D., Manyenga, D., Misukonis, M.A., Arnelle, D.R., Hollis, D., McDonald, M.I., & Granger, D.L. (1996). Nitric oxide in Tanzanian children with malaria: inverse relationship between malaria severity and nitric oxide production/nitric oxide synthase type 2 expression. *The Journal of experimental medicine*, Vol. 184, No. 2, (Aug 1996), pp. 557-567, ISSN 0022-1007

Antic, D., Perunicic Jovanovic, M., Dencic Fekete, M., & Cokic, V.P. Assessment of bone marrow microvessel density in chronic lymphocytic leukemia. (2010). *Applied immunohistochemistry & molecular morphology*, Vol. 18, No. 4, (Jul 2010), pp. 353-356, ISSN 1533-4058

Antic, D., Mihaljevic, B., Cokic, V., Fekete, M.D., Djurasevic, T.K., Pavlovic, S., Milic, N., & Elezovic, I. (2011). Patients with early stage chronic lymphocytic leukemia: new risk stratification based on molecular profiling. *Leukemia & Lymphoma*, Vol. 524, No. 7, (Jul 2011), pp. 1394-1397, ISSN 1029-2403

Asano, H., Li, X.S., & Stamatoyannopoulos, G. (1999). FKLF, a novel Krüppel-like factor that activates human embryonic and fetal beta-like globin genes. *Molecular and cellular biology*, Vol. 19, No. 5, (May 1999), pp. 3571-3579, ISSN 0270-7306

Asano, H., Li, X.S., & Stamatoyannopoulos, G. (2000). FKLF-2: a novel Krüppel-like transcriptional factor that activates globin and other erythroid lineage genes. *Blood*, Vol. 95, No.6, (Jun 2000), pp.3578-3584, ISSN 0006-4971

Ascensao, J.L., Vercellotti, G.M., Jacob, H.S., & Zanjani, E.D. (1984). Role of endothelial cells in human hematopoiesis: modulation of mixed colony growth in vitro. *Blood*, Vol. 63, No. 3, (Mar 1984), pp. 553-558, ISSN 0006-4971

Azzouzi, I., Moest, H., Winkler, J., Fauchère, J.C., Gerber, A.P., Wollscheid, B., Stoffel, M., Schmugge, M., & Speer, O. (2011). MicroRNA-96 Directly Inhibits γ-Globin Expression in Human Erythropoiesis. *PLoS One*, Vol. 6, No.7, (2011), e22838, ISSN 1932-6203

Bae, S.W., Kim, H.S., Cha, Y.N., Park, Y.S., Jo, S.A., & Jo, I. (2003). Rapid increase in endothelial nitric oxide production by bradykinin is mediated by protein kinase A signaling pathway. *Biochemical and Biophysical Research Communications*, Vol. 306, No. 4, (Jul 2003), pp. 981-987, ISSN 0006-291X

Bailey, L., Kuroyanagi, Y., Franco-Penteado, C.F., Conran, N., Costa, F.F., Ausenda, S., Cappellini, M.D., & Ikuta, T. (2007). Expression of the gamma-globin gene is sustained by the cAMP-dependent pathway in beta-thalassaemia. *British Journal of Haematology*, Vol. 138, No. 3, (Aug 2007), pp. 382-395, ISSN 0007-1048

Baliga, B.S., Haynes, J. Jr, Obiako, B., & Mishra, N. (2010). Combined effects of arginine and hydroxyurea on BFU-E derived colony growth and HbF synthesis in erythroid progenitors isolated from sickle cell blood. *Cellular and Molecular Biology (Noisy-le-grand)*, Vol. 56, Suppl, (Jun 2010), pp. OL1290-1298, ISSN 1165-158X

Basu, P., Morris, P.E., Haar, J.L., Wani, M.A., Lingrel, J.B., Gaensler, K.M., & Lloyd, J.A. (2005). KLF2 is essential for primitive erythropoiesis and regulates the human and murine embryonic {beta}-like globin genes in vivo. *Blood*, Vol. 106, No. 7, (Oct 2005), pp. 2566-2571, ISSN 0006-4971

Beleslin-Cokic, B.B., Cokic, V.P., Yu, X., Weksler, B.B., Schechter, A.N., & Noguchi, C.T. (2004). Erythropoietin and hypoxia stimulate erythropoietin receptor and nitric oxide production by endothelial cells. *Blood*, Vol. 104, No. 7, (Oct 2004), pp. 2073-2080, ISSN 0006-4971

Beleslin-Cokic, B.B., Cokic, V.P., Wang, L., Piknova, B., Teng, R., Schechter, A.N., & Noguchi, C.T. (2011). Erythropoietin and hypoxia increase erythropoietin receptor and nitric oxide levels in lung microvascular endothelial cells. *Cytokine*, Vol. 54, No. 2, (May 2011), pp. 129-135, ISSN 1096-0023

Bianchi, N., Zuccato, C., Lampronti, I., Borgatti, M., & Gambari, R. (2009). Expression of miR-210 during erythroid differentiation and induction of gamma-globin gene expression. *BMB Reports*, Vol. 42, No. 8, (Aug 2009), pp. 493-499, ISSN 1976-6696

Bieker, J.J., & Southwood, C.M. (1995). The erythroid Kruppel-like factor transactivation domain is a critical component for cell-specific inducibility of a beta-globin promoter. *Molecular and Cellular Biology*, Vol. 15, No. 2, (Feb 1995), pp. 852-860, ISSN 0270-7306

Bogdan, C. (2001). Nitric oxide and the immune response. *Nature Immunology*, Vol. 2, No. 10, (Oct 2001), pp. 907-916, ISSN 1529-2908

Boo, Y.C., Sorescu, G., Boyd, N., Shiojima, I., Walsh, K., Du, J., & Jo, H. (2002). Shear stress stimulates phosphorylation of endothelial nitricoxide synthase at Ser1179 by Akt-independent mechanisms: role of protein kinase A. *The Journal of Biological Chemistry*, Vol. 277, No. 5, (Feb 2002), pp. 3388-3396, ISSN 0021-9258

Borg, J., Papadopoulos, P., Georgitsi, M., Gutiérrez, L., Grech, G., Fanis, P., Phylactides, M., Verkerk, A.J., van der Spek, P.J., Scerri, C.A., Cassar, W., Galdies, R., van Ijcken, W., Ozgür, Z., Gillemans, N., Hou, J., Bugeja, M., Grosveld, F.G., von Lindern, M., Felice, A.E., Patrinos, G.P., & Philipsen, S. (2010). Haploinsufficiency for the erythroid transcription factor KLF1 causes hereditary persistence of fetal hemoglobin. *Nature Genetics*, Vol. 42, No. 9, (Sep 2010), pp. 801-805, ISSN 1546-1718

Brüne, B., & Zhou, J. (2007). Hypoxia-inducible factor-1alpha under the control of nitric oxide. *Methods in Enzymology*, Vol. 435, (2007), pp. 463-478, ISSN 0076-6879

Butt, E., Bernhardt, M., Smolenski, A., Kotsonis, P., Fröhlich, L.G., Sickmann, A., Meyer, H.E., Lohmann, S.M., & Schmidt, H.H. (2000). Endothelial nitric-oxide synthase (type III) is activated and becomes calcium independent upon phosphorylation by cyclic nucleotide-dependent protein kinases. *The Journal of Biological Chemistry*, Vol. 275, No. 7, (Feb 2000), pp. 5179-5187, ISSN 0021-9258

Casteel, D., Suhasini, M., Gudi, T., Naima, R., & Pilz, R.B. (1998). Regulation of the erythroid transcription factor NF-E2 by cyclic adenosine monophosphate- dependent protein kinase. *Blood*, Vol. 91, No. 9, (May 1998), pp. 3193-3201, ISSN 0006-4971

Chen, L.Y., & Mehta, J.L. (1998). Evidence for the presence of L-arginine-nitric oxide pathway in human red blood cells: relevance in the effects of red blood cells on platelet function. *Journal of Cardiovascular Pharmacology*, Vol. 32, No. 1, (Jul 1998), pp. 57-61, ISSN 0160-2446

Chénais, B., Molle, I., & Jeannesson, P. (1999). Inhibitory effect of nitric oxide on chemically induced differentiation of human leukemic K562 cells. *Biochemical Pharmacology*, Vol. 58, No. 5, (Sep 1999), pp. 773-778, ISSN 0006-2952

Cheung, P., Allis, C.D., & Sassone-Corsi, P. Signaling to chromatin through histone modifications. *Cell*, Vol. 103, No. 2, (Oct 2000), pp. 263-271, ISSN 0092-8674

Choi, J.W., Pai, S.H., Kim, S.K., Ito, M., Park, C.S., & Cha, Y.N. Iron deficiency anemia increases nitric oxide production in healthy adolescents. *Annals of Hematology*, Vol. 81, No. 1, (Jan 2002), pp. 1-6, ISSN 0939-5555

Cobb, R.R., Felts, K.A., Parry, G.C., & Mackman, N. (1996). Proteasome inhibitors block VCAM-1 and ICAM-1 gene expression in endothelial cells without affecting nuclear translocation of nuclear factor-kappa B. *European Journal of Immunology*, Vol. 26, No. 4, (Apr 1996), pp. 839-845, ISSN 0014-2980

Cokic, V.P., Smith, R.D., Beleslin-Cokic, B.B., Njoroge, J.M., Miller, J.L., Gladwin, M.T., & Schechter, A.N. (2003). Hydroxyurea induces fetal hemoglobin by the nitric oxide-dependent activation of soluble guanylyl cyclase. *Journal of Clinical Investigation*, Vol. 111, No. 2, (Jan 2003), pp. 231-239, ISSN 0021-9738

Cokic, V.P., Beleslin-Cokic, B.B., Tomic, M., Stojilkovic, S.S., Noguchi, C.T., & Schechter, A.N. (2006). Hydroxyurea induces the eNOS-cGMP pathway in endothelial cells. *Blood*, Vol. 108, No. 1, (Jul 2006), pp. 184-191, ISSN 0006-4971

Cokic, V.P., Beleslin-Cokic, B.B., Noguchi, C.T., & Schechter, A.N. (2007). Hydroxyurea increases eNOS protein levels through inhibition of proteasome activity. *Nitric Oxide: Biology and Chemistry*, Vol. 16, No. 3, (May 2007), pp. 371-378, ISSN 1089-8603

Cokic, V.P., Andric, S.A., Stojilkovic, S.S., Noguchi, C.T., & Schechter, A.N. (2008). Hydroxyurea nitrosylates and activates soluble guanylyl cyclase in human erythroid cells. *Blood*, Vol. 111, No. 3, (Feb 2008), pp. 1117-1123, ISSN 0006-4971

Cokic, V.P., & Schechter, A.N. (2008). Effects of nitric oxide on red blood cell development and phenotype. *Current Topics in Developmental Biology*, Vol. 82, (2008), pp. 169-215, ISSN 0070-2153

Cokic, V.P., Beleslin-Cokic, B.B., Smith, R.D., Economou, A.P., Wahl, L.M., Noguchi, C.T., & Schechter, A.N. (2009). Stimulated stromal cells induce gamma-globin gene expression in erythroid cells via nitric oxide production. *Experimental Hematology*, Vol. 37, No. 10, (Oct 2009), pp. 1230-1237, ISSN 1873-2399

Conran, N., Oresco-Santos, C., Acosta, H.C., Fattori, A., Saad, S.T., & Costa, F.F. (2004). Increased soluble guanylate cyclase activity in the red blood cells of sickle cell patients. *British Journal of Haematology*, Vol. 124, No. 4, (Feb 2004), pp. 547-554, ISSN 0007-1048

Cosby, K., Partovi, K.S., Crawford, J.H., Patel, R.P., Reiter, C.D., Martyr, S., Yang, B.K., Waclawiw, M.A., Zalos, G., Xu, X., Huang, K.T., Shields, H., Kim-Shapiro, D.B., Schechter, A.N., Cannon, R.O. 3rd, & Gladwin, M.T. (2003). Nitrite reduction to nitric oxide by deoxyhemoglobin vasodilates the human circulation. *Nature Medicine*, Vol. 9, No. 12, (Dec 2003), pp. 1498-1505, ISSN 1078-8956

Dasgupta, T., Fabry, M.E., & Kaul, D.K. (2010). Antisickling property of fetal hemoglobin enhances nitric oxide bioavailability and ameliorates organ oxidative stress in transgenic-knockout sickle mice. *American Journal of Physiology*, Vol. 298, No. 2, (Feb 2010), R394-402, ISSN 1522-1490

Davis, T.A., Robinson, D.H., Lee, K.P., & Kessler, S.W. (1995). Porcine brain microvascular endothelial cells support the in vitro expansion of human primitive hematopoietic bone marrow progenitor cells with a high replating potential: requirement for cell-to-cell interactions and colony-stimulating factors. *Blood*, Vol. 85, No. 7, (Apr 1995), pp. 1751-1761, ISSN 0006-4971

De Caterina, R., Libby, P., Peng, H.B., Thannickal, V.J., Rajavashisth, T.B., Jr., Gimbrone, M.A., Shin, W.S., & Liao, J.K. (1995). Nitric oxide decreases cytokine induced endothelial activation. Nitric oxide selectively reduces endothelial expression of adhesion molecules and proinflammatory cytokines. *The Journal of Clinical Investigation*, Vol. 96, No. 1, (Jul 1995), pp. 60-68, ISSN 0021-9738

Donze, D., Townes, T.M., & Bieker, J.J. (1995). Role of erythroid Kruppel-like factor in human gamma- to beta-globin gene switching. *The Journal of Biological Chemistry*, Vol. 270, No. 4, (Jan 1995), pp. 1955-1959, ISSN 0021-9258

Dumitriu, B., Dy, P., Smits, P., & Lefebvre, V. (2006). Generation of mice harboring a Sox6 conditional null allele. *Genesis*, Vol. 44, No. 5, (May 2006), pp. 219-224, ISSN 1526-954X

Ferro, A., Queen, L.R., Priest, R.M., Xu, B., Ritter, J.M., Poston, L., Ward, J.P. (1999). Activation of nitric oxide synthase by beta 2-adrenoceptors in human umbilical vein endothelium in vitro. *British Journal of Pharmacology*, Vol. 126, No. 8, (Apr 1999), pp. 1872-1880, ISSN 0007-1188

Fujishima, N., Hirokawa, M., Aiba, N., Ichikawa, Y., Fujishima, M., Komatsuda, A., Suzuki, Y., Kawabata, Y., Miura, I., & Sawada, K. (2004). Gene expression profiling of human erythroid progenitors by micro-serial analysis of gene expression. *International Journal of Hematology*, Vol. 80, No. 3, (Oct 2004), pp. 239-245, ISSN 0925-5710

Gabbianelli, M., Testa, U., Morsilli, O., Pelosi, E., Saulle, E., Petrucci, E., Castelli, G., Giovinazzi, S., Mariani, G., Fiori, M.E., Bonanno, G., Massa, A., Croce, C.M., Fontana, L., & Peschle, C. (2010). Mechanism of human Hb switching: a possible role of the kit receptor/miR 221-222 complex. *Haematologica*, Vol. 95, No. 8, (Aug 2010), pp. 1253-1260, ISSN 1592-8721

Galarneau, G., Palmer, C.D., Sankaran, V.G., Orkin, S.H., Hirschhorn, J.N., & Lettre, G. (2010). Fine-mapping at three loci known to affect fetal hemoglobin levels explains additional genetic variation. *Nature Genetics*, Vol. 42, No. 12, (Dec 2010), pp. 1049-1051, ISSN 1546-1718

Gibbons, R.J., Picketts, D.J., Villard, L., & Higgs, D.R. (1995). Mutations in a putative global transcriptional regulator cause X-linked mental retardation with alpha-thalassemia (ATR-X syndrome). *Cell*, Vol. 80, No. 6, (Mar 1995), pp. 837-845, ISSN 0092-8674

Goh, S.H., Josleyn, M., Lee, Y.T., Danner, R.L., Gherman, R.B., Cam, M.C., & Miller, J.L. (2007). The Human Reticulocyte Transcriptome. *Physiological Genomics*, Vol. 30, No. 2, (Jul 2007), pp. 172-178, ISSN 1531-2267

Gregory, R.C., Taxman, D.J., Seshasayee, D., Kensinger, M.H., Bieker, J.J., & Wojchowski, D.M. (1996). Functional interaction of GATA1 with erythroid Krüppel-like factor and Sp1 at defined erythroid promoters. *Blood,* Vol. 87, No. 5, (Mar 1996), pp. 1793-1801, ISSN 0006-4971

Grosveld, F., van Assendelft, G.B., Greaves, D.R., & Kollias, G. (1987). Position-independent, high-level expression of the human beta-globin gene in transgenic mice. *Cell*, Vol. 51, No. 6, (Dec 1987), pp. 975-985, ISSN 0092-8674

Gubin, A.N., Njoroge, J.M., Bouffard, G.G., & Miller, J.L. (1999). Gene Expression in Proliferating Human Erythroid Cells. *Genomics*, Vol. 59, No. 2, (Jul 1999), pp. 168-177, ISSN 0888-7543

Guo-wei, Z., Rui-feng, Y., Xiang, L., Mitchell, W.J., De-pei, L., & Chih-chuan, L. (2010). NF-E2: a novel regulator of alpha-hemoglobin stabilizing protein gene expression. *Chinese Medical Sciences Journal*, Vol. 25, No. 4, (Dec 2010), pp. 193-198, ISSN 1001-9294

Hanspal, M., & Hanspal, J.S. (1994). The association of erythroblasts with macrophages promotes erythroid proliferation and maturation: a 30-kD heparin-binding protein is involved in this contact. *Blood*, Vol. 84, No. 10, (Nov 1994), pp. 3494-3504, ISSN 0006-4971

Harju-Baker, S., Costa, F.C., Fedosyuk, H., Neades, R., & Peterson, K.R. (2008). Silencing of Agamma-globin gene expression during adult definitive erythropoiesis mediated by GATA-1-FOG-1-Mi2 complex binding at the -566 GATA site. *Molecular and Cellular Biology*, Vol. 28, No. 10, (May 2008), pp. 3101-3113, ISSN 1098-5549

Hawkes, M., Opoka, R.O., Namasopo, S., Miller, C., Thorpe, K.E., Lavery, J.V., Conroy, A.L., Liles, W.C., John, C.C., & Kain, K.C. (2011). Inhaled nitric oxide for the adjunctive therapy of severe malaria: protocol for a randomized controlled trial. *Trials*, Vol. 12, (Jul 2011), pp. 176, ISSN 1745-6215

Haynes, J. Jr., Baliga, B.S., Obiako, B., Ofori-Acquah, S., & Pace, B. (2004). Zileuton induces hemoglobin F synthesis in erythroid progenitors: role of the L-arginine-nitric oxide signaling pathway. *Blood*, Vol. 103, No. 10, (May 2004), pp. 3945-3950, ISSN 0006-4971

He, X., Gonzalez, V., Tsang, A., Thompson, J., Tsang, T.C., & Harris, D.T. (2005). Differential Gene Expression Profiling of CD34+ CD133+ Umbilical Cord Blood Hematopoietic Stem Progenitor Cells. *Stem Cells and Development*, Vol. 14, No. 2, (Apr 2005), pp. 188-198, ISSN 1547-3287

Head, C.A., Swerdlow, P., McDade, W.A., Joshi, R.M., Ikuta, T., Cooper, M.L., & Eckman, J.R. (2010). Beneficial effects of nitric oxide breathing in adult patients with sickle cell crisis. *American Journal of Hematology*, Vol. 85, No. 10, (Oct 2010), pp. 800-802, ISSN 1096-8652

Higgs, D.R., Sharpe, J.A., & Wood, W.G. (1998). Understanding alpha globin gene expression: a step towards effective gene therapy. *Seminars in Hematology*, Vol. 35, No. 2, (Apr 1998), pp. 93-104, ISSN 0037-1963

Hikiji, H., Shin, W. S., Oida, S., Takato, T., Koizumi, T., & Toyo-oka, T. (1997). Direct action of nitric oxide on osteoblastic differentiation. *FEBS Letters*, Vol. 410, No. 2-3, (Jun 1997), pp. 238-242, ISSN 0014-5793

Ikuta, T., Ausenda, S., & Cappellini, M.D. (2001). Mechanism for fetal globin gene expression: role of the soluble guanylate cyclase-cGMP-dependent protein kinase pathway. *Proceedings of the National Academy of Sciences of the USA*, Vol. 98, No. 4, (Feb 2001), pp. 1847-1852, ISSN 0027-8424

Ikuta, T., Thatte, H.S., Tang, J.X., Mukerji, I., Knee, K., Bridges, K.R., Wang, S., Montero-Huerta, P., Joshi, R.M., & Head, C.A. (2011). Nitric oxide reduces sickle hemoglobin polymerization: potential role of nitric oxide-induced charge alteration in depolymerization. *Archives of Biochemistry and Biophysics*, Vol. 510, No. 1, (Jun 2011), pp. 53-61, ISSN 1096-0384

Inoue, A., Kuroyanagi, Y., Terui, K., Moi, P., & Ikuta, T. (2004). Negative regulation of gamma-globin gene expression by cyclic AMP-dependent pathway in erythroid cells. *Experimental Hematology*, Vol. 32, No. 3, (Mar 2004), pp. 244-253, ISSN 0301-472X

Iyamu, E.W., Cecil, R., Parkin, L., Woods, G., Ohene-Frempong, K., & Asakura, T. Modulation of erythrocyte arginase activity in sickle cell disease patients during hydroxyurea therapy. (2005). *British Journal of Haematology*, Vol. 131, No. 3, (Nov 2005), pp. 389-394, ISSN 0007-1048

Jeffers, A., Xu, X., Huang, K.T., Cho, M., Hogg, N., Patel, R.P., & Kim-Shapiro, D.B. (2005). Hemoglobin mediated nitrite activation of soluble guanylyl cyclase. *Comparative Biochemistry and Physiology. Part A, Molecular and Integrative Physiology*, Vol. 142, No. 2, (Oct 2005), pp. 130-135, ISSN 1095-6433

Jensen, M., Attemberg, H., Schneider, C.H., & Walter, J.U. (1982). The developmental change in the G gamma and A gamma globin proportions in hemoglobin F. *European Journal of Pediatrics*, Vol. 138, No. 4, (Jul 1982), pp. 311-314, ISSN 0340-6199

Jiang, J., Best, S., Menzel, S., Silver, N., Lai, M.I., Surdulescu, G.L., Spector, T.D.,& Thein, S.L. (2006). cMYB is involved in the regulation of fetal hemoglobin production in adults. *Blood*, Vol. 108, No. 3, (Aug 2006), pp. 1077-1083, ISSN 0006-4971

Jovcic, G., Bugarski, D., Krstic, A., Vlaski, M., Petakov, M., Mojsilovic, S., Stojanovic, N., & Milenkovic, P. (2007). The effect of interieukin-17 on hematopoietic cells and cytokine release in mouse spleen. *Physiological Research*, Vol. 56, No. 3, (2007), pp. 331-339, ISSN 0862-8408

Jubelin, B.C., & Gierman, J.L. (1996). Erythrocytes may synthesize their own nitric oxide. *American Journal of Hypertension*, Vol. 9, No. 12, (Dec 1996), pp. 1214-1219, ISSN 0895-7061

Kameoka, J., Yanai, N., & Obinata, M. (1995). Bone marrow stromal cells selectively stimulate the rapid expansion of lineage-restricted myeloid progenitors. *Journal of Cellular Physiology*, Vol. 164, No. 1, (Jul 1995), pp. 55-64, ISSN 0021-9541

Kang, E.S., Ford, K., Grokulsky, G., Wang, Y.B., Chiang, T.M., & Acchiardo, S.R. (2000). Normal circulating adult human red blood cells contain inactive NOS proteins. *Journal of Laboratory and Clinical Medicine*, Vol. 135, No. 6, (Jun 2000), pp. 444-451, ISSN 0022-2143

Keefer, J.R., Schneidereith, T.A., Mays, A., Purvis, S.H., Dover, G.J., & Smith, K.D. (2006). Role of cyclic nucleotides in fetal hemoglobin induction in cultured CD34+ cells. *Experimental Hematology*, Vol. 34, No. 9, (Sep 2006), pp. 1151-1161, ISSN 0301-472X

Kihm, A.J., Kong, Y., Hong, W., Russell, J.E., Rouda, S., Adachi, K., Simon, M.C., Blobel, G.A., & Weiss, M.J. (2002). An abundant erythroid protein that stabilizes free alpha-haemoglobin. *Nature*, Vol. 417, No. 6890, (Jun 2002), pp. 758-763, ISSN 0028-0836

Kleinbongard, P., Schulz, R., Rassaf, T., Lauer, T., Dejam, A., Jax, T., Kumara, I., Gharini, P., Kabanova, S., Ozuyaman, B., Schnurch, H.G., Godecke, A., Weber, A.A., Robenek, M., Robenek, H., Bloch, W., Rosen, P., & Kelm, M. (2006). Red blood cells express a functional endothelial nitric oxide synthase. *Blood*, Vol. 107, No. 7, (Apr 2006), pp. 2943-2951, ISSN 0006-4971

Kodeboyina, S., Balamurugan, P., Liu, L., & Pace, B.S. (2010). cJun modulates Ggamma-globin gene expression via an upstream cAMP response element. *Blood cells, molecules & diseases*, Vol. 44, No. 1, (Jan 2010), pp. 7-15, ISSN 1096-0961

Kovacevic-Filipovic, M., Petakov, M., Hermitte, F., Debeissat, C., Krstic, A., Jovcic, G., Bugarski, D., Lafarge, X., Milenkovic, P., Praloran, V., & Ivanovic, Z. (2007). Interleukin-6 (IL-6) and low O2 concentration (1%) synergize to improve the maintenance of hematopoietic stem cells (pre-CFC). *Journal of Cellular Physiology*, Vol. 212, No. 1, (Jul 2007), pp. 68-75, ISSN 0021-9541

Krstic, A., Ilic, V., Mojsilovic, S., Jovcic, G., Milenkovic, P., & Bugarski, D. (2009). p38 MAPK signaling mediates IL-17-induced nitric oxide synthase expression in bone marrow cells. *Growth Factors*, Vol. 27, No. 2, (Apr 2009), pp. 79-90, ISSN 1029-2292

Krstic, A., Vlaški, M., Hammoud, M., Chevaleyre, J., Duchez, P., Jovcic, G., Bugarski, D., Milenkovic, P., Bourin, P., Boiron, J.M., Praloran, V., & Ivanovic, Z. (2009). Low O2 concentrations enhance the positive effect of IL-17 on the maintenance of erythroid progenitors during co-culture of CD34+ and mesenchymal stem cells. *European Cytokine Network*, Vol. 20, No. 1, (Mar 2009), pp. 10-16, ISSN 1148-5493

Krstic, A., Santibanez, J.F., Okic, I., Mojsilovic, S., Kocic, J., Jovcic, G., Milenkovic, P., & Bugarski, D. (2010). Combined effect of IL-17 and blockade of nitric oxide biosynthesis on haematopoiesis in mice. *Acta Physiologica (Oxford, England)*, Vol. 199, No. 1, (May 2010), pp. 31-41, ISSN 1748-1716

Kucukkaya, B., Ozturk, G., & Yalcintepe, L. (2006). Nitric oxide levels during erythroid differentiation in K562 cell line. *Indian Journal of Biochemistry and Biophysics*, Vol. 43, No. 4, (Aug 2006), pp. 251-253, ISSN 0301-1208

Kuroyanagi, Y., Kaneko, Y., Muta, K., Park, B.S., Moi, P., Ausenda, S., Cappellini, M.D., & Ikuta, T. (2006). cAMP differentially regulates gamma-globin gene expression in erythroleukemic cells and primary erythroblasts through c-Myb expression. *Biochemical and Biophysical Research Communications*, Vol. 344, No. 3, (Jun 2006), pp. 1038-1047, ISSN 0006-291X

Kwan, H.Y., Huang, Y., & Yao, X. (2000). Store-operated calcium entry in vascular endothelial cells is inhibited by cGMP via a protein kinase G-dependent mechanism.*The Journal of Biological Chemistry*, Vol. 275, No. 10, (Mar 2000), pp. 6758-6763, ISSN 0021-9258

Leonard, M., Brice, M., Engel, J.D., & Papayannopoulou T. (1993). Dynamics of GATA transcription factor expression during erythroid differentiation. *Blood*, Vol. 82, No. 4, (Aug 1993), pp. 1071-1079, ISSN 0006-4971

Lodish, H.F., & Jacobsen, M. (1972). Regulation of hemoglobin synthesis. Equal rates of translation and termination of-and-globin chains. *The Journal of Biological Chemistry*, Vol. 247, No. 11, (Jun 1972), pp. 3622-3629, ISSN 0021-9258

Lopansri, B.K., Anstey, N.M., Weinberg, J.B., Stoddard, G.J., Hobbs, M.R., Levesque, M.C., Mwaikambo, E.D., & Granger, D.L. (2003). Low plasma arginine concentrations in children with cerebral malaria and decreased nitric oxide production. *Lancet*, Vol. 361, No. 9358, (Feb 2003), pp. 676-678, ISSN 0140-6736

Lou, T.F., Singh, M., Mackie, A., Li, W., & Pace, B.S. (2009). Hydroxyurea generates nitric oxide in human erythroid cells: mechanisms for gamma-globin gene activation. *Experimental Biology and Medicine (Maywood)*, Vol. 234, No. 11, (Nov 2009), pp. 1374-1382, ISSN 1535-3699

Lu, J., Guo, S., Ebert, B.L., Zhang, H., Peng, X., Bosco, J., Pretz, J., Schlanger, R., Wang, J.Y., Mak, R.H., Dombkowski, D.M., Preffer, F.I., Scadden, D.T., & Golub, T.R. (2008). MicroRNA-mediated control of cell fate in megakaryocyte-erythrocyte progenitors. *Developmental Cell*, Vol. 14, No. 6, (Jun 2008), pp. 843-853, ISSN 1878-1551

Lugnier, C., Keravis, T., & Eckly-Michel, A. (1999). Cross talk between NO and cyclic nucleotide phosphodiesterases in the modulation of signal transduction in blood vessel. *Journal of Physiology and Pharmacology*, Vol. 50, No. 4, (Dec 1999), pp. 639-652, ISSN 0867-5910

Maciejewski, J. P., Selleri, C., Sato, T., Cho, H. J., Keefer, L. K., Nathan, C. F., & Young, N. S. (1995). Nitric oxide suppression of human hematopoiesis in vitro. Contribution to inhibitory action of interferon-gamma and tumor necrosis factor-alpha. *The Journal of Clinical Investigation*, Vol. 96, No. 2, (Aug 2005), pp.1085-1092, ISSN 0021-9738

Majka, M., Janowska-Wieczorek, A., Ratajczak, J., Ehrenman, K., Pietrzkowski, Z., Kowalska, M.A., Gewirtz, A.M., Emerson, S.G., & Ratajczak, M.Z. (2001). Numerous growth factors, cytokines, and chemokines are secreted by human CD34(+) cells, myeloblasts, erythroblasts, and megakaryoblasts and regulate normal hematopoiesis in an autocrine/paracrine manner. *Blood*, Vol. 97, No. 10, (May 2001), pp. 3075-3085, ISSN 0006-4971

Maley, J.H., Lasker, G.F., & Kadowitz, P.J. (2010). Nitric oxide and disorders of the erythrocyte: emerging roles and therapeutic targets. *Cardiovascular & hematological disorders drug targets*, Vol. 10, No. 4, (Dec 2010), pp. 284-291, ISSN 1871-529X

Michell, B.J., Chen, Z., Tiganis, T., Stapleton, D., Katsis, F., Power, D.A., Sim, A.T., & Kemp, B.E. (2001). Coordinated control of endothelial nitric-oxide synthase phosphorylation by protein kinase C and the cAMP dependent protein kinase. The Journal of biological chemistry, Vol. 276, No. 21, (May 2001), pp. 17625-17628, ISSN 0021-9258

Migliaccio, G., Migliaccio, A.R., Petti, S., Mavilio, F., Russo, G., Lazzaro, D., Testa, U., Marinucci, M., & Peschle, C. (1986). Human embryonic hemopoiesis. Kinetics of progenitors and precursors underlying the yolk sac-liver transition. The Journal of Clinical Investigation, Vol. 78, No. 1, (Jul 1986), pp. 51-60, ISSN 0021-9738

Miller, I.J., & Bieker, J.J. (1993). A novel, erythroid cell-specific murine transcription factor that binds to the CACCC element and is related to the Krüppel family of nuclear proteins. Molecular and cellular biology, Vol.13, No. 5, (May 1993), pp. 2776-2786, ISSN 0270-7306

Morris, C.R., Vichinsky, E.P., van Warmerdam, J., Machado, L., Kepka-Lenhart, D., Morris, S.M. Jr, & Kuypers, F.A. (2003). Hydroxyurea and arginine therapy: impact on nitric oxide production in sickle cell disease. Journal of pediatric hematology/oncology, Vol. 25, No. 8, (Aug 2003), pp. 629-634, ISSN 1077-4114

Nahavandi, M., Tavakkoli, F., Wyche, M.Q., Perlin, E., Winter, W.P., & Castro, O. (2002). Nitric oxide and cyclic GMP levels in sickle cell patients receiving hydroxyurea. British journal of haematology, Vol. 119, No. 3, (Dec 2002), pp. 855-857, ISSN 0007-1048

Nahavandi, M., Tavakkoli, F., Millis, R.M., Wyche, M.Q., Habib, M.J., & Tavakoli, N. (2006) Effects of hydroxyurea and L-arginine on the production of nitric oxide metabolites in cultures of normal and sickle erythrocytes. Hematology, Vol. 11, No. 4, (Aug 2006), pp. 291-294, ISSN 1607-8454

Ng, Y.Y., van Kessel, B., Lokhorst, H.M., Baert, M.R., van den Burg, C.M., Bloem, A.C., & Staal, F.J. (2004). Gene-expression profiling of CD34+ cells from various hematopoietic stem-cell sources reveals functional differences in stem cell activity. Journal of leukocyte biology, Vol. 75, No. 2, (Feb 2004), pp. 314-323, ISSN 0741-5400

Nienhuis, A.W., & Benz, E.J. (1977). Regulation of hemoglobin synthesis during the development of the red cell. The New England journal of medicine, Vol. 297, No. 24, (Dec 1977), pp. 1318-1328, ISSN 0028-4793

Noh, S.J., Miller, S.H., Lee, Y.T., Goh, S.H., Marincola, F.M., Stroncek, D.F., Reed, C., Wang, E., & Miller, J.L. (2009). Let-7 microRNAs are developmentally regulated in circulating human erythroid cells. Journal of translational medicine, Vol. 7:98, (Nov 2009), ISSN 1479-5876

Oh, I.H., Lau, A., & Eaves, C.J. (2000). During ontogeny primitive (CD34+CD38-) hematopoietic cells show altered expression of a subset of genes associated with early cytokine and differentiation responses of their adult counterparts. Blood, Vol. 96, No. 13, (Dec 2000), pp. 4160-4168, ISSN 0006-4971

Ohneda, O., & Bautch, V.L. (1997). Murine endothelial cells support fetal liver erythropoiesis and myelopoiesis via distinct interactions. British journal of haematology, Vol. 98, No. 4, (Sep 1997), pp. 798-808, ISSN 0007-1048

Orkin, S.H. (1992). GATA-binding transcription factors in hematopoietic cells. Blood, Vol. 80, No. 3, (Aug 1992), pp. 575-581, ISSN 0006-4971

Pazin, M.J., & Kadonaga, J.T. (1997). What's up and down with histone deacetylation and transcription? *Cell*, Vol. 89, No. 3, (May 1997), pp. 325-328, ISSN 0092-8674

Perrine, S.P., Mankidy, R., Boosalis, M.S., Bieker, J.J., & Faller, D.V. (2009). Erythroid Kruppel-like factor (EKLF) is recruited to the gamma-globin gene promoter as a co-activator and is required for gamma-globin gene induction by short-chain fatty acid derivatives. *European journal of haematology*, Vol. 82, No. 6, (Jun 2009), pp. 466-476, ISSN 1600-0609

Persons, D.A., Allay, J.A., Allay, E.R., Ashmun, R.A., Orlic, D., Jane, S.M., Cunningham, J.M., & Nienhuis, A.W. (1999). Enforced expression of the GATA-2 transcription factor blocks normal hematopoiesis. *Blood*, Vol. 93, No. 2, (Jan 1999), pp. 488-499, ISSN 0006-4971

Peschle, C., Migliaccio, A.R., Migliaccio, G., Petrini, M., Calandrini, M., Russo, G., Mastroberardino, G., Presta, M., Gianni, A.M., & Comi, P. (1984). Embryonic fetal Hb switch in humans: studies on erythroid bursts generated by embryonic progenitors from yolk sac and liver. *Proceedings of the National Academy of Sciences of the USA*, Vol. 81, No. 8, (Apr 1984), pp. 2416-2420, ISSN 0027-8424

Pevny, L., Lin, C.S., D'Agati, V., Simon, M.C., Orkin, S.H., & Costantini, F. (1995). Development of hematopoietic cells lacking transcription factor GATA-1. *Development*, Vol. 121, No. 1, (Jan 1995), pp. 163-172, ISSN 0950-1991

Pruzina, S., Hanscombe, O., Whyatt, D., Grosveld, F., & Philipsen, S. (1991). Hypersensitive site 4 of the human beta globin locus control region. *Nucleic acids research*, Vol. 19, No. 7, (Apr 1991), pp. 1413-1419, ISSN 0305-1048

Pullamsetti, S.S., Savai, R., Schaefer, M.B., Wilhelm, J., Ghofrani, H.A., Weissmann, N., Schudt, C., Fleming, I., Mayer, K., Leiper, J., Seeger, W., Grimminger, F., & Schermuly, R.T. (2011). cAMP phosphodiesterase inhibitors increases nitric oxide production by modulating dimethylarginine dimethylaminohydrolases. *Circulation*, Vol. 123, No. 11, (Mar 2011), pp. 1194-1204, ISSN 1524-4539

Ramakrishnan, V., & Pace, B.S. (2011). Regulation of γ-globin gene expression involves signaling through the p38 MAPK/CREB1 pathway. *Blood cells, molecules & diseases*, Vol. 47, No. 1, (Jun 2011), pp. 12-22, ISSN 1096-0961

Ratajczak, J., Majka, M., Kijowski, J., Baj, M., Pan, Z.K., Marquez, L.A., Janowska-Wieczorek, A., & Ratajczak, M.Z. (2001). Biological significance of MAPK, AKT and JAK-STAT protein activation by various erythropoietic factors in normal human early erythroid cells. *British journal of haematology*, Vol. 115, No.1, (Oct 2001), pp. 195-204, ISSN 0007-1048

Reiser, G. (1992). Nitric oxide formation caused by Ca^{2+} release from internal stores in neuronal cell line isenhanced by cyclic AMP. *European journal of pharmacology*, Vol. 227, No. 1, (Sep 1992), pp. 89-93, ISSN 0014-2999

Risinger, J.I., Maxwell, G.L., Chandramouli, G.V., Aprelikova, O., Litzi, T., Umar, A., Berchuck, A., & Barrett, J.C. (2003). Microarray analysis reveals distinct gene expression profiles among different histologic types of endometrial cancer. *Cancer research*, Vol. 63, No. 1, (Jan 2003), pp. 6-11, ISSN 0008-5472

Rogers, H.M., Yu, X., Wen, J., Smith, R., Fibach, E., & Noguchi, C.T. (2008). Hypoxia alters progression of the erythroid program. *Experimental hematology*, Vol. 36, No. 1, (Jan 2008), pp. 17-27, ISSN 0301-472X

Salhany, J.M. (2010). Reaction of nitrite with human fetal oxyhemoglobin: a model simulation study with implications for blood flow regulation in sickle cell disease (SCD). *Blood cells, molecules & diseases*, Vol. 44, No. 2, (Apr 2010), pp111-114, ISSN 1096-0961

Sankaran, V.G., Menne, T.F., Xu, J., Akie, T.E., Lettre, G., Van Handel, B., Mikkola, H.K., Hirschhorn, J.N., Cantor, A.B., & Orkin, S.H. (2008). Human fetal hemoglobin expression is regulated by the developmental stage-specific repressor BCL11A. *Science*, Vol. 322, No. 5909, (Dec 2008), pp. 1839-1842, ISSN 1095-9203

Setchenska, M.S., Arnstein, H.R., & Vassileva-Popova, J.G. (1981). Cyclic AMP phosphodiesterase activity during differentiation of rabbit erythroid bone marrow cells. *The Biochemical journal*, Vol. 196, No. 3, (Jun 1981), pp. 887-892, ISSN 0264-6021

Shami, P.J., & Weinberg, J.B. (1996). Differential effects of nitric oxide on erythroid and myeloid colony growth from CD34+ human bone marrow cells. *Blood*, Vol. 87, No. 3, (Feb 1996), pp. 977-982, ISSN 0006-4971

Stamatoyannopoulos, G. (2005). Control of globin gene expression during development and erythroid differentiation. *Experimental hematology*, Vol. 33, No. 3, (Mar 2005), pp. 259-271, ISSN 0301-472X

Stangl, V., Lorenz, M., Meiners, M., Ludwig, A., Bartsch, C., Moobed, M., Vietzke, A., Kinkel, H.T., Baumann, G., & Stangl, K. (2004). Long-term up-regulation of eNOS and improvement of endothelial function by inhibition of the ubiquitin-proteasome pathway. *The FASEB journal*, Vol. 18, No. 2, (Feb 2004), pp. 272-279, ISSN 1530-6860

Steidl, U., Kronenwett, R., Rohr, U.P., Fenk, R., Kliszewski, S., Maercker, C., Neubert, P., Aivado, M., Koch, J., Modlich, O., Bojar, H., Gattermann, N., & Haas, R. (2002). Gene expression profiling identifies significant differences between the molecular phenotypes of bone marrow-derived and circulating human CD34+ hematopoietic stem cells. *Blood*, Vol. 99, No. 6, (Mar 2002), pp. 2037-2044, ISSN 0006-4971

Su, K.H., Shyue, S.K., Kou, Y.R., Ching, L.C., Chiang, A.N., Yu, Y.B., Chen, C.Y., Pan, C.C., & Lee, T.S. (2011). β common receptor integrates the erythropoietin signaling in activation of endothelial nitric oxide synthase. *Journal of cellular physiology*, (Feb 2011), doi: 10.1002/jcp.22678, ISSN 1097-4652

Suhasini, M., Boss, G.R., Pascual, F.E., & Pilz, R.B. (1995). Nitric oxide-releasing agents and cGMP analogues inhibit murine erythroleukemia cell differentiation and suppress erythroid-specific gene expression: correlation with decreased DNA binding of NF-E2 and altered c-myb mRNA expression. *Cell growth & differentiation*, Vol. 6, No. 12, (Dec 1995), pp. 1559-1566, ISSN 1044-9523

Sullivan, K.J., Kissoon, N., Sandler, E., Gauger, C., Froyen, M., Duckworth, L., Brown, M., & Murphy, S. (2010). Effect of oral arginine supplementation on exhaled nitric oxide concentration in sickle cell anemia and acute chest syndrome. *Journal of pediatric hematology/oncology*, Vol. 32, No. 7, (Oct 2010), pp. 249-258, ISSN 1536-3678

Tamura, K., Sudo, T., Senftleben, U., Dadak, A.M., Johnson, R., & Karin, M. (2000). Requirement for p38α in erythropoietin expression: a role for stress kinases in erythropoiesis. *Cell*, Vol. 102, No. 2, (Jul 2000), pp. 221-231, ISSN 0092-8674

Tanimoto, K., Liu, Q., Grosveld, F., Bungert, J., & Engel, J.D. (2000). Context dependent EKLF responsiveness defines the developmental specificity of the human epsilon-globin gene in erythroid cells of YAC transgenic mice. *Genes & development*, Vol. 14, No. 21, (Nov 2000), pp. 2778-2794, ISSN 0890-9369

Tsang, A.P., Visvader, J.E., Turner, C.A., Fujiwara, Y., Yu, C., Weiss, M.J., Crossley, M., & Orkin, S.H. (1997). FOG, a multitype zinc finger protein, acts as a cofactor for transcription factor GATA-1 in erythroid and megakaryocytic differentiation. *Cell*, Vol. 90, No. 1, (Jul 1997), pp. 109-119, ISSN 0092-8674

Vaandrager, A.B., & de Jonge, H.R. (1996). Signalling by cGMP-dependent protein kinases. *Molecular and cellular biochemistry*, Vol. 157, No. 1-2, (Apr 1996), pp. 23-30, ISSN 0300-8177

Vakoc, C.R., Letting, D.L., Gheldof, N., Sawado, T., Bender, M.A., Groudine, M., Weiss, M.J., Dekker, J., & Blobel. G.A. (2005). Proximity among distant regulatory elements at the beta-globin locus requires GATA-1 and FOG-1. *Molecular cell*, Vol. 17, No. 3, (Feb 2005), pp. 453-462, ISSN 1097-2765

Wen, J., Huang, S., Rogers, H., Dickinson, L.A., Kohwi-Shigematsu, T., & Noguchi, C.T. (2005). SATB1 family protein expressed during early erythroid differentiation modifies globin gene expression. *Blood*, Vol. 105, No. 8, (Apr 2005), pp. 3330-3339, ISSN 0006-4971

Wong, J.C., & Fiscus, R.R. (2011). Essential roles of the nitric oxide (no)/cGMP/protein kinase G type-Ia (PKG-Ia) signaling pathway and the atrial natriuretic peptide (ANP)/cGMP/PKG-Ia autocrine loop in promoting proliferation and cell survival of OP9 bone marrow stromal cells. *Journal of cellular biochemistry*, Vol. 112, No. 3, (Mar 2011), pp. 829-39, ISSN 1097-4644

Xu, B., Li, J., Gao, L., & Ferro, A. (2000). Nitric oxide-dependent vasodilatation of rabbit femoral artery by beta(2)-adrenergic stimulation or cyclic AMP elevation in vivo. *British journal of pharmacology*. Vol. 129, No. 5, (Mar 2000), pp. 969-974, ISSN 0007-1188

Xu, J., Sankaran, V.G., Ni, M., Menne, T.F., Puram, R.V., Kim, W., & Orkin, S.H. (2010). Transcriptional silencing of {gamma}-globin by BCL11A involves long-range interactions and cooperation with SOX6. *Genes & development*. Vol. 24, No. 8, (Apr 2010), pp. 783-798, ISSN 1549-5477

Yeo, T.W., Lampah, D.A., Gitawati, R., Tjitra, E., Kenangalem, E., McNeil, Y.R., Darcy, C.J., Granger, D.L., Weinberg, J.B., Lopansri, B.K., Price, R.N., Duffull, S.B., Celermajer, D.S., & Anstey, N.M. (2007). Impaired nitric oxide bioavailability and L-arginine reversible endothelial dysfunction in adults with falciparum malaria. *The Journal of experimental medicine*, Vol. 204, No. 11, (Oct 2007), pp. 2693-2704, ISSN 1540-9538

Zanini, G.M., Cabrales, P., Barkho, W., Frangos, J.A., & Carvalho, L.J. (2011). Exogenous nitric oxide decreases brain vascular inflammation, leakage and venular resistance during Plasmodium berghei ANKA infection in mice. *Journal of neuroinflammation*. (Jun 2011) Vol. 8, pp 66, ISSN 1742-2094

Zhou, D., Liu, K., Sun, C.W., Pawlik, K.M., & Townes, T.M. (2010). KLF1 regulates BCL11A expression and gamma- to beta-globin gene switching. *Nature genetics*, Vol 42, No 9, (Sep 2010), 742-744, ISSN 1546-1718.

Zhu, J., Chin, K., Aerbajinai, W., Trainor, C., Gao, P., & Rodgers, G.P. (2011). Recombinant erythroid Kruppel-like factor fused to GATA1 up-regulates delta- and gamma-globin expression in erythroid cells. *Blood*, Vol. 117, No 11, (Mar 2011), pp. 3045-3052 ISSN 1528-0020

Zuhrie, S.R., Pearson, J.D., & Wickramasinghe, S.N. (1988). Haemoglobin synthesis in K562 erythroleukaemia cells is affected by intimate contact with monolayers of various human cell types. *Leukemia research*, Vol. 12, No. 7, (Nov 1988), pp.567-574, ISSN 0145-2126

5

Asymmetric Division in the Immuno-Hematopoietic System

Daniel Jimenez-Teja, Nadia Martin-Blanco and Matilde Canelles
Instituto de Parasitología y Biomedicina, CSIC, P. T. Ciencias de la Salud, Granada
Spain

1. Introduction

Asymmetric division is a process by which stem cells asymmetrically segregate certain proteins, called "cell fate determinants", in order to generate two functionally different cells. Normally, one of the daughter cells terminally differentiates while the other retains stem cell properties and continues proliferating. Asymmetric division has been found in virtually all developing systems where stem cells need to simultaneously proliferate and generate differentiated cells: brain, skin, gut, mammary gland, hematopoiesis, also in plants and algae. As a consequence of these studies, it has been established that, by virtue of asymmetric division, both developing and adult organs maintain the delicate equilibrium between proliferation and differentiation. The recent discovery of links to cancer has added momentum to an already very dynamic research area. This review article will discuss the latest developments in the asymmetric division field, with a focus on the immuno-hematopoietic system.

2. Historical perspective

The hypothesis about the existence of asymmetric division was postulated in 1878 based on studies of leech development, where certain cytoplasmic domains of the egg are differentially segregated to the descendants (Whitman, 1878). In the 1980s asymmetric division was described and analyzed in many other organisms, like yeasts, nematode, algae and *Drosophila* (see Horvitz and Herskowitz 1992 for a comprehensive review). At this stage, it was thought that each organism had a different means to undergo asymmetric division. Daughter cells acquired the differences that made them differentiate into various lineages either intrinsically (by differential inheritance of cytoplasmic or chromosomal factors) or extrinsically, by differential segregation of soluble factors. Intrinsic differences were described in expression of transcription factors, chromatin components, nucleases, receptors, cytoskeletal proteins and others; however, at this point it was not clear which of them were involved in generating asymmetry or were subject to asymmetric segregation themselves to influence differentiation. Extrinsic asymmetric cell division seemed to be the result of either direct cell-cell contact, or secretion of soluble factors. We will focus on intrinsic asymmetric division, which has been most widely studied.

In the 1990s, *Drosophila* asymmetric division was analyzed in detail and visualized by confocal microscopy (Rhyu, Jan, and Jan 1994). Two proteins with antagonistic function,

Numb and Notch, were pointed out as the main characters in this complicated process. This was followed by the description of asymmetric division in mammalian brain, with a similar mechanism and also involving asymmetric segregation of Numb (Zhong et al. 1996). At this point, Numb function was unknown, however it was discovered that it could bind (and antagonize) the transmembrane receptor Notch. During the following years, efforts in the two main invertebrate model systems, C. elegans and Drosophila, were focused on the mechanisms to set up cell polarity previous to division, spindle positioning and asymmetric localization of cell fate determinants (Betschinger and Knoblich 2004). Studies on vertebrates showed that many of the proteins involved were conserved, and that there may be a general mechanism for asymmetric division, conserved from the most ancient organisms up to our own brain and muscles. These discoveries resulted on a shift of research in the direction of vertebrates and, concretely, mammalians, and soon asymmetric division was first described in the hematopoietic system (Wu et al. 2007; Schroeder 2007). Studies in Drosophila were still ahead, thus the first link between cancer and asymmetric division was discovered in Drosophila earlier than in mammalians (Caussinus and Gonzalez 2005). In the following years, an important role for phosphorylation of cell fate determinants during mitosis was described (Wirtz-Peitz, Nishimura, and Knoblich 2008). Additionally, the mechanisms for asymmetric inheritance of centrioles (mediated by microtubules), DNA and vesicles were discovered [reviewed in (Neumuller and Knoblich 2009)]. It was realized that, although the proteins involved in asymmetric division are conserved, their roles are different in vertebrates. However, Drosophila studies were vey helpful in the case of the link to cancer, and a molecular mechanism involving Numb and p53 was discovered (Colaluca et al. 2008). The challenge for the next decade will be to integrate all this knowledge at the systems level to understand how asymmetric division works in health and disease, with enormous implications for stem cell research.

3. Molecular mechanisms of asymmetric division

Although the mechanism of asymmetric cell division has been intensively studied, there is no general model of how it occurs, because the data have been obtained studying different organisms that normally have their own specificity. Besides, different techniques, depending on the field, have been used to obtain the data, making it difficult to discern real differences from those arising as a result of using different techniques. Another problem, even when dealing with a single model system, is that there are data on asymmetric segregation of different proteins and organelles of the cell, but these data are not connected either temporally or mechanistically. A considerable effort to unify this knowledge into a common model has been made by J. Knoblich, who has continually summarized the data from diverse model systems in a series of excellent reviews [specifically (Knoblich 2010) (Neumuller and Knoblich 2009) are of great help in understanding the underlying mechanisms of asymmetric division]. We will first summarize the current knowledge on how different components of the cell are asymmetrically segregated.

Membrane adaptors- The first stage of asymmetric division in Drosophila neuroblasts is polarization of the cell fate determinants Numb (an endocytic adaptor) and Miranda (an adaptor that recruits other proteins to the membrane), as a result of asymmetric phosphorylation by aPKC (Wirtz-Peitz, Nishimura, and Knoblich 2008). If Numb and Miranda are phosphorylated by aPKC, they cannot localize to the membrane and exert their function (Wirtz-Peitz, Nishimura, and Knoblich 2008). During interphase, aPKC is bound to

PAR6 and Numb to L(2)GL, which allows Numb to be at the membrane. When the cell enters mitosis, Aurora A phosphorylates PAR6, resulting in L(2)GL phosphorylation and decoupling from Numb, allowing the adaptor PAR3 to bind simultaneously to both Numb and aPKC. Numb is then phosphorylated by aPKC and excluded from the membrane as a consequence (Smith et al. 2007; Wirtz-Peitz, Nishimura, and Knoblich 2008). Since aPKC is asymmetrically positioned in a constitutive fashion, this automatically results in asymmetric membrane distribution of Numb. This mechanism seems to be conserved in mammalians.

Vesicular compartments- Both endocytic adaptors (like Numb) and vesicles have been described to segregate asymmetrically both in *Drosophila* and mammalians (Zhong et al. 1996; Le Borgne and Schweisguth 2003). Most transmembrane receptors are subject to constant internalization, degradation and recycling, and the balance between these defines signaling levels at each moment. It is also known that receptors inside the endosomes do not only undergo degradation, but are also able to signal, sometimes even at a stronger level than on the membrane (Miaczynska and Bar-Sagi, 2010). This indicates that asymmetric segregation of vesicular compartments is a means to enhance signaling by certain receptors in one of the daughter cells at the expense of the other. Interestingly, such asymmetric segregation of vesicles or proteins involved in endocytosis has been shown to exist in the hematopoietic system (Aguado et al. 2010; Giebel and Beckmann 2007).

Microtubules- During telophase, microtubules play a role in spindle orientation and maintenance of Numb and Miranda asymmetric segregation, although the mechanism is not completely understood (Knoblich 2010).

Centrioles- It has been shown that centrioles are asymmetrically segregated in neuroblasts (the old centriole normally remains with the cell retaining progenitor potential) and this may play a role in cell fate determination (Yamashita et al. 2007).

DNA- There is evidence in some model systems of asymmetric DNA segregation, where the "template" DNA strand is retained by the less differentiated cell. This seems to be true for intestinal epithelium (Potten et al. 1978), muscle (Shinin et al. 2006), and neural stem cells (Karpowicz et al. 2005) but not for hair follicle (Sotiropoulou, Candi, and Blanpain 2008) or hematopoietic (Kiel et al. 2007) stem cells. However, it is not clear whether these disparities arise from looking at cells with different specifics in terms of lag between divisions.

Ribosomal components- In *Drosophila*, the cell that retains stem cell properties has been shown to present both increased size and enhanced protein synthesis. This seems to be related to asymmetric segregation of ribosomes (Neumuller et al. 2008) and other factors involved in protein synthesis (Fichelson et al. 2009). This has not yet been demonstrated in mammalians, but nevertheless is very intriguing and may be the mechanism by which the capacity to keep proliferating is asymmetrically inherited by just one of the precursors during development.

At this point, the data indicate that the main mechanism of asymmetric division consists on asymmetric inheritance of diverse proteins and subcellular structures, which in its turn helps to enhance the difference between the two daughter cells, so that one can retain stem cell capabilities while the other terminally differentiates. In this way, asymmetric segregation of endocytic adaptors, vesicles and microtubules may contribute to differential signaling in the two daughter cells, while differential inheritance of centrioles, DNA and ribosomes may help preserve stem cell capabilities in just one of the cells.

Two other important aspects that influence asymmetric division are polarization and spindle orientation during cell division. Polarization has been most extensively studied in *C. elegans*, where a complex formed by the proteins Par-3, Par-6 and aPKC are already polarized during interphase (Suzuki and Ohno 2006). This mechanism is conserved in *Drosophila* and is involved in all processes that depend on cell polarity. The mentioned complex is located in the apical part of the cell and, in mammalian cells, is combined with Cadherin and mediates adhesion. Thus, when the spindle forms during cell division, its orientation is crucial to determine symmetry or asymmetry. If the spindle is positioned perpendicular to the Par complex, the cell divides asymmetrically, and the daughter cell that inherits the complex remains a stem cell (probably through adhesion to the stem cell niche), while the other daughter cell abandons the cell niche and differentiates. On the contrary, if the spindle axis parts the Par complex, both daughter cells inherit it and the division is symmetric (Knoblich 2010; Fig. 1).

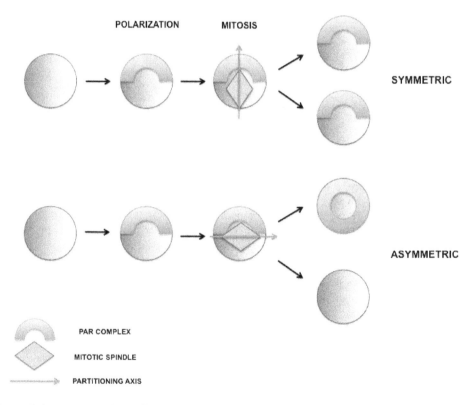

Fig. 1. Polarization and spindle orientation during symmetric or asymmetric division in *C. elelgans*.

Undoubtedly, in the future all these facts will be unified in a single model explaining how and when things happen during asymmetric division, independently of individual differences among the various model systems used to obtain the data.

4. Asymmetric division during normal hematopoiesis

Hematopoiesis is the process by which about $7x10^9$ blood cells are replaced everyday and per kg to maintain the Hematopoietic Stem Cell (HSC) pool in an organism. On the other hand, a HSC can be defined as a clonogenic cell that has the capacity to self-renew and differentiate into the progenitors of mature blood cells through a symmetric or an asymmetric division, respectively.

The hematopoietic system in mammalians shows a hierarchical structure. There is a wide range of distinct mature cells, such as erythrocytes, megacaryocytes, myeloid cells, mast cells, NK cells, monocytes, B and T cells, and others (Figure 2). All these different cells share a common progenitor cell, the Hematopoietic Stem Cell (HSC). HSCs can divide trough a symmetric process to self-renew or through an asymmetric division process to generate daughter cells with different fates: one daughter cell with the same fate as the progenitor cell, and the second one with Multipotent Progenitor cell fate (MPP). Later, MPPs go downstream through the hierarchy and can divide into three different Oligopotent Progeitors (OPPs). These three different OPPs are Common Lymphoid Progenitors (CLPs), megakaryocyte/erythrocyte progenitors (MEPs) and Common Myeloid Progenitors (CMPs). The last type of OPPs can generate other OPPs such as granulocyte/macrophage progenitors (GMPs) or MEPs. Then, these OPPs derive in a wide range of Lineage Restricted Progenitors, such as pro-B lymphoid cells, pro-T lymphoid cells, pro-NK cells, etc., to finally generate Mature Effector Cells (platelets, dendritic cells, macrophages, erytorocytes, NK, B & T cells, etc). It must be emphasized that multipotency is lost during this process, therefore, the potency to generate two daughter cells with different fates is reduced from HSCs to mature effector cells (Seita and Weissman 2010).

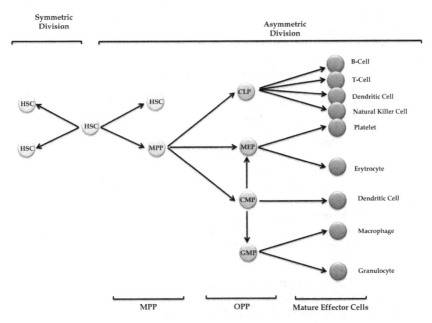

Fig. 2. Schematic representation of precursor decisions during hematopoiesis.

In symmetric divisions, identical copies of the progenitor cell are generated, maintaining the pool of HSCs. On the other hand, asymmetric divisions contribute to generate diversity. Although it is accepted that the capacity to generate cells with different fates is an intrinsic property of HSCs, and studies with fluorescent proteins have shown that several determinant factors can be asymmetrically distributed during mitosis (Congdon and Reya 2008), the environment has an important role in asymmetric division, as well. Thus, several studies have indicated that the stroma plays an important role in differentiation of HSCs into all blood cell types (Purton and Scadden 2008). In this study, different cell lineages with various fates were obtained culturing the HSCs in the presence of different stromas. Other studies indicate that osteoblasts and endothelial cells act as stem cell niches and may play an important role in progenitor diversity generation. Some experiments show that when HSCs are cultured in the presence of osteoblasts asymmetric division is induced, and symmetric division is more frequent when HSCs are cultured on stromal cells. In addition, experiments where HSCs were cultured in presence or not of Lnk, trombopoeitin (TPO) and several interleukins such as IL-3, IL-6 and IL-11 showed effects in self-renewal and differentiation processes. For instance, Lnk is considered a negative regulator of self-renewal while TPO is a negative regulator of differentiation. In addition, there are other cell types with a potential role as regulators of the HSC niche. One of them is the sympathetic nervous system (Katayama et al. 2006). Therefore, it seems that asymmetric division is an important process for hematopoiesis, although the molecular details remain to be elucidated.

5. Role of cell fate determinants in hematopoietic malignant proliferation

The plasma membrane receptor Notch in directly implicated in the proliferative/ differentiative balance of stem cells. Thus, deregulation in Notch signaling is related with several diseases, such as cancer. An increase in Notch signaling results in the development of adenocarcinomas in lung and mammary gland (Allen et al. 2010; Farnie and Clarke 2007). Notch1 can be found in many hematopoietic tissues, such as peripheral T and B cells, neutrophils and bone marrow precursors (Stier et al. 2002), and activation of Notch1 increases self-renewal of HSCs while inhibiting the generation of mature cells. This supports previous *in vitro* studies where Notch activation produced immortalized clones of multipotent cells (Stier et al. 2002; Varnum-Finney et al. 2000), however Notch1 did not completely block the generation of mature cells.

The first proof of the relationship between Notch signaling and cancer was found in acute T lymphoblastic leukemia (T-ALL), and afterwards Notch signaling was shown to be involved in generation of solid tumors, including melanoma, colorectal cancer, breast cancer, non-small cell lung carcinoma and others (Ranganathan, P., et al. 2011). Currently, Notch signaling is receiving increased attention in the development of new therapies against cancer. Some studies have shown that its ligands (specifically Dll4, involved in angiogenesis and T cell fate specification) are overexpressed in different kinds of cancer (Stylianou S, et al. 2006). As a result, several ways of inhibiting Notch signaling are being tested at different levels:

Synthetic inhibitors. The Notch pathway is inhibited by small compounds, which arrest the proteolysis of Notch receptors by the γ-secretases-presenilin complex or interfere with the activity of the Notch intracellular domain. The most common γ-secretases (GSIs) are DAPT and DBZ (dibenzazepine). In addition, specific inhibitors for Dll4-Notch signaling have been developed as well. Although different versions of these inhibitors can be found, all of them present the same disadvantage. Initially, these drugs were developed to arrest proteolysis of the amyloid precursor protein (APP) in Alzheimer's disease and therefore, they are not specific and normally interfere with a wide range of different pathways. On the other hand, dnMAML1, a dominant negative of Mastermind-like 1 (MAML1) represents a more selective option. dnMAML1 blocks the transduction of the four known Notch receptors (Notch 1-4). Although dnMAML1 is a potent inhibitor, it shows low levels of cell permeability; for this reason, similar compounds with a better cell permeability have been developed. All these inhibitors down-regulate Notch signaling and have shown good results in treating T-ALL.

Endogenous inhibitors. Endogenous inhibitors, such as Fwb (an E3 ligase), Cbl, Numb and Numblike can be used to regulate Notch signaling by targeting Notch receptors, however, an important disadvantage is their poor specifity. On the other hand, soluble inhibitors such as the extracellular domains of Jagged1, DLk1 and EGFL7 can offer a more specific alternative. However, it must be considered that the mechanism of these inhibitors is not well known and their role in Notch signaling must be studied in detail.

Antibodies. Antibodies against Notch receptors can be used to regulate Notch signaling. Some antibodies have been already developed against Notch1 and Notch3 receptors (Asano N., et al. 2008, Elyaman W., et al 2007, Jurynczyk M., et al 2008, Maekawa Y., et al 2003, Schaller MA., et al. 2007 and Li K., et al. 2008). Antibodies can block specific Notch receptors with a high selectivity, leaving other Notch receptors activated. For example, an anti-Dll4 antibody has been developed against Dll4-Notch signaling and it is showing promising perspectives in anti-angiogenic cancer therapy because of its low toxicity (Ridgway J, et al. 2006). A similar strategy uses molecules called decoys. Decoys are soluble extracellular domains of Notch receptors or ligands. They compete with Notch receptors, inhibiting Notch signaling by binding to endogenous molecules. These associations do not trigger Notch signaling because of lacking the transmembrane region. Notch signaling in endothelial cells has been inhibited using a decoy of Notch1, successfully reducing tumor growth. Other decoys of Dll1, Dll4 and Jagged1 have been successfully developed (Funahashi Y., et al. 2008, Varnum-Finney B., et al. 2000 and Small D., et al. 2001). However, decoys show an important disadvantage. It has been observed that they can be switched from inhibitors into activators easily. The association of decoys with extracellular matrix can produce an activator and trigger Notch proteolysis and activation. The process by which a decoy can be transformed into an activator is not yet fully understood, and this feature makes decoys unpredictable and not valid as therapeutics (Hicks C., et al. 2002).

Notch is regulated by Numb, and loss of this regulation has been described in more than 50% of human mammary carcinomas. When Numb is lost, Notch signaling is increased, and the balance between self-renewal and differentiation is affected, which results in uncontrolled proliferation. Loss of Numb may be due to ubiquitylation and subsequent proteosomal degradation.

Recent studies carried out by Colaluca et al. (Colaluca et al. 2008) showed that Numb plays an important role in the regulation of the protein p53, also called TP53, an important tumor suppressor involved in 50% of breast cancers and in 70% of colon cancers. Numb binds to p53 and the E3 ubiquitin ligase HDM2 (or MDMD2 ligase) to form a triple complex, inhibiting p53 ubiquitylation and, therefore, its degradation. As a consequence, p53 levels are higher and the apparition of breast cancer is diminished. When there is loss of Numb, p53 degradation is higher, allowing higher expression of Notch, which results in chemoresistance to the drugs used to combat the disease and in uncontrolled cellular proliferation. Besides, p53 regulates the expression of genes implicated in cell-cycle arrest and apoptosis upon cellular stress. Additionally, it acts as transcriptional factor. Therefore, it seems clear that there is a relationship between Numb deregulation and uncontrolled cellular proliferation via the tumor suppressor p53. However, the mechanism by which Numb regulates p53 remains still unclear (Carter and Vousden 2008).

In some cases, such as in breast cancers, deficiency in Numb expression is due to an increase in ubiquitylation resulting in higher proteasomal degradation. This may be related to increased levels or activity of E3-ligases such as LNK, Siah-1 and MDM2. Another explanation for Numb loss may be ubiquitylation after over-phosphorylation. Restoration of Numb normal levels could be achieved pharmacologically using substances with antiproteasomal activity such as PS-341 or enzymatic inhibitors of Numb degradation (Pece et al. 2004). These investigations have a clear practical application: hopefully, in the future some of the resulting knowledge will be applied to the clinic.

6. Asymmetric division in the immune system

During immune system development and function, progenitor cells undergo a series of proliferation and differentiation processes in order to generate the different mature cell populations that protect the body from foreign pathogens. T cells develop in the thymus from bone marrow precursors through a series of intermediate stages. Double negative cells (DN) undergo some division rounds before differentiating into double positive cells (DP), afterwards T cell progenitors do not divide again in the thymus: only after exiting the thymus and populating the periphery will mature T cells be able to proliferate again. During the immune response, naive T lymphocytes (T lymphocytes recently created that have not encountered antigen) are activated by antigen-presenting cells. Naive T cell activation, through the T cell receptor (TCR), leads to proliferation and differentiation, triggering a massive expansion of differentiated effector cells, as well as a small number of memory cells (these will remain undifferentiated until subsequent antigen encounters). Thus, after T cell activation, a single naïve T cell is able to generate many different T cell types in order to orchestrate an effective immune response (Stemberger et al. 2007). How can a single cell generate all the T lymphocyte types that are required for immunity? This question has fascinated immunologists over the past years. Several models have been suggested to explain the generation of subset diversity during the immune response. Some studies suggest a progressive differentiation model (Sallusto, Geginat, and Lanzavecchia 2004), while others suggest an early bifurcation between effector and memory phenotypes, more consistent with asymmetric division, but the question remains controversial. Despite asymmetric division being the most widespread process that regulates the generation of a variety of cell types, this process has only started to be studied in the immune system in the last few years, and it still remains controversial.

Nothing suggests, *a priori*, that the widespread principle of asymmetric division should not be applied to the thymus, where DN cell proliferation does regulate the total number of cells in the whole organ, and during this process, precursor cells resulting from such divisions must decide between differentiation and proliferation. In this respect, three different aspects should have been studied before making statements about the role of asymmetrically segregated cell fate determinants in thymocytes. First, demonstration of the existence of asymmetric division itself (including an assessment of the effect of manipulating asymmetric division); second, identification of cell fate determinants that are asymmetrically segregated and their signaling pathways; finally, elucidation of the mechanisms that lead to asymmetric localization of these determinants, including external cues that regulate cell polarization, as well as intracellular processes that mediate asymmetric segregation of proteins and organelles (as has been described before for studies of both *Drosophila* and mammalian neural system).

However, the first studies related to asymmetric division in the thymus used either transgenic or knockout mice to over-express or delete Numb (French et al. 2002; Anderson et al. 2005; Wilson et al. 2007). In these studies, investigators used classical assessments of thymocyte differentiation in order to determine whether or not Numb played a role in thymocyte differentiation (they never examined asymmetric division). The conclusion drawn by the three studies was that Numb plays no role in thymus differentiation. However, there are three important considerations that were not taken into account. First, both Numb and its homologue Numblike are expressed in mammalians (the thymus included), and if their levels are reduced so that just 1% of endogenous levels of either Numb or Numblike remain in the cells, this is still enough to maintain normal asymmetric division (Petersen et al. 2002; Petersen et al. 2006). Second, four different isoforms of Numb are expressed in mammalians (Dho et al. 1999). Third, knockout studies in the immune system must be taken with caution, since there is accumulating evidence that the absence of phenotype does not necessarily mean that the protein does not have a function (Saveliev and Tybulewicz 2009). If Numb acts as a cell fate determinant during asymmetric division in the thymus, one would expect an effect in precursor proliferation rate and the total number of thymocytes, however none of these were examined in these first studies. Nevertheless, the existence of three studies claiming no role for Numb in the thymus predisposed the whole field against the notion of asymmetric division.

Fortunately, over the past few years, the first studies on asymmetric division in the thymus and peripheral T lymphocytes performed following a more logical order (i.e., examining in the first place asymmetric segregation of determinants) have provided exciting data about asymmetric division in the immune system (Aguado et al. 2010; Chang et al. 2007). In the first study, our group showed by confocal microscopy that Numb is segregated asymmetrically during thymocyte division. By inhibiting Numb (using a dominant negative), or overexpressing it, we showed that functional Numb levels determine DN thymocyte proliferation rate and, ultimately, thymus size. Furthermore, we showed that Numb can regulate pre-TCR localization and signaling, acting as an endocytic protein. As a result, a model was proposed where thymocytes divide by asymmetric division to generate one daughter cell that inherits Numb and keeps precursor properties and a second that does not inherit Numb and receives pre-TCR signaling as a consequence, which results in differentiation (Fig. 3). The second study showed that peripheral CD8+ T cells do indeed undergo asymmetric division, and this process regulates the choice between effector and memory differentiation (Chang et al. 2007). The authors showed that after the first naïve CD8+ T cell division, the proximal and distal daughter cells have different phenotypes. Thus, proximal daughter cells expressed low CD62L levels and higher CD69, CD43 and CD25 levels. Furthermore, when these cells were transferred into naïve secondary recipients, they provided protection against acute infection, but poor long-term protection, a profile consistent with the effector lineage. However, distal daughters expressed high levels of CD62L and lower levels of CD69, CD43, CD25 and CD44 and these cells provided a good long-term protection *in vivo*, a profile more consistent with the central memory cells. This is clear evidence that asymmetric division occurs, at least during the first division.

As we have explained before, for asymmetric division to occur, the progenitor cell needs to receive an external cue to dictate the axis of polarity, recruit cell fate determinants and align the mitotic spindle with a correct position that ensures asymmetric segregation of the determinants. During mature T cell division, the axis of polarity and mitotic spindle alignment are established by the formation of the immunological synapse. The immunological synapse has been extensively studied as a site of clustered signaling molecules, and can be considered as a marker of the polarized T cell and a mechanism for asymmetric division regulation. Recent studies showed that asymmetric cell division is not observed either during non antigen–dependent activation or the second and subsequent cell divisions following antigen stimulation, and that the polarity cue for asymmetric cell division requires the contact with antigen-presenting cells (Chang et al. 2007; Oliaro et al. 2010; Fig. 3). One problem with this model is that if it is just the first division that is

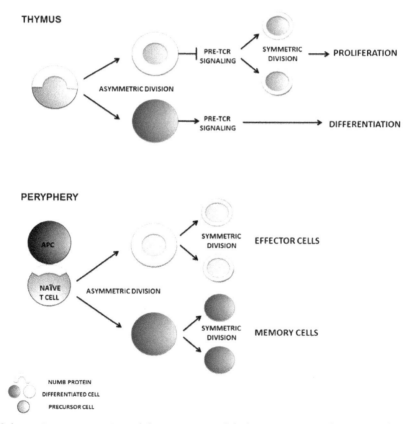

Fig. 3. Schematic representation of the current models for asymmetric division in thymus and periphery.

asymmetric during the immune response, and all the subsequent divisions are symmetric, it is not clear how the final numbers of memory and effector cells are achieved. In any case, these data on thymus and peripheral T cells demonstrate that the immunological system is not a remarkable exception to the principle of asymmetric division as the universal mechanism to ensure a correct balance between expansion and differentiation during development. The mechanistic details on how asymmetric division is orchestrated in the immune system in order to achieve correct numbers of mature cells will surely be elucidated soon.

7. Future directions of the field

Asymmetric division has transitioned from being an intriguing but unexplained anomaly of neural development into a fertile field where scientists working on different developmental biology areas converge to exchange methods and ideas. The recently discovered link to cancer stresses out the importance of these studies in the immuno-hematopoietic system.

An important current challenge for the field of asymmetric division is unification of knowledge. A general model for the functioning of asymmetric division that applies to all organisms and tissues needs to be postulated, even if it is very schematic at the beginning. Next, unification of methods should be achieved: the same phenomenon in different organisms should not be studied using different techniques simply because researchers of different areas feel more comfortable with a certain approach. To avoid this, more joint scientific meetings on asymmetric division must be organized, so that researchers can exchange views and knowledge, besides funding should be available for those willing to assume the risk of applying new techniques to old model systems. If the field does not evolve in this way, it risks loosing its current novelty and drive. Hopefully, new exciting discoveries will keep the area alive, and the many open questions about how organisms and tissues orchestrate growth and differentiation will be answered soon.

8. References

Aguado, R., N. Martin-Blanco, M. Caraballo, and M. Canelles. 2010. The endocytic adaptor Numb regulates thymus size by modulating pre-TCR signaling during asymmetric division. *Blood* 116 (10):1705-14.

Allen, T. D., E. M. Rodriguez, K. D. Jones, and J. M. Bishop. 2010. Activated notch1 induces lung adenomas in mice and cooperates with myc in the generation of lung adenocarcinoma. *Cancer Res* 71 (18):6010-8.

Anderson, A. C., E. A. Kitchens, S. W. Chan, C. St Hill, Y. N. Jan, W. Zhong, and E. A. Robey. 2005. The Notch regulator Numb links the Notch and TCR signaling pathways. *J Immunol* 174 (2):890-7.

Asano N., Watanabe T., Kitani A., et al. 2008. Notch1 signaling and regulatory T cell function. J Immunol 180: 2796–804.

Betschinger, J., and J. A. Knoblich. 2004. Dare to be different: asymmetric cell division in *Drosophila, C. elegans* and vertebrates. *Curr Biol* 14 (16):R674-85.

Carter, S., and K. H. Vousden. 2008. A role for Numb in p53 stabilization. *Genome Biol* 9 (5):221.

Caussinus, E., and C. Gonzalez. 2005. Induction of tumor growth by altered stem-cell asymmetric division in *Drosophila melanogaster*. *Nat Genet* 37 (10):1125-9.

Chang, J. T., V. R. Palanivel, I. Kinjyo, F. Schambach, A. M. Intlekofer, A. Banerjee, S. A. Longworth, K. E. Vinup, P. Mrass, J. Oliaro, N. Killeen, J. S. Orange, S. M. Russell, W. Weninger, and S. L. Reiner. 2007. Asymmetric T lymphocyte division in the initiation of adaptive immune responses. *Science* 315 (5819):1687-91.

Colaluca, I. N., D. Tosoni, P. Nuciforo, F. Senic-Matuglia, V. Galimberti, G. Viale, S. Pece, and P. P. Di Fiore. 2008. NUMB controls p53 tumour suppressor activity. *Nature* 451 (7174):76-80.

Congdon, K. L., and T. Reya. 2008. Divide and conquer: how asymmetric division shapes cell fate in the hematopoietic system. *Curr Opin Immunol* 20 (3):302-7.

Dho, S. E., M. B. French, S. A. Woods, and C. J. McGlade. 1999. Characterization of four mammalian numb protein isoforms. Identification of cytoplasmic and membrane-associated variants of the phosphotyrosine binding domain. *J Biol Chem* 274 (46):33097-104.

Elyaman W., Bradshaw E. M., Wang Y., et al. 2007. JAGGED1 and delta1 differentially regulate the outcome of experimental autoimmune encephalomyelitis. J Immunol 179: 5990–98.

Farnie, G., and R. B. Clarke. 2007. Mammary stem cells and breast cancer--role of Notch signalling. *Stem Cell Rev* 3 (2):169-75.

Fichelson, P., C. Moch, K. Ivanovitch, C. Martin, C. M. Sidor, J. A. Lepesant, Y. Bellaiche, and J. R. Huynh. 2009. Live-imaging of single stem cells within their niche reveals that a U3snoRNP component segregates asymmetrically and is required for self-renewal in *Drosophila*. *Nat Cell Biol* 11 (6):685-93.

French, M. B., U. Koch, R. E. Shaye, M. A. McGill, S. E. Dho, C. J. Guidos, and C. J. McGlade. 2002. Transgenic expression of numb inhibits notch signaling in immature thymocytes but does not alter T cell fate specification. *J Immunol* 168 (7):3173-80.

Funahashi Y., Hernandez S. L., Das I., et al. 2008. A notch1 ectodomain construct inhibits endothelial notch signaling, tumor growth, and angiogenesis. Cancer Res 68: 4727–35.

Giebel, B., and J. Beckmann. 2007. Asymmetric cell divisions of human hematopoietic stem and progenitor cells meet endosomes. *Cell Cycle* 6 (18):2201-4.

Hicks C., Ladi E., Lindsell C., et al. 2002. A secreted Delta1-Fc fusion protein functions both as an activator and inhibitor of Notch1 signaling. J Neurosci Res 68: 655–67.

Horvitz, H. R., and I. Herskowitz. 1992. Mechanisms of asymmetric cell division: two Bs or not two Bs, that is the question. *Cell* 68 (2):237-55.

Jurynczyk M., Jurewicz A., Raine C. S., et al. 2008. Notch3 inhibition in myelin-reactive T cells down-regulates protein kinase C theta and attenuates experimental autoimmune encephalomyelitis. J Immunol 180: 2634– 40.

Karpowicz, P., C. Morshead, A. Kam, E. Jervis, J. Ramunas, V. Cheng, and D. van der Kooy. 2005. Support for the immortal strand hypothesis: neural stem cells partition DNA asymmetrically in vitro. *J Cell Biol* 170 (5):721-32.

Katayama, Y., M. Battista, W. M. Kao, A. Hidalgo, A. J. Peired, S. A. Thomas, and P. S. Frenette. 2006. Signals from the sympathetic nervous system regulate hematopoietic stem cell egress from bone marrow. *Cell* 124 (2):407-21.

Kiel, M. J., S. He, R. Ashkenazi, S. N. Gentry, M. Teta, J. A. Kushner, T. L. Jackson, and S. J. Morrison. 2007. Haematopoietic stem cells do not asymmetrically segregate chromosomes or retain BrdU. *Nature* 449 (7159):238-42.

Knoblich, J. A. 2010. Asymmetric cell division: recent developments and their implications for tumour biology. *Nat Rev Mol Cell Biol* 11 (12):849-60.

Le Borgne, R., and F. Schweisguth. 2003. Unequal segregation of Neuralized biases Notch activation during asymmetric cell division. *Dev Cell* 5 (1):139-48.

Li K., Li Y., Wu W., et al. 2008. Modulation of Notch signaling by antibodies specific for the extracellular negative regulatory region of NOTCH3. J Biol Chem 283: 8046–54.

Maekawa Y., Tsukumo S., Chiba S., et al. 2003. Delta1-Notch3 inter- actions bias the functional differentiation of activated CD4þ T cells. Immunity 19: 549–59.

Miaczynska, M., and D. Bar-Sagi. 2010. Signaling endosomes: seeing is believing. *Curr Opin Cell Biol* 22 (4):535-40.

Neumuller, R. A., and J. A. Knoblich. 2009. Dividing cellular asymmetry: asymmetric cell division and its implications for stem cells and cancer. *Genes Dev* 23 (23):2675-99.

Neumuller, R. A., J. Betschinger, A. Fischer, N. Bushati, I. Poernbacher, K. Mechtler, S. M. Cohen, and J. A. Knoblich. 2008. Mei-P26 regulates microRNAs and cell growth in the *Drosophila* ovarian stem cell lineage. *Nature* 454 (7201):241-5.

Oliaro, J., V. Van Ham, F. Sacirbegovic, A. Pasam, Z. Bomzon, K. Pham, M. J. Ludford-Menting, N. J. Waterhouse, M. Bots, E. D. Hawkins, S. V. Watt, L. A. Cluse, C. J. Clarke, D. J. Izon, J. T. Chang, N. Thompson, M. Gu, R. W. Johnstone, M. J. Smyth, P. O. Humbert, S. L. Reiner, and S. M. Russell. 2010. Asymmetric cell division of T cells upon antigen presentation uses multiple conserved mechanisms. *J Immunol* 185 (1):367-75.

Pece, S., M. Serresi, E. Santolini, M. Capra, E. Hulleman, V. Galimberti, S. Zurrida, P. Maisonneuve, G. Viale, and P. P. Di Fiore. 2004. Loss of negative regulation by Numb over Notch is relevant to human breast carcinogenesis. *J Cell Biol* 167 (2):215-21.

Petersen, P. H., H. Tang, K. Zou, and W. Zhong. 2006. The enigma of the numb-Notch relationship during mammalian embryogenesis. *Dev Neurosci* 28 (1-2):156-68.

Petersen, P. H., K. Zou, J. K. Hwang, Y. N. Jan, and W. Zhong. 2002. Progenitor cell maintenance requires numb and numblike during mouse neurogenesis. *Nature* 419 (6910):929-34.

Potten, C. S., W. J. Hume, P. Reid, and J. Cairns. 1978. The segregation of DNA in epithelial stem cells. *Cell* 15 (3):899-906.

Purton, L. E., and D. T. Scadden. 2008. The hematopoietic stem cell niche.

Rhyu, M. S., L. Y. Jan, and Y. N. Jan. 1994. Asymmetric distribution of numb protein during division of the sensory organ precursor cell confers distinct fates to daughter cells. *Cell* 76 (3):477-91.

Sallusto, F., J. Geginat, and A. Lanzavecchia. 2004. Central memory and effector memory T cell subsets: function, generation, and maintenance. *Annu Rev Immunol* 22:745-63.

Saveliev, A., and V. L. Tybulewicz. 2009. Lymphocyte signaling: beyond knockouts. *Nat Immunol* 10 (4):361-4.

Schaller M. A., Neupane R., Rudd B. D., et al. 2007. Notch ligand Delta-like 4 regulates disease pathogenesis during respiratory viral infections by modulating Th2 cytokines. J Exp Med 204: 2925–34.

Schroeder, T. 2007. Asymmetric Cell Division in Normal and Malignant Hematopoietic Precursor Cells. *Cell Stem Cell* 1 (5):479-481.

Seita, J., and I. L. Weissman. 2010. Hematopoietic stem cell: self-renewal versus differentiation. *Wiley Interdiscip Rev Syst Biol Med* 2 (6):640-53.

Shinin, V., B. Gayraud-Morel, D. Gomes, and S. Tajbakhsh. 2006. Asymmetric division and cosegregation of template DNA strands in adult muscle satellite cells. *Nat Cell Biol* 8 (7):677-87.

Small D., Kovalenko D., Kacer D., et al. 2001. Soluble Jagged 1 represses the function of its transmembrane form to induce the formation of the Src- dependent chord-like phenotype. J Biol Chem 276: 32022–30.

Smith, C. A., K. M. Lau, Z. Rahmani, S. E. Dho, G. Brothers, Y. M. She, D. M. Berry, E. Bonneil, P. Thibault, F. Schweisguth, R. Le Borgne, and C. J. McGlade. 2007. aPKC-mediated phosphorylation regulates asymmetric membrane localization of the cell fate determinant Numb. *EMBO J* 26 (2):468-80.

Sotiropoulou, P. A., A. Candi, and C. Blanpain. 2008. The majority of multipotent epidermal stem cells do not protect their genome by asymmetrical chromosome segregation. *Stem Cells* 26 (11):2964-73.

Stemberger, C., K. M. Huster, M. Koffler, F. Anderl, M. Schiemann, H. Wagner, and D. H. Busch. 2007. A single naive CD8+ T cell precursor can develop into diverse effector and memory subsets. *Immunity* 27 (6):985-97.

Stier, S., T. Cheng, D. Dombkowski, N. Carlesso, and D. T. Scadden. 2002. Notch1 activation increases hematopoietic stem cell self-renewal in vivo and favors lymphoid over myeloid lineage outcome. *Blood* 99 (7):2369-78.

Suzuki A. and Ohno S. 2006. The PAR-aPKC systme: lessons in polarity. *J.Cell Sci.* 119: 979-987.

Varnum-Finney, B., L. Xu, C. Brashem-Stein, C. Nourigat, D. Flowers, S. Bakkour, W. S. Pear, and I. D. Bernstein. 2000. Pluripotent, cytokine-dependent, hematopoietic stem cells are immortalized by constitutive Notch1 signaling. *Nat Med* 6 (11):1278-81.

Whitman, C.. 1878. The embryology of *Clepsine*. *Q.J. Microsc. Sci.* 18: 215.

Wilson, A., D. L. Ardiet, C. Saner, N. Vilain, F. Beermann, M. Aguet, H. R. Macdonald, and O. Zilian. 2007. Normal hemopoiesis and lymphopoiesis in the combined absence of numb and numblike. *J Immunol* 178 (11):6746-51.

Wirtz-Peitz, F., T. Nishimura, and J. A. Knoblich. 2008. Linking cell cycle to asymmetric division: Aurora-A phosphorylates the Par complex to regulate Numb localization. *Cell* 135 (1):161-73.

Wu, M., H. Y. Kwon, F. Rattis, J. Blum, C. Zhao, R. Ashkenazi, T. L. Jackson, N. Gaiano, T. Oliver, and T. Reya. 2007. Imaging hematopoietic precursor division in real time. *Cell Stem Cell* 1 (5):541-54.

Yamashita, Y. M., A. P. Mahowald, J. R. Perlin, and M. T. Fuller. 2007. Asymmetric inheritance of mother versus daughter centrosome in stem cell division. *Science* 315 (5811):518-21.

Zhong, W., J. N. Feder, M. M. Jiang, L. Y. Jan, and Y. N. Jan. 1996. Asymmetric localization of a mammalian numb homolog during mouse cortical neurogenesis. *Neuron* 17 (1):43-53.

6

Mechanisms of αIIbβ3 Biogenesis in the Megakaryocyte: A Proteomics Approach

Amanda Chen[1], Haiqiang Yu[2], Haiteng Deng[2] and W. Beau Mitchell[1]
[1]Laboratory of Platelet Biology, New York Blood Center
[2]Proteomics Resources Center, The Rockefeller University
USA

1. Introduction

Platelets play a central role in hemostasis and thrombosis, initiating clot formation in response to vessel wall damage. Platelet aggregates are formed at sites of injury by the binding and crosslinking of the integrin αIIbβ3 to fibrinogen, von Willebrand factor and other soluble ligands. Platelets also form pathological thrombi, and the resulting arterial occlusion can lead to myocardial infarction or stroke. Inhibition of αIIbβ3 binding can decrease the formation of pathologic thrombi, and αIIbβ3 has become an important pharmacological target. Anti-αIIbβ3 therapies have been highly successful in preventing death following myocardial infarction and percutaneous arterial stent placement.(Topol, Lincoff et al. 2002; De Luca, Ucci et al. 2009) However, attempts to design novel, orally available anti-αIIbβ3 agents have been hampered by what appears to be paradoxical activation of αIIbβ3 by the drug, in some cases leading to an increased risk of mortality in patients who received the drug.(Quinn, Plow et al. 2002)

A novel approach to manipulating αIIbβ3 would be to perturb its post-translational processing and trafficking within the megakaryocyte, prior to platelet formation. Like most membrane proteins, αIIbβ3 is formed by concerted processes of protein sorting and trafficking. Some of the mechanisms underlying αIIbβ3 biogenesis and expression in megakaryocytes have been described, such as the calnexin cycle of protein quality control.(King and Reed 2002; Tiwari, Italiano et al. 2003; El.Golli, Issertial et al. 2005; Lo, Li et al. 2005) Clues to the stringent protein quality control of αIIbβ3 biogenesis come from the study of patients with defective or absent αIIbβ3, who manifest the mucocutaneous bleeding disorder Glanzmann thrombasthenia. A subset of patients with mutations in the αIIb gene produce full-length αIIb that retains the ability to form a complex with β3 but is retained within the cell and degraded, resulting in disease. These patients demonstrate the existence of stringent quality control mechanisms acting post-translationally to control αIIbβ3 biogenesis and expression. A clearer understanding of these mechanisms may lead to new possibilities of anti-integrin therapy.

Toward the goal of identifying proteins involved in αIIbβ3 biogenesis we performed a proteomic analysis of proteins interacting with αIIb in megakaryocytes cultured from human umbilical cord blood (UCB) and in HEK293 cells expressing αIIb and β3.

Megakaryocyte proteins were captured by poly-histidine tagged αIIb, or by photoreactive crosslinking followed by immunoprecipitation with anti-αIIb mAbs, and analyzed by mass spectrometry.

The αIIb and b3 subunits are synthesized as a single-chain precursors in the chaperone-rich folding environment of the endoplasmic reticulum (ER) (Fig 1). The precursor αIIb, pro-αIIb, is glycosylated under control of the calnexin cycle of protein folding. The β3 precursor is also glycosylated but does not appear to interact with the calnexin cycle. The two precursors heterodimerize to briefly form pro-αIIbβ3, and then pro-αIIb is cleaved by one or more members of the furin family of proteases in the Golgi. Cleavage of pro-αIIb to mature αIIb marks the exit of αIIb from the ER, and this cleavage occurs only when pro-αIIb is in complex with β3.(Bray, Rosa et al. 1986; Rosa and McEver 1989) Both αIIb and β3 are synthesized in excess of what will finally be processed to mature αIIbβ3. The calnexin cycle exerts stringent quality control over αIIb production and up to one half of all pro-αIIb is targeted to the proteasome for degradation in megakaryocytes. Excess β3 is degraded by a non-proteasomal mechanism. Inhibition of the proteasome in megakaryocytes resulted in a build-up of pro-αIIb that was not being degraded, but had no apparent effect on the level of mature αIIb in the αIIbβ3 complex. Thus, the expression level of mature αIIbβ3 is not simply a result of the stoichiometry of production vs. degradation. Rather there appears to be a concerted mechanism that controls how much pro-αIIbβ3 will be converted into mature αIIbβ3, and this mechanism is not grossly responsive to excessive levels of pro-αIIb or β3.

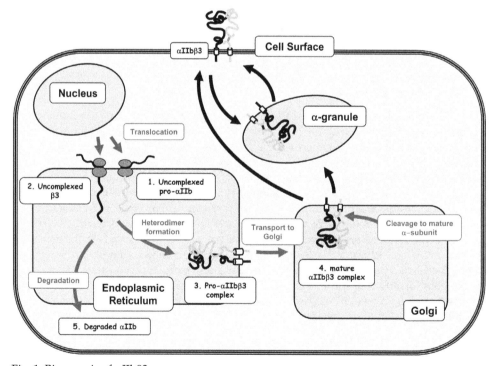

Fig. 1. Biogenesis of αIIbβ3

We hypothesized that whatever proteins underlie this mechanism must be interacting with pro-αIIb and/or pro-αIIbβ3 complex, but not with the mature αIIbβ3 complex. We chose a proteomics approach to identify these interacting proteins. In order to enrich our assay for proteins that preferentially bound pro-αIIb or pro-αIIbβ3, we used an αIIb subunit harboring R858G and R859G mutations that eliminates furin cleavage and traps αIIb in its pro-αIIb form.(Kolodziej, Vilaire et al. 1991) This αIIbR858G/R859G construct can form a complex with β3, but only in small amounts compared to normal αIIbβ3. In addition, while some of the mutant αIIbβ3 complexes reach the cell surface and can mediate adherence to immobilized fibrinogen, the proportion of αIIbR858G/R859G reaching the surface is very small compared to normal αIIb.(Kolodziej, Vilaire et al. 1991) Thus, αIIbR858G/R859G is a "nearly normal" mutant αIIb subunit that is primarily retained within the cell, making it a useful bait to capture the proteins involved in that process.

The hsp40 type chaperone protein, DNAJC10, was captured by both the normal αIIb and αIIbR858G/R859G subunits, and was evaluated as a putative αIIb interacting protein.. We report that DNAJC10 interacted with pro-αIIb and β3 in megakaryocytes, and appears to promote the degradation of pro-αIIb. Notably, while αIIbβ3-DNAJC10 interaction was evident in megakaryocytes, specific interaction was not detectable in HEK293 cells transfected with αIIb cDNA, suggesting megakaryocyte specificity. Knockdown of DNAJC10 by siRNA increased αIIbβ3 surface expression in UCB derived megakaryocytes, indicating that DNAJC10 negatively regulates αIIbβ3 surface expression. Thus, DNAJC10-αIIb interaction represents a novel post-translational mechanism regulating αIIbβ3 surface expression.

2. Materials and methods

2.1 Antibodies

The antibodies used in this study were: 10E5 (anti-αIIbβ3 complex); B1B5 (anti-αIIb);7H2 and B36 (anti-β3) (all 4 generous gifts from Dr Barry Coller); CA3 (anti-αIIb), anti-V5 epitope, and anti-Myc epitope (all three Millipore, Temecula,CA); anti-DNAJC10 (Genetex, Irvine, CA); M148 (anti-αIIb) (Santa Cruz Biotechnology, Santa Cruz, CA); mouse IgG, and rabbit IgG (both Jackson ImmunoResearch Inc, West Grove, PA).

2.2 Human Umbilical Cord Blood culture

This study used human UCB from the US National Cord Blood Bank that was deemed not suitable for clinical use due to low white blood cell number. Mothers who donate their UCB to the National Cord Blood Bank sign a consent giving permission to donate the UCB to research if it is inadequate for clinical use and will be discarded. Because the donated units are completely de-identified and are not collected prospectively specifically for research, the New York Blood Center Institutional Review Board (IRB), which oversees research ethics at the National Cord Blood Bank, considers their use exempt from IRB review. Human UCB was prepared as previously described.(Mitchell, Li et al. 2006) Briefly, leukocytes were separated from 1-3 units of human UCB judged to be inadequate for clinical purposes (generously provided by the New York Blood Center) by Dextran 70 sedimentation (Amersham Biosciences, Piscataway, NJ) for 1h, and then enriched for CD34+ progenitor cells by negative selection using a combination of antibodies against maturation/lineage-specific markers (RosetteSep, StemCell Technologies, Vancouver, BC) concomitant with density sedimentation using Ficoll-Paque Plus (Amersham Biosciences, Piscataway, NJ). These cells were cultured in serum-free medium (StemCell Technologies, Vancouver, BC) with 50 ng/ml thrombopoietin (TPO) plus 1 ng/ml SCF (both Millipore, Temecula,CA) for 3 days in 10 cm dishes in a 37°C incubator. At this point a portion of the cells will have died. The remaining living population of larger cells was gently washed and replated in fresh media with the same cytokines in 10 cm dishes and left until use (Day 8 or 9). Fresh media was added on day 6. We have previously reported that under these conditions the UCB differentiate into a population of large cells with > 90% expressing $\alpha IIb\beta 3$, > 80% expressing GPIb, about 50% expressing $\alpha 2\beta 1$.(Mitchell, Li et al. 2007) For experimental use the cells were gently harvested, pelleted at 300 rpm for 5 min, or let settle by gravity, and gently resuspended in the appropriate buffer.

2.3 HEK293 cell culture

HEK293 cell lines (American Type Culture Collection (ATCC), Manassas, VA) that stably expressed human $\alpha IIb\beta 3$ receptors were established as previously described.(Mitchell, Li et al. 2006) Transfections were performed using Lipofectamine 2000 (Gibco-BRL, Carlsbad, CA) according to the manufacturer's instructions, followed by selection in media containing 500 µg/ml G418 for 2-4 weeks. To obtain a population of cells uniformly expressing high levels of $\alpha IIb\beta 3$, cells were labeled with the mAb 10E5 (anti-$\alpha IIb\beta 3$) and sorted using a MoFlo cell sorter (Beckman Coulter, Fullerton, CA).

2.4 Immunoprecipitation and biosynthetic labeling

Samples were prepared as previously described and all steps were performed on ice unless otherwise stated.(Mitchell, Li et al. 2006) Briefly, cells (either day 8 megakaryocytes derived from UCB cells or HEK293 cells) were lysed in 1% Brij 98 lysis buffer containing protease inhibitors and 20uM N-methylmaleimide (NEM). Lysates were precleared with protein-G Sepharose beads (Amersham Biosciences, Piscataway, NJ), and then equivalent amounts of protein, usually 400 µg, were incubated one h at 4°C with one or more of the antibodies listed above (4 µg/reaction). Samples were incubated with protein-G Sepharose beads for one h at 4°C, washed twice, and incubated with SDS sample buffer for 10 min at 100°C. Reduced samples contained 10% beta mercaptoethanol (Sigma, Thermo Scientific, Rockford, IL). Samples were subjected to SDS-PAGE on 7% gels, and the gels were either stained for mass spectrometry identification (described below) or transferred to PVDF membranes for immunoblotting. Non-specific binding was determined by performing parallel immunoprecipitation with mouse or rabbit IgG in each experiment. In preliminary experiments, the production of $\alpha IIbR858G/R859G$ and $\beta 3$ was confirmed in the transfected HEK293 cell line by immunoprecipitation with both anti-αIIb and anti-$\beta 3$ mAbs followed by immunoblot. For biosynthetic labeling, cells were incubated for 30 min at 37°C in methionine/cysteine-free medium, followed by pulse-labeling for 15 min at 37°C in medium containing ^{35}S-methionine/cysteine (300 µCi/10 cm plate). The pulse was terminated by incubation in medium containing unlabeled methionine/cysteine (1 mg/ml each) and the cells were incubated at 37 °C until lysis in 1% Triton-X 100 lysis buffer. Following cell lysis, supernatants were prepared as above. Gels were dried and exposed to film. For inhibition of the proteasome cells were incubated in the proteasome inhibitor MG132 (10 μM)(Sigma_Aldrich, St Louis, MO) in normal growth medium at 37C and then immediately lysed.

2.5 Histidine-tag/Nickel bead pulldown assay

HEK293 cells expressing poly-histidine tagged αIIb cDNA (in vector pEF1/V5-His) and β3 cDNA (in vector pcDNA3.1)(Mitchell, Li et al. 2007) were lysed in 1% Triton, 150 mM NaCl, 10 mM imidazole buffer (lysis buffer) on ice for 30 m, centrifuged for 30m at 4C, and then the supernatant was reacted with 50 μl of a 6:4 slurry of Ni beads:imidazole buffer (Qiagen, Inc. Valencia, CA) to bind the histidine-tagged subunits to the nickel beads. After incubating for 30 m the beads were washed four times with 10 mM imidazole lysis buffer by using a magnetic chamber to isolate the beads. Next, fresh whole cell lysates (1 mL) of UCB-derived megakaryocytes in 1% Triton, 150 mM NaCl, 10 mM imidazole buffer were incubated with the washed, Ni-bound αIIb for 1 h, and then the beads were washed twice with 1 mL lysis buffer containing 20 mM imidazole. Ni-bound proteins were eluted with 250 mM imidazole and the entire eluate was subjected to SDS-PAGE on a 7% gel followed by staining with Imperial Stain (Pierce, Thermo Scientific, Rockford, IL). Control experiments were run in parallel in which no megakaryocyte lysate was added to the beads, but all other steps remained the same. These controls aimed to identify the remaining HEK293 cell proteins still bound to either the beads or to αIIb after the washing steps, before incubation with megakaryocyte lysate. Experimental and control gels were run simultaneously, and the lanes were excised and analyzed by mass spectrometry.

2.6 Photocrosslinking amino acids

UCB cells were cultured as described above for eight days, then were washed and incubated for 24 hours in leucine- and methionine- free medium containing photoreactive methionine and leucine, dialyzed FBS (both Pierce, Thermo Scientific, Rockford, IL), and 50 ng/ml TPO (Millipore, Temecula,CA). The cells were exposed to 345 nm UV light for 15 minutes to crosslink the photoreactive amino acids, and harvested immediately, according to manufacturer's instructions. Whole cell lysates were immunoprecipitated with antibodies specific for αIIb or β3, and the proteins were separated by SDS-PAGE using the same protocol as for the histidine-tag affinity capture. Controls were simultaneously immunoprecipitated with non-immune IgG. Experimental and control lanes were excised and analyzed by mass spectrometry.

2.7 RNAi

HEK293 cells stably expressing high levels of αIIb and β3 were transfected with 100 nM siRNA duplexes (Dharmacon, Thermo Scientific, Rockford, IL and Qiagen, Valencia, CA) using Dharmafect-1 reagent (Dharmacon, Thermo Scientific, Rockford, IL), then analyzed by flow cytometry using a FacsCanto (Becton Dickenson,) at 48-96 h after transfection. Cultured UCB cells were transfected twice, on culture days 3 and 5, with 100 nM of siRNA duplexes or controls also using Dharmafect-1 reagent, and then analyzed 48 – 72 h later by flow cytometry. In order to identify individual transfected cells by FACS, cells were co-transfected with 10 nM of fluorescent-labeled non-coding siRNA (Qiagen, Valencia, CA). In some experiments, Cy3-labeled siRNA duplexes were used (Dharmacon, Thermo Scientific, Rockford, IL). Controls were: no treatment, transfection reagent but no siRNA duplex, Cy3-labeled negative control siRNA duplex only (Qiagen), siControl non targeting siRNA duplex, and siRNA duplex against cyclophillin B (positive control) (both Dharmacon).

2.8 Quantitative RT-PCR

For analysis of RNA content, cells were collected in RNAlater (Applied Biosystems, Foster City, CA) and RNA was purified using the RNEasy mini kit (Qiagen, Valencia, CA). For some analyses, siRNA transfected cells were sorted for expression of the fluorescent marker using a MoFlo sorter, and the sorted cells were subjected to QRT-PCR. Analysis was performed on an ABI 7900 or an ABI 7700 thermocycler/ fluorescence analyzer (Applied Biosystems, Foster City, CA) using the SYBR green probe (Qiagen or Invitrogen) and Quantitect primer assays (Qiagen). Relative mRNA levels were calculated using the ΔΔCt method that corrects for GAPDH expression in all samples. Fold-reduction was corrected for percent transfection in each experiment.

2.9 Immunofluorescence analysis

Mks were cytospun onto poly L-lysine-coated glass coverslips and fixed in methanol for 5 minutes at RT. Cells were then washed with saponin buffer (PBS containing 0.02% BSA, 0.005% saponin), then blocked with saponin buffer for 1 hour at RT. Cells were then incubated with the primary antibody diluted in saponin buffer for 1 hour at RT. After washing with PBS, cells were incubated with the appropriate conjugated secondary antibody in PBS for 1 hour at RT. Specimens were mounted with Prolong gold (Invitrogen). Images were acquired using a Zeiss LSM 510 META (Axiovert 200M Inverted Microscope Stand) confocal laser scanning microsope through a 100x objective. Each set of staining conditions was repeated 3 times. Background fluorescence was measured by incubating fixed cells with the secondary antibody only and then acquiring images with the exact settings used to obtain the experimental images.

2.10 Mass spectrometry data analysis

The protein gel bands were excised from the SDS-PAGE. The gel bands were reduced with 10 mM of DTT and alkylated with 55 mM iodoacetamide, and then digested with Sequence Grade Modified Trypsin (Promega, Madison, Wisconsin) in ammonium bicarbonate buffer at 37° overnight.(Kumarathasan, Mohottalage et al. 2005) The digestion products were extracted twice with 0.1% trifluoroacetic acid and 50% Acetonitrile and 1.0% trifluoroacetic acid respectively. The extracted mixture was dried by Speed-Vac and redisolved in 10 μL 0.1% trifluoroacetic acid. Half of the extracts were injected by LC-MS/MS analysis. For LC-MS/MS analysis, each digestion product was separated by a 60 min gradient elution with the Dionex U3000 capillary/nano-HPLC system (Dionex, Sunnyvale, California) at a flow rate of 0.250 μL/min that is directly interfaced with the Thermo-Fisher LTQ-Obritrap mass spectrometer (Thermo Fisher, San Jose, California) operated in data-dependent scan mode. The analytical column was a home-made fused silica capillary column (75 μm ID, 100 mm length; Upchurch, Oak Harbor, Washington) packed with C-18 resin (300 A, 5 μm, Varian, Palo Alto, California). Mobile phase A consisted of 0.1% formic acid, and mobile phase B consisted of 100% acetonitrile and 0.1% formic acid. The 60 min gradients with 250 nL/min flow rate for B solvent went from 0 to 55% in 34 minutes and then in 4 min to 80%. The B solvent stayed at 80% for another 8 min and then decreased to 5% in 8 min. Another 6 min was used for equilibration, loading and washing. The mass acquisition method was one FT-MS scan followed by 6 subsequent MS/MS scan in the ion trap. The FT-MS scan was acquired at resolution 30,000 in the Orbi-trap. The six most intense peaks from the FT full scan were selected in the ion trap for MS/MS. The selected ions were excluded for further selection for 180 seconds. The following search parameters were used in all MASCOT searches: maximum of 1 missed trypsin cleavages, cysteine carbamidomethylation, methionine oxidation. The maximum error tolerance for MS scans was 10 ppm for MS and 1.0 Da for MS/MS respectively. Proteins were designated as "hits" if they matched at least 2 distinctive peptides with a MASCOT score of at least 40. For proteins matching the same sets of peptides, only the protein with the greater percentage of coverage was selected. In the one case where 2 isoforms could not be distinguished (HSP70A/B), both proteins are reported. Proteins identified in the control gels were considered "negative," and these proteins were removed from further analysis. The interaction data were further analyzed using the Cytoscape(Cline, Smoot et al. 2007) software and publically available protein interaction databases (e.g. INTACT, NCBI, UniProt) to generate a network of first-degree interactions with αIIb. The network was further expanded to include proteins that were previously reported to interact with αIIb and known interactions between any of the proteins identified in our primary assays.

2.11 Statistical analysis

Flow cytometry data was summarized as the geographic mean fluorescence intensity (MFI) of antibody binding, and normalized to the MFI of control siRNA treated cells, so that the experimental MFI is expressed as a percentage of the control MFI. The overall percent change of the replicates was expressed as the average percent change +/- the confidence interval. The two-sided, paired t-test was used to determine whether there were differences in antibody binding between the different experimental groups. In the siRNA experiments, relative mRNA levels were calculated using the $\Delta\Delta Ct$ method that corrects for GAPDH expression.

3. Results

3.1 The αIIb interactome

Proteins putatively interacting with αIIb were isolated from UCB derived megakaryocytes and from HEK293 cells expressing αIIbβ3, and these proteins were analyzed by mass spectrometry. Samples were processed by the two methods depicted in **Figure 2**. In the first method, recombinant αIIb or αIIbR858G/R859G subunits bearing a polyhistidine tag were expressed in HEK293 cells along with normal β3. The cells were lysed with 1% Triton buffer, and the lysates were reacted with Ni beads that bind polyhistidine. The Ni beads were washed using a magnetic separator to reduce non-specific binding to the Ni-bound αIIb, and then incubated with fresh whole cell lysate of umbilical cord blood derived megakaryocyte. Since we are interested in the early process of αIIbβ3 formation and intracellular trafficking we used megakaryocytes at day 8 or 9 of culture; at that point in our system αIIbβ3 is highly expressed but there is not yet any proplatelet formation. The Ni-bound histidine-tagged αIIb and αIIb-bound proteins were washed twice and then were eluted from the Ni beads with 250 mM imidazole in a 1% Triton buffer. Simultaneous control experiments were performed without megakaryocyte lysate in order to identify proteins non-specifically binding to either the Ni beads or the polyhistidine tag. The proteins thus collected were separated by one dimensional SDS-PAGE on a 7% gel. After staining, the experimental and control lanes were cut out and analyzed by mass spectrometry. This entire process was repeated in three separate experiments with normal αIIb, and in four separate experiments with αIIbR858G/R859G.

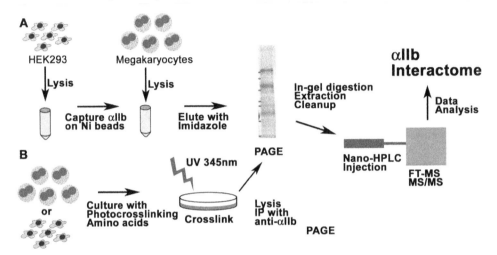

Fig. 2. Methods used to isolate and identify αIIb-interacting proteins. A): Polyhistidine-tagged αIIb subunits were captured on Ni beads and then incubated with whole cell lysate of day 8 UCB-derived megakaryocytes. Protein complexes thus captured were processed as described in the text, and then the proteins were identified by FT-MS and MS/MS. B) Crosslinking experiments were performed on day 8 UCB-derived megakaryocytes and transfected HEK293 cells. Cells were fed photoactivatable methionine and leucine, exposed to UV light and lysed immediately. Samples were processed for mass spectrometry as described.

The second strategy used photo-activated amino acids to crosslink αIIb to its binding partners (**Figure 2B**). UCB-derived megakaryocytes were starved for methionine and leucine, then fed photo-activatable methionine and leucine overnight, and then exposed to UV light to crosslink the amino acids of neighboring proteins. The megakaryocytes were immediately lysed and the αIIb-bound proteins were immunoprecipitated by anti-αIIb mAb. These proteins were separated by one dimensional SDS-PAGE and then the appropriate bands were cut out and analyzed by mass spectrometry. Because we were looking only for proteins crosslinked to αIIb, only the portions of the bands with $M_r > 120$ (M_r of the mature αIIb subunit) were analyzed. Five separate crosslinking experiments were performed with UCB-derived megakaryocytes and two on HEK293 cells expressing αIIbR858G/R859G and normal β3.

Minimum criteria for protein inclusion in data analysis were at least 2 distinctive peptides with a MASCOT score of at least 40, and absence of the protein in the control lanes. Importantly, since we were interested in proteins that are more abundant in the megakaryocyte than in HEK293 cells, even proteins known to interact with αIIbβ3, such as talin, were removed from the final results because they were present in the control lanes. Proteins identified in the Ni bead extraction experiments that are known to harbor natural polyhistidine sequences (such as the DEAH boxes) that could independently bind to the Ni beads were also excluded. Combining the results of both methods, 98 proteins were identified as potentially interacting with the normal αIIb subunit, and 79 proteins were identified as putatively interacting with the αIIbR858G/R859G subunit (Table 1). These 163 proteins putatively constitute a portion of the αIIb interactome, a network of protein-protein interactions relevant to the trafficking and function of αIIb in megakaryocytes (**Figure 3**).

Proteins Captured with αIIbR858G/R859G

Gene Symbol	Entrez Gene ID	SwissProt Acc No.	Protein Acc No.	Description	# Pep	% Cov	#. Expt
MYH9	4627	P35579 Q60FE2	gi|12667788	MYOSIN, HEAVY POLYPEPTIDE 9, NON-MUSCLE	70	45	4
LMNA	4000	P02545	gi|5031875	LAMIN A/C	37	61	3
HNRNPL*	3191	P14866 A6NIT8 Q6NTA2	gi|11527777	HETEROGENEOUS NUCLEAR RIBONUCLEOPROTEIN L	33	53	4
STIM1	6786	Q13586	gi|21070997	STROMAL INTERACTION MOLECULE 1	28	46	2
CKAP4	10970	Q07065	gi|19920317	CYTOSKELETON-ASSOCIATED PROTEIN 4	27	55	2
HSP90AB1	3326	P08238	gi|154146191	HEAT SHOCK PROTEIN 90kDa ALPHA, CLASS A MEMBER 1	21	36	1
SF3A1	10291	Q15459	gi|53831995	SPLICING FACTOR 3A, SUBUNIT 1, 120kDa	16	32	1
HSPA1A*	3303	B3KTT5 P08107 A8K5I0	gi|5123454	HEAT SHOCK 70kDa PROTEIN 1A	15	34	3
ATXN2L*	11273	Q8WWM7 A8K1R6	gi|119572372	ATAXIN 2-LIKE	14	20	2
MYH10	4628	Q6PK16 P35580 Q9BWG0	gi|41406064	MYOSIN, HEAVY POLYPEPTIDE 10, NON-MUSCLE	13	9	1
DNAJC10*	54431	Q8IXB1	gi|24308127	DNAJ (HSP40) HOMOLOG, SUBFAMILY C, MEMBER 10	13	21	3
PSPC1	55269	Q8WXF1	gi|109240550	PARASPECKLE COMPONENT 1	13	35	3
SFPQ	6421	P23246 Q86VG2	gi|119627829	SPLICING FACTOR PROLINE/GLUTAMINE-RICH (POLYPYRIMIDINE TRACT BINDING PROTEIN ASSOCIATED)	12	35	1
SF1*	7536	Q14820	gi|42544123	SPLICING FACTOR 1	12	20	2

Symbol	Number	Accession	gi	Protein			
		Q15637		HEAT SHOCK 70kDa PROTEIN 5 (GLUCOSE-REGULATED PROTEIN, 78kDa)			
HSPA5*	3309	P11021	gi|119608027		11	37	4
HLF2	4057	P02788	gi|16198357	LACTOTRANSFERRIN	11	30	1
MYH11	4629	P35749 Q3MNF1 Q3MIV8 Q3MNF0	gi|119574312	MYOSIN, HEAVY POLYPEPTIDE 11	11	9	1
LTBP1	4052	Q14766 B7ZLY3	gi|46249414	LATENT TRANSFORMING GROWTH FACTOR BETA BINDING PROTEIN 1	10	8	2
PKM2*	5315	P14618	gi|127795697	PYRUVATE KINASE, MUSCLE	10	28	1
RAVER1*	125950	Q8IY67	gi|123173757	RAVER1	10	29	2
XIRP2	129446	A4UGR9 Q8NE71 Q2L6I2	gi|61696134	CARDIOMYOPATHY ASSOCIATED 3	10	16	1
ABCF1	23	A2BF75	gi|21759807	ATP-BINDING CASSETTE, SUB-FAMILY F (GCN20), MEMBER 1	9	14	1
POTEF	728378	A5A3E0	gi|153791352	POTE ANKYRIN DOMAIN FAMILY, F	9	8	1
HSP90AA1	3320	P07900 Q86SX1	gi|153792590	HEAT SHOCK PROTEIN 90kDa ALPHA, CLASS A MEMBER 1	8	13	3
ITGA2B*	3674	P08514	gi|119571981	INTEGRIN, ALPHA 2B (PLATELET GLYCOPROTEIN IIB OF IIB/IIIA COMPLEX, ANTIGEN CD41)	8	17	2
TF*	7018	Q06AH7 P02787	gi|110590597	TRANSFERRIN	8	18	2
SAP 62	8175	A0PJA6	gi|21361376	SPLICING FACTOR 3A, SUBUNIT 2, 66kDa	8	19	1
LYZ	4069	Q05DF2 Q15428	gi|4930023	LYSOZYME (RENAL AMYLOIDOSIS)	7	70	1
SMAD4	4089	P61626 B2R4C5 Q13485	gi|4885457	SMAD, MOTHERS AGAINST DPP HOMOLOG 4 (DROSOPHILA)	7	12	2
HSP90B1	7184	P14625	gi|4507677	HEAT SHOCK PROTEIN 90kDa BETA (GRP94), MEMBER 1	7	12	2
CANX	821	P27824	gi|10716563	CALNEXIN	6	13	1
LRP2	4036	Q7Z5C1 P98164 Q7Z5C0 A6NE14 P49368	gi|32816595	LOW DENSITY LIPOPROTEIN-RELATED PROTEIN 2	6	1	1
CCT3	7203	B3KX11	gi|14124984	CHAPERONIN CONTAINING TCP1, SUBUNIT 3 (GAMMA)	6	21	2
HSPA1L	3305	P34931	gi|21759781	HEAT SHOCK 70kDa PROTEIN 1-LIKE	5	15	2
NCL	4691	P19338	gi|189306	NUCLEOLIN	5	6	1

		B3KM80					
PIP	5304	P12273	gi|4505821	PROLACTIN-INDUCED PROTEIN	5	31	1
SLPI	6590	P03973	gi|4507065	SECRETORY LEUKOCYTE PEPTIDASE INHIBITOR	5	28	1
		P09493 Q9Y427					
TPM1	7168	O15513	gi|854189	TROPOMYOSIN 1 (ALPHA)	5	10	1
HECTD1	25831	Q9ULT8	gi|118498337	HECT DOMAIN CONTAINING 1	5	5	3
LACRT	90070	Q9GZZ8	gi|15187164	LACRITIN	5	30	1
ACTG3	71	P63261	gi|178045		4	12	1
DMBT1	1755	Q9UGM3	gi|169218264	DELETED IN MALIGNANT BRAIN TUMORS 1	4	11	1
FLG	2312	P20930	gi|62122917	FILAGGRIN	4	2	1
		P61978					
HNRNPK	3190	Q6IBN1	gi|55958544	HETEROGENEOUS NUCLEAR RIBONUCLEOPROTEIN K	4	11	2
		B3KTV0					
HSPA8*	3312	P11142	gi|5729877	HEAT SHOCK 70kDa PROTEIN 8	4	8	1
KPNB1	3837	Q14974	gi|119615215	KARYOPHERIN (IMPORTIN) BETA 1	4	8	1
LCN1	3933	P31025	gi|4504963	LIPOCALIN 1	4	30	1
LMAN1*	3998	P49257	gi|5031873	LECTIN, MANNOSE-BINDING, 1	4	15	1
		P07478					
PRSS2	5645	Q5NV56	gi|74353564	PROTEASE, SERINE, 2 (TRYPSIN 2)	4	15	1
ALDH18A1	5832	P54886	gi|76779856	ALDEHYDE DEHYDROGENASE 18 FAMILY, MEMBER A1	4	5	1
NPM3	10360	O75607	gi|5801867	NUCLEOPHOSMIN/NUCLE OPLASMIN, 3	4	12	1
WAC	51322	Q9BTA9	gi|55664165	WW DOMAIN CONTAINING ADAPTOR WITH COILED-COIL	4	5	1
ANKRD24	170961	Q8TF*21	gi|16418357	ANKYRIN REPEAT DOMAIN 24	4	5	1
		Q96HY3 P62158					
CALM1	801	B4DJ51	gi|61680528	CALMODULIN	3	18	1
		Q02388		COLLAGEN, TYPE VII, ALPHA 1 (EPIDERMOLYSIS BULLOSA, DYSTROPHIC, DOMINANT AND			
COL7A1	1294	Q59F16	gi|119585300	RECESSIVE)	3	1	1
HSPD1	3329	P10809	gi|14326412	HEAT SHOCK 60kDa PROTEIN 1	3	15	2
		P23368		MALIC ENZYME 2, NAD(+)-			
ME2	4200	Q9BWL6	gi|5822326	DEPENDENT	3	5	2
PEX1	5189	O43933	gi|4505725	PEROXISOMAL BIOGENESIS FACTOR 1	3	2	1
PRKAA1	5562	Q13131	gi|29124503	PROTEIN KINASE, AMP-ACTIVATED, ALPHA 1	3	5	1

Gene Symbol	Entrez Gene ID	SwissProt Acc No.	Protein Acc No.	Description	# Pep	% Cov	# Exp
H6PD	9563	O95479	gi|51859374	CATALYTIC SUBUNIT HEXOSE-6-PHOSPHATE DEHYDROGENASE (GLUCOSE 1-DEHYDROGENASE)	3	3	2
PDIA4	9601	Q549T6 P13667	gi|37182276	PROTEIN DISULFIDE ISOMERASE FAMILY A, MEMBER 4	3	2	1
COLEC10	10584	Q9Y6Z7	gi|5453619	COLLECTIN SUB-FAMILY MEMBER 10 (C-TYPE LECTIN)	3	12	1
FOXJ3	22887		gi|114555879	FORKHEAD BOX J3	3	4	1
ARS2	51593	Q9BXP5	gi|33150698	ARS2 PROTEIN	3	5	1
FOXJ2	55810	Q9P0K8	gi|8923842	FORKHEAD BOX J2	3	4	1
UBAP2	55833	Q5T6F2 Q9P0H6	gi|22325364	UBIQUITIN ASSOCIATED PROTEIN 2	3	3	1
KIAA1529*	57653	Q9P1Z9	gi|7959325	KIAA1529	3	2	3
LRRC8E	80131	B3KR78	gi|801893	LEUCINE RICH REPEAT CONTAINING 8 FAMILY, MEMBER E	3	3	1
QRICH2	84074	Q9H0J4	gi|14149793	GLUTAMINE RICH 2	3	3	1
DPP9*	91039	Q86TI2 Q1ZZB8	gi|119589606	DIPEPTIDYL-PEPTIDASE 9	3	4	2
LPLUNC1	92747	Q8TDL5	gi|40807482	NASOPHARGYNEAL RELATED	3	6	1
DOK7	285489	Q18PE1	gi|119602869	HYPOTHETICAL PROTEIN FLJ33718	3	4	1
SLFN14	342618	P0C7P3	gi|193788704	ORTHOLOG OF MOUSE SCHLAFEN 10	3	5	1
ENO1	2023	P06733	gi|4503571	ENOLASE 1	2	6	1
XRCC5	7520	P13010	gi|119590969	X-RAY REPAIR COMPLEMENTING DEFECTIVE REPAIR IN CHINESE HAMSTER CELLS 5 (DOUBLE-STRAND-BREAK REJOINING; KU AUTOANTIGEN, 80kDa)	2	4	1
WDR1	9948	O75083	gi|12652891	WD REPEAT DOMAIN 1	2	6	1
NLRP1	22861	Q9C000 Q9H5Z7	gi|37927559	NLR FAMILY, PYRIN DOMAIN CONTAINING 1	2	1	1
PPA2	27068	Q9H2U2 A6NKL9	gi|119612395	PYROPHOSPHATASE (INORGANIC) 2	2	1	1
VPS35	55737	Q96QK1	gi|7022978	VACUOLAR PROTEIN SORTING 35	2	2	1

Proteins Captured with normal αIIb

Gene Symbol	Entrez Gene ID	SwissProt Acc No.	Protein Acc No.	Description	# Pep	% Cov	# Exp
ITGB3*	3690	P05106	gi|183531	INTEGRIN, BETA 3 (PLATELET GLYCOPROTEIN IIIA, ANTIGEN CD61)	25	42	7

Symbol	GeneID	UniProt	gi	Description			
TUBB2C	7284	P49411	gi|20809886	TUBULIN, BETA 2C	17	35	1
DHTKD1	55526	Q96HY7	gi|119606733	DEHYDROGENASE E1 AND TRANSKETOLASE DOMAIN CONTAINING 1	15	36	1
GLUD1	2746	P00367 P14868	gi|183056	GLUTAMATE DEHYDROGENASE 1	15	67	3
DARS	1615	P78371	gi|45439306	ASPARTYL-TRNA SYNTHETASE	14	60	3
LMAN1*	3998	P49257	gi|5031873	LECTIN, MANNOSE-BINDING, 1	12	36	1
PRKAB1	5564	Q9Y478	gi|4506061	PROTEIN KINASE, AMP-ACTIVATED, BETA 1 NON-CATALYTIC SUBUNIT	12	38	1
HSPA5*	3309	P11021	gi|16507237	HEAT SHOCK 70kDa PROTEIN 5 (GLUCOSE-REGULATED PROTEIN, 78kDa)	11	30	1
SCN10A	6336	P08246 P43626 P43628 P43632	gi|110835709	SODIUM CHANNEL, VOLTAGE-GATED, TYPE X, ALPHA	11	5	1
TUBB	10383	P68371	gi|7106439	TUBULIN, BETA 5	11	44	4
TUBB4	23071	Q9BS26	gi|21361322	TUBULIN, BETA 4	10	26	1
ALDH18A1	5832	P54886	gi|76779856	ALDEHYDE DEHYDROGENASE 18 FAMILY, MEMBER A1	9	18	2
DNAJC10*	54431	Q8IXB1	gi|24308127	DNAJ (HSP40) HOMOLOG, SUBFAMILY C, MEMBER 10	9	21	4
EXOSC10	5394	Q01780 P05156	gi|50301239	EXOSOME COMPONTENT 10	9	8	1
UGP1	10352	Q9UGM6	gi|48255966	UDP-GLUCOSE PYROPHOSPHORYLASE 1	9	33	1
ADPGK	83440	Q9BRR6	gi|31542509	ADP-DEPENDENT GLUCOKINASE	8	22	1
ALAD	210	P13716	gi|248839	AMINOLEVULINATE, DELTA-, DEHYDRATASE	8	22	1
CCT2	10576	P78371	gi|5453603	CHAPERONIN CONTAINING TCP1, SUBUNIT 2 (BETA)	8	39	1
CCT4	10575	P50991	gi|38455427	CHAPERONIN CONTAINING TCP1, SUBUNIT 4 (DELTA)	8	28	1
FARS2	10667	O95363	gi|62898407	PHENYLALANINE-TRNA SYNTHETASE 2	8	24	1
HSPA1A*	3303	B3KTT5	gi|5123454	HEAT SHOCK 70kDa PROTEIN 1A	8	19	1
HSPA1B	3304	P08107	gi|167466173	HEAT SHOCK 70kDa PROTEIN 1B	8	21	1
HSPA9	3313	P38646	gi|12653415	HEAT SHOCK 70kDa PROTEIN 9B (MORTALIN-2)	8	17	2
NUDT19	390916	A8MXV4	gi|157739940	NUDIX (NUCLEOSIDE DIPHOSPHATE LINKED MOIETY X)-TYPE MOTIF 19	8	36	1

Symbol	Gene ID	UniProt	gi	Description			
AKR7A2	8574	O43488	gi|41327764	ALDO-KETO REDUCTASE FAMILY 7, MEMBER A2 (AFLATOXIN ALDEHYDE REDUCTASE)	7	37	1
CHD9	80205	Q3L8U1	gi|95147342	CHROMODOMAIN HELICASE DNA BINDING PROTEIN 9	7	2	1
FAM175B	23172		gi|148529023	UNKNOWN PROTEIN LOC23172	7	14	1
KIF14	9928	Q15058	gi|7661878	KINESIN FAMILY MEMBER 14	7	4	1
NT5DC2	22978	A8K6K2	gi|12597653	5'-NUCLEOTIDASE DOMAIN CONTAINING 2	7	36	2
P15RS	55197	Q96P16	gi|142385371	REGULATION OF NUCLEAR pre-mRNA DOMAIN CONTAINING 1A	7	20	1
PDLIM1	9260	Q9Y3C6 Q9NR12	gi|13994151	PDZ AND LIM DOMAIN 1 (ENIGMA)	7	37	1
PM20D2	135293	Q8IYS1	gi|58082085	AMINOACYLASE 1-LIKE 2	7	15	1
POLDIP2	26073	Q9Y2S7 Q9BVV8	gi|7661672	POLYMERASE (DNA-DIRECTED), DELTA INTERACTING PROTEIN 2	7	26	1
TF*	7018	P02787	gi|553788	TRANSFERRIN	7	12	1
ACTN4	604638		gi|2804273	ACTININ, ALPHA 4	6	9	1
ATXN2L*	11273	Q8WWM7	gi|119572372	ATAXIN 2-LIKE	6	9	1
CCT7	10574	Q99832	gi|62896515	CHAPERONIN CONTAINING TCP1, SUBUNIT 7 (ETA)	6	23	1
CNDP2	55748	Q96KP4	gi|8922698	CNDP DIPEPTIDASE 2 (METALLOPEPTIDASE M20 FAMILY)	6	11	1
FLJ12529	79869	Q8N684	gi|24432016	PRE-MRNA CLEAVAGE FACTOR I, 59 kDa SUBUNIT	6	12	1
PBEF1	10135	P43490	gi|55960735	PRE-B-CELL COLONY ENHANCING FACTOR 1	6	4	1
PPP1R9A	55607	Q9ULJ8	gi|261244899	PROTEIN PHOSPHATASE 1, REGULATORY (INHIBITOR) SUBUNIT 9A, 5 isoforms	6	5	1
RB1CC1	9821	Q8TDY2	gi|134304845	RB1-INDUCIBLE COILED-COIL 1	6	3	1
SERBP1	26135	Q8NC51 Q9H707	gi|66346679	SERPINE1 MRNA BINDING PROTEIN 1	6	16	1
TXNDC4	23352	Q8WXW3 Q5T4S7 Q9NP58	gi|119579327	THIOREDOXIN DOMAIN CONTAINING 4 (ENDOPLASMIC RETICULUM)	6	35	3
ACLY	47	P53396	gi|38569423	ATP CITRATE LYASE	5	3	1
ACTB	60	Q1KLZ0	gi|14250401	ACTIN, BETA	5	22	3
CTTN	2017		gi|2498954	CORTACTIN	5	4	1
CUL-5	8065	Q93034	gi|67514034	CULLIN 5	5	5	1
FHL1	2273	Q13642	gi|3851650	FOUR AND A HALF LIM	5	3	1

Gene	ID	UniProt	gi	Description			
GPHN	10243	Q9NQX3	gi|10880983	DOMAINS 1 GEPHYRIN ISOFORM 1	5	8	1
HNRPH1	3187	P31943	gi|5031753	HETEROGENEOUS NUCLEAR RIBONUCLEOPROTEIN H1	5	16	1
HSPA8*	3312	P11142	gi|10880983	HEAT SHOCK 70kDa PROTEIN 8	5	8	3
IDH3A	3419	P50213	gi|5031777	ISOCITRATE DEHYDROGENASE 3 (NAD+) ALPHA	5	13	1
PRKAG1	5571	P54619	gi|2230863	PROTEIN KINASE, AMP-ACTIVATED, GAMMA 1 NON-CATALYTIC SUBUNIT	5	27	1
RILPL1	353116	Q5EBL4	gi|30315660	RAB INTERACTING LYSOSOMAL PROTEIN-LIKE 1	5	12	1
SAP130	79595	Q9H0E3	gi:25579126	SIN3A-ASSOCIATED PROTEIN, 130kDa	5	3	1
WARS2	80139	Q9H7S9	gi|7710154	TRYPTOPHANYL TRNA SYNTHETASE 2	5	19	1
ADCY6	112	O43306	gi|168480141	ADENYLATE CYCLASE 6	4	3	1
C5orf25	375484	Q8NDZ2	gi|196259795	FLJ44216 PROTEIN	4	8	1
CARS2	79587	Q9HA77	gi|119618821	HYPOTHETICAL PROTEIN FLJ39378	4	10	1
CIT	11113	O14578	gi|32698687	CITRON (RHO-INTERACTING, SERINE/THREONINE KINASE 21)	4	2	1
EEF2K	29904	O00418	gi|9558749	EUKARYOTIC ELONGATION FACTOR-2 KINASE	4	4	1
FLJ22184	80164	Q9H6K5	gi|239757129	HYPOTHETICAL PROTEIN FLJ22184	4	5	1
FLNA	2316	P21333	gi|57284166	FILAMIN A, ALPHA (ACTIN BINDING PROTEIN 280)	4	2	2
FRMPD1	22844	Q5SYB0	gi|239582740	FERM AND PDZ DOMAIN CONTAINING 1	4	3	1
GOPC	57120	Q9HD26	gi|9966877	GOLGI ASSOCIATED PDZ AND COILED-COIL MOTIF CONTAINING	4	12	1
HMGCS1	3157	Q01581	gi|53734504	3-HYDROXY-3-METHYLGLUTARYL-COENZYME A SYNTHASE 1 (SOLUBLE)	4	14	1
HNRNPL*	3191	P14866	gi|133274	HETEROGENEOUS NUCLEAR RIBONUCLEOPROTEIN L	4	11	2
HTRA2	27429	O43464	gi|21614538	HTRA SERINE PEPTIDASE 2	4	16	1
NAGK	55577	Q9UJ70	gi|6491737	N-ACETYLGLUCOSAMINE KINASE	4	10	1
PKM2*	5315	P14618	gi|31416989	PYRUVATE KINASE,	4	16	1

Gene		UniProt	gi	Protein			
				MUSCLE			
		Q05940					
PRDX3	10935	P30048	gi|14250063	PEROXIREDOXIN 3	4	20	1
SF1*	7536	Q15637	gi|46362557	SPLICING FACTOR 1	4	5	1
TIMM50	92609	Q3ZCQ8	gi|48526509	TRANSLOCASE OF INNER MITOCHONDRIAL MEMBRANE 50 HOMOLOG	4	6	1
AER61	285203		gi|39930530	GLUCOSYLTRANSFERASE AER61 C3orf64	3	6	1
CSNK2A2	1459	Q14012	gi|4503097	CASEIN KINASE 2, ALPHA PRIME POLYPEPTIDE	3	6	1
DPP9*	91039	Q86TI2	gi|114657671	DIPEPTIDYL-PEPTIDASE 9	3	2	1
DVL2	1856	O14641	gi|55665917	DISHEVELLED, DSH HOMOLOG 2 (DROSOPHILA)	3	2	1
ELMO1	9844	O60895	gi|86788139	ENGULFMENT AND CELL MOTILITY 1	3	5	1
GAPDH	2597	P04406 Q16678	gi|31645	GLYCERALDEHYDE-3-PHOSPHATE DEHYDROGENASE	3	18	1
KIAA0895	23366	Q8NCT3	gi|154426319	KIAA0895 PROTEIN	3	6	1
LUC7L2	51631	Q9Y383	gi|4929587	CGI-59 PROTEIN	3	5	1
MPO	4353	P05164	gi|88180	MYELOPEROXIDASE	3	5	2
PEG10	23089	Q86TG7	gi|94421473	PATERNALLY EXPRESSED 10	3	11	1
RPLP0	6175	P05388 Q9NQX7	gi|12654583	RIBOSOMAL PROTEIN, LARGE, P0	3	12	1
SEC13	6396	A8MV37	gi|119584482	SEC13-LIKE 1 (S. CEREVISIAE)	3	11	1
SEC23A	10484	Q15436 Q92736	gi|22477159	SEC23 HOMOLOG A (S. CEREVISIAE)	3	3	1
SHROOM3	57619	Q8TF72	gi|57284166	SHROOM3 F-ACTIN BINDING PROTEIN	3	2	4
UBR4	23352		gi|9367763	ZINC FINGER, UBR1 TYPE 1	3	3	1
A2M	2	P01023	gi|177872	ALPHA-2-MACROGLOBULIN	2	1	1
ABCA13	154664	Q86UQ4	gi|8928549	ATP-BINDING CASSETTE, SUB-FAMILY A (ABC1), MEMBER 13	2	5	2
CORO1A	11151	P31146	gi|5902134	CORONIN, ACTIN BINDING PROTEIN, 1A	2	4	1
KIAA1529*	57653	Q9P1Z9	gi|7959325	KIAA1529	2	2	4
MAP3K7IP2	23118	Q9NYJ8	gi|14149669	MITOGEN-ACTIVATED PROTEIN KINASE KINASE KINASE 7 INTERACTING PROTEIN 2	2	2	1
RANBP10	57610	Q6VN20	gi|40538736	RAN BINDING PROTEIN 10	2	4	1
RAVER1*	125950	Q8IY67	gi|123173757	RAVER1	2	4	1
TUBA1A	203068	P07437	gi|340021	TUBULIN, ALPHA	2	2	3
ZNF703	80139		gi|13376610	ZINC FINGER PROTEIN 703	2	3	1

Table 1. Proteins captured with αIIb in megakaryocytes and HEK293 cells. Results are separated according to the αIIb subunit they were captured with. Column labels: Gene

Symbol, EntrezGene ID, Protein Accession Number and Description are from the NCBI database. SwissProt Accession Number is from the UniProt database. Number of Unique Peptides is cumulative from all experiments. Coverage percent is cumulative for all experiments. Tally is shown of the total number of experiments in which a protein was identified (No Expts), and whether captured by histidine tag/Ni affinity (Ni-His) or by crosslinking (X-link). Presence or absence in a recently published expression study (HaemAtlas) is indicated. * Proteins captured by both normal and mutant αIIb subunits.

3.2 Gene Ontology analysis

Gene Ontology (GO) analysis using the DAVID Bioinformatics Resources(Dennis, Sherman et al. 2003; Huang, Sherman et al. 2008) revealed enrichment for protein functions related to processing and trafficking, and ER, Golgi or vesicle components (Figure 3). Comparison of the proteins isolated with the normal αIIb subunits *vs* with the αIIbR858G/R859G subunits showed similar distributions of their localization and molecular functions (**Table 2**). Notably, the αIIbR858G/R859G subunits captured a greater percentage of these types of proteins, suggesting that a greater percentage of the αIIbR858G/R859G subunits were associated with the ER, Golgi and vesicles. Comparison of our data set to a recently published analysis of gene expression in megakaryocytes(Watkins, Gusnanto et al. 2009) showed that approximately 70% of the proteins identified herein as potentially interacting with αIIb were identified as expressed in the megakaryocyte transcriptome.

GO function/location	% of total proteins	
	αIIb	αIIbR858G/R859G
Protien transport	31	49
Stress Caperone	21	34
Vesicle part	6	14
ER or Golgi part	19	21
Organelle part	27	41
Cytoskeleton	21	29
ATP/GTP binding	31	45

Table 2. Distribution of captured proteins into Gene Ontology categories. Some proteins appear in more than one category.

Despite the similarity in distributions into GO categories pertaining to protein processing and localization, there were only 14 proteins in common between the normal αIIb and αIIbR858G/R859G captured proteins (**Table 1**). This may indicate a difference in the relative amount of time spent by the normal and mutant subunits in the protein processing environment. One protein, DNAJC10, was captured in all experiments by both αIIb and αIIbR858G/R859G. Like other DNAJ proteins, DNAJC10 contains a binding domain for the chaperone BiP, but is unique in that its second domain has four protein-disulfide-isomerase (PDI) consensus sequences. (Cunnea, Miranda-Vizuete et al. 2003; Dong, Bridges et al. 2008) Because disulfide bond rearrangement is important for both biogenesis and function of αIIbβ3, we investigated the putative interaction between αIIb and DNAJC10. To our knowledge, DNAJC10 has not previously been reported to interact with αIIb or β3.

3.3 DNAJC10 interacts with αIIbβ3 during biogenesis

DNAJC10 coimmunoprecipitated with αIIb and β3 from UCB derived megakaryocytes using anti-αIIb mAbs 10E5, B1B5, M148 and CA3, and the anti β3 mAb 7H2. DNAJC10 either interacted with αIIb and β3 directly or was part of a complex with them (**Figure 3**). Because DNAJC10 was captured by the αIIbR858G/R859G subunit, we explored the possibility that DNAJC10 interacted with αIIb prior to αIIbβ3 complex formation and αIIb cleavage to its mature form. We have previously shown that pro-αIIb is degraded by the proteasome and that proteasome inhibition leads to an increase of pro-αIIb within the cells. (Mitchell, Li et al. 2006) The undegraded pro-αIIb is trapped in a "pre-degradation" state in which normally transient protein interactions, which usually lead to degradation, may become more long-lived and may be captured by co-immunoprecipitation. Incubation of megakaryocytes with MG132 resulted in increased DNAJC10 co-immunoprecipitation with αIIb by all mAbs, but particularly M148 and CA3. Thus, DNAJC10 may associate with αIIb early in biogenesis, before excess pro-αIIb is targeted to the proteasome.

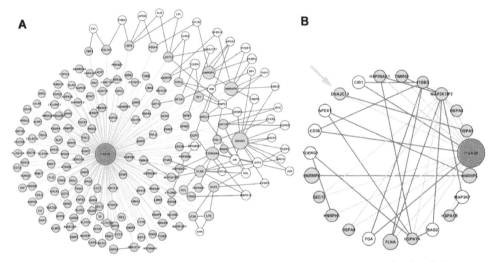

Fig. 3. Network derived from Table 1 data. Proteins are represented as nodes (circles) labeled with their gene symbol, and putative protein interactions with αIIb are indicated by thin green connecting lines. Thick blue lines and blues circles represent interactions or proteins, respectively, retrieved from online databases (Intact and NCBI) using the Cytoscape software. Arrow indicates DNAJC10. Figure prepared using Cytoscape.

To test this possibility we used a panel of conformation-specific mAbs that we have previously used to track the conformational changes of αIIb as it proceeds through biogenesis (**Figure 3**).(Mitchell, Li et al. 2007) Specifically: mAb10E5 binds to the αIIb head region and recognizes both the pro-αIIbβ3 and mature αIIbβ3 complex; mAb 7E3 binds to the β3 head region and also recognizes both the pro- and mature complex; mAb B1B5 binds to the αIIb tail and preferentially recognizes pro-αIIb and pro-αIIbβ3 complex, and mAb M148 preferentially recognizes mature αIIbβ3 but its epitope is not known.(Mitchell, Li et al.

2007) To determine whether DNAJC10 interacts with αIIb during a specific stage of biogenesis, αIIb was immunoprecipitated from megakaryocytes in the presence of MG132 using this panel of conformation-specific mAbs. DNAJC10 was most strongly coimmunoprecipitated by mAb B1B5, suggesting that DNAJC10 preferentially interacts with pro-αIIb or the pro-αIIbβ3 complex. In contrast, DNAJC10 coimmunoprecipitated less well with mAb M148, suggesting less interaction with mature αIIb. DNAJC10 also interacted with the precursor and/or mature αIIbβ3 complex, since it coimmunoprecipitated with the complex-specific mAb10E5. Since the ratio of pro-αIIbβ3 to mature αIIbβ3 is small in megakaryocytes,(Mitchell, Li et al. 2007) this binding pattern is consistent with DNAJC10 having bound preferentially to the small amount of pro-αIIbβ3 present in the cells. Together these findings suggest that DNAJC10 preferentially interacted with pro-αIIb and the pro-αIIbβ3 complex, rather than the mature complex.

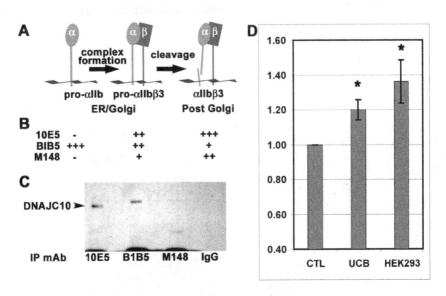

Fig. 4. Interaction of DNAJC10 with αIIbβ3 during biogenesis. A) Schematic of changing conformations of αIIbβ3 as it progresses through biogenesis. B) Changing specificity of 3 mAbs against αIIb as it progresses through distinct conformations during biogenesis. B1B5 preferentially recognizes pro-αIIb, while M148 shows preference for mature αIIb, and 10E5 recognizes the heterodimer complex.C) Immunoprecipitation and Western blot of proteins isolated from megakaryocytes, as described in text. DNAJC10 coimmunoprecipitated preferentially with αIIb that was pulled down by 10E5 and B1B5, but not M148, suggesting that DNAJC10 preferentially interacts with pro-αIIb and pro-αIIbβ3. The last lane is an IgG control. D) siRNA mediated knockdown of DNAJC10 increased surface expression of αIIbβ3 as measured by flow cytometry using an Alexa647-labeled anti-αIIbβ3 mAb (10E5). Expression was increased by 25 +\- 11% (p=0.02, n=4) in UCB-derived megakaryocytes (UCB) and by 35 +\- 12% (p=0.01, n=3) in HEK293 cells (HEK293) compared to control siRNA transfection (CTL).

3.4 DNAJC10 depletion increases surface expression of αIIbβ3

To determine whether the αIIb-DNAJC10 interaction had physiological relevance, we assessed its impact on the surface expression of αIIbβ3 in megakaryocytes. siRNA mediated knockdown of DNAJC10 was performed on both human megakaryocytes derived from UCB and on HEK293 cells expressing normal αIIb and β3. At least an 80% decrease in RNA level was achieved (data not shown). Knockdown of DNAJC10 increased αIIbβ3 surface expression on megakaryocytes by 25% +/- 11% (n = 4, p = 0.02), and on HEK293 cells expressing αIIbβ3 by 35% +/- 12% (n=4, p = 0.01) (**Figure 3D**).

3.5 Intracellular localization of DNAJC10 in megakaryocytes

DNAJC10 was localized within megakaryocytes by immunofluorescence microscopy (Figure 5). The distribution of DNAJC10 was compared to that of αIIb, β3, and the ER and Golgi compartments. Both αIIb and β3 were distributed throughout the ER as well as on the cell surface. DNAJC10 had a diffuse punctate distribution in the periphery of the cell, away from the nucleus, and colocalized with only a portion of αIIb and β3, consistent with their presumably transient interaction. There was partial overlap between the ER marker calnexin and DNAJC10, suggesting that part of the DNAJC10 distribution is outside the ER or at least

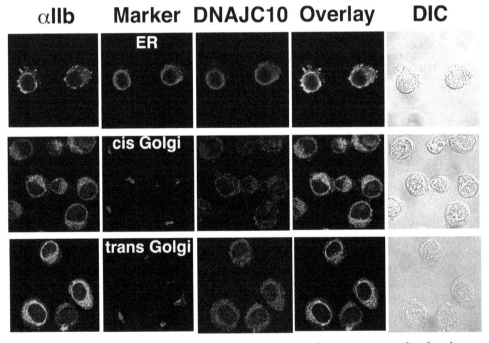

Fig. 4. Intracellular localization of DNAJC10. Cultured megakaryocytes were fixed and immunostained as described in the text. DNAJC10 (Blue) exhibited a punctate staining in the periphery of the cells, away from the nucleus. There was partial overlap of DNAJC10 with calnexin (Red) staining. αIIb (Green) was distributed throughout the ER and cell surface. While αIIb partially colocalized with the cis- and trans-Golgi, DNAJC10 did not.

separate from the distribution of calnexin in the ER. This finding was surprising since DNAJC10 has the ER-retention signal KDEL. DNAJC10 did not localize with markers for the cis- or trans-Golgi compartments.

4. Discussion

We have used a proteomics approach to identify novel proteins interacting with αIIb in megakaryocytes. Two different constructs of αIIb, representing normal αIIb and pro-αIIb subunits, were used to capture proteins interacting with both nascent and mature subunits. Megakaryocytes were derived from human UCB and used on day 8, which in our system yields high expression αIIbβ3 on the surface but no proplatelet formation.(Mitchell, Li et al. 2006) In all, 163 proteins were identified as potentially interacting with αIIb subunits; 98 were captured with normal αIIb and 79 with aIIbR858/G859G, with 14 overlapping (Table 1). Day 8 megakaryocytes express very high amounts of αIIb, most of which is mature αIIbβ3, resulting in a relatively small proportion of nascent αIIb. However, a large proportion of the mutant aIIbR858/G859G subunits are retained within the cell and degraded. Thus the difference between the two protein lists could partly be due to their differences in localization within the cell. This may be reflected in the larger proportion of ER and Golgi related proteins that were captured with the mutant subunit (**Table 2**). Only a few intracellular proteins have been reported to interact with αIIb and αIIbβ3, most notably talin, calnexin, and calreticulin (Intact and NCBI). Our two-step protein capture method was designed to isolate proteins with low affinity binding to αIIb, such as calnexin, while screening out higher affinity binding proteins, such as talin and β3. In accord with this expectation, both talin and β3 were identified in both the control and experimental lanes, and so were excluded from the final interaction list, while calnexin and calreticulin were identified only in the experimental lanes. Surprisingly, while DNAJC10 readily coimmunoprecipitates with αIIbβ3 from megakaryocytes, we have been unable to replicate this finding in HEK293 cells transfected with αIIb and β3, despite an abundance of DNAJC10 in HEK293 cells (data not shown). While this is in no way conclusive, it is suggestive of cell-specific interaction of αIIbβ3 and DNAJC10 in megakaryocytes. Comparison of our experimental results with previously reported platelet proteomic data and αIIbβ3 interaction data showed good correlation. About 70% of the proteins identified in our screens were reported as "present" in platelets in the Haem Atlas, a proteomic analysis of platelet protein content(Watkins, Gusnanto et al. 2009).

Two protein capturing strategies were used, each with strengths and weaknesses. The two-cell pull-down assay using Ni beads to capture poly-histidine-tagged αIIb, allowed the use of mutant cDNA constructs, such as αIIbR858G/R859G, as bait. However, by introducing a protein synthesized in HEK293 cells as bait, there was the potential for false positive identification of proteins that associated with αIIb in the HEK293 cells but not in megakaryocytes. Since the interactions of chaperone proteins are typically of low affinity, these proteins were most likely cleared by the washing steps and did not appear in the control lanes. Another source of false positives was non-specific binding to the Ni beads. Proteins with poly-His sequences (such as DEAH boxes) or naturally occurring Ni binding activity (such as keratin) could have bound to the beads, constituting false positives. However, virtually all of these potential false positives appeared in the control lanes as well and were excluded from analysis. The photoreactive crosslinking assay was intended to capture proteins in situ with αIIb in megakaryocytes. While crosslinking experiments typically produce high numbers of false positives, in our experiments we identified low numbers of proteins from both the experimental and control lanes. The low yield may be due in part to the short crosslinking time used. We found that more than 15 minutes of UV exposure caused excessive protein degradation, while shorter exposure resulted in low crosslinking activity.

Of the proteins captured using both αIIb and αIIbR858G/R859G the Hsp40-type chaperone protein, DNAJC10 (ERdj5), was notable due to its disulfide isomerase activity, since both αIIb and β3 require disulfide bond rearrangement for both biogenesis and function. (Shen, Meunier et al. 2002; Cunnea, Miranda-Vizuete et al. 2003; Dong, Bridges et al. 2008) Among its several functions, the ER chaperone protein BiP protects nearly-folded proteins against aggregation by binding to exposed hydrophobic patches.(Hendershot 2004) The Hsp40 chaperones bind to BiP and increase its efficiency of ATP hydrolysis, which allows BiP to release its substrate. DNAJC10 has been shown to be induced during ER stress, and may assist in delivering misfolded ER proteins to the proteasome for degradation.(Shen, Meunier et al. 2002; Cunnea, Miranda-Vizuete et al. 2003; Dong, Bridges et al. 2008)

DNAJC10 coimmunoprecipitated with both αIIb and β3 subunits in megakaryocytes, suggesting that it may bind the αIIbβ3 complex. The immunoprecipitation pattern obtained using a panel of conformation-specific mAbs(Mitchell, Li et al. 2007) indicated that DNAJC10 preferentially interacted with pro-αIIb or pro-αIIbβ3 rather than mature αIIbβ3. Together these findings suggest that DNAJC10 interacted with pro-αIIb up to the point of complex formation, but not after pro-αIIb cleavage (Figure 2). Thus DNAJC10 appears to be present and interacting with αIIb at a critical decision point during αIIbβ3 biogenesis, i.e. when pro-αIIb will either form the mature αIIbβ3 complex or be targeted to degradation.

Surprisingly, the distribution of DNAJC10, which has a KDEL ER-localization signal, was not confined to the ER, as judged by the distribution of calnexin. To determine if DNAJC10 was cycling to the Golgi and back, as many ER packaging proteins do, we looked for colocalization of DNAJC10 with cis and trans Golgi markers, and found none. The identity of the organelle(s) where DNAJC10 resides remains to be determined.

Depletion of DNAJC10 by siRNA resulted in an increase in surface expression of αIIbβ3 on both human megakaryocytes and transfected HEK293 cells (**Figure 2D**) Since DNAJC10 depletion led to an increase in αIIbβ3 surface expression, it appears to be a negative regulator of αIIbβ3 surface expression. These findings make DNAJC10 an interesting and potentially targetable protein for perturbing αIIbβ3 biogenesis.

5. Conclusion

While the details of DNAJC10-αIIb interaction remain to be investigated, the current findings provide proof of principle that manipulation of early events in αIIb biogenesis can result in altered expression levels of the mature αIIbβ3 receptor, thereby setting a precedent for a novel approach to integrin-related therapy. These studies also support the validity of the data set, although other putative interactions must be explored for greater validation. We hope that the data set created will be a useful tool for studying integrin and megakaryocyte biology.

By deciphering the αIIbβ3 biogenesis pathway we hope to gain an inroad into controlling the level of αIIbβ3 expression on platelets with the long-term goal of developing novel anti-thrombotic therapies. These types of therapy would not just inactivate the circulating platelets, but would modulate the megakaryocytes to make less adhesive platelets. One can imagine a scenario where patients at high risk of heart attack or stroke could be maintained on a drug that decreases their platelet αIIbβ3 expression. Below a certain level of expression, platelet activation and aggregation would be diminished but not completely eliminated, resulting in an overall decrease in platelet thrombus formation but not complete loss of platelet function. This type of therapy could potentially have a greater safety profile than current therapies that summarily inactivate circulating platelets.

This study also assembles some of the wide range of research methods available to hematology research. No single technique could have discovered, validated and explored the function of DNAJC10 in megakaryocytes: rather, a broad range of methods was required. This wide variety is part of what makes research exciting and underscores the benefits of collaboration.

6. Acknowledgement

We are grateful to Willem Ouwehand for helpful discussions and suggestions for data analysis, and to the National Cord Blood Bank at the New York Blood Center for providing the UCB. This work was supported in part by research funding from NIH grant KO8HL68622 (WBM).

7. References

Bray, P. F., J. P. Rosa, et al. (1986). "Biogenesis of the platelet receptor for fibrinogen: Evidence for separate precursors for glycoproteins IIb and IIIa." Proc Natl Acad Sci USA 83: 1480-1484.

Cline, M. S., M. Smoot, et al. (2007). "Integration of biological networks and gene expression data using Cytoscape." Nat. Protocols 2(10): 2366-2382.

Cunnea, P. M., A. Miranda-Vizuete, et al. (2003). "ERdj5, an Endoplasmic Reticulum (ER)-resident Protein Containing DnaJ and Thioredoxin Domains, Is Expressed in Secretory Cells or following ER Stress." Journal of Biological Chemistry 278(2): 1059-1066.

De Luca, G., G. Ucci, et al. (2009). "Benefits from small molecule administration as compared with abciximab among patients with ST-segment elevation myocardial infarction treated with primary angioplasty: a meta-analysis." J Am Coll Cardiol 53(18): 1668-73.

Dennis, G., B. Sherman, et al. (2003). DAVID: Database for Annotation, Visualization, and Integrated Discovery. Genome Biol 4(5):P3.

Dong, M., J. P. Bridges, et al. (2008). "ERdj4 and ERdj5 Are Required for Endoplasmic Reticulum-associated Protein Degradation of Misfolded Surfactant Protein C." Molecular Biology of the Cell 19(6): 2620-2630.

El.Golli, N., O. Issertial, et al. (2005). "Evidence for a Granule Targeting Sequence within Platelet Factor 4." Journal of Biological Chemistry 280(34): 30329-30335.

Hendershot, L. M. (2004). "The ER function BiP is a master regulator of ER function." Mt Sinai J Med 71(5): 289-97.

Huang, D. W., B. T. Sherman, et al. (2008). "Systematic and integrative analysis of large gene lists using DAVID bioinformatics resources." Nat. Protocols 4(1): 44-57.

King, S. M. and G. L. Reed (2002). "Development of platelet secretory granules." Seminars in Cell & Developmental Biology 13(4): 293-302.

Kolodziej, M. A., G. Vilaire, et al. (1991). "Study of the endoproteolytic cleavage of platelet glycoprotein IIb using oligonucleotide-mediated mutagenesis." J Biol Chem 266: 23499-23504.

Kumarathasan, P., S. Mohottalage, et al. (2005). "An optimized protein in-gel digest method for reliable proteome characterization by MALDI-TOF-MS analysis." Anal Biochem 346(1): 85-9.

Lo, B., L. Li, et al. (2005). "Requirement of VPS33B, a member of the Sec1/Munc18 protein family, in megakaryocyte and platelet {alpha}-granule biogenesis." Blood 106(13): 4159-4166.

Mitchell, W. B., J. Li, et al. (2006). "alphaIIbbeta3 biogenesis is controlled by engagement of alphaIIb in the calnexin cycle via the N15-linked glycan." Blood 107(7): 2713-2719.

Mitchell, W. B., J. Li, et al. (2007). "Mapping early conformational changes in alphaIIb and beta3 during biogenesis reveals a potential mechanism for alphaIIbbeta3 adopting its bent conformation." Blood 109(9): 3725-32.

Quinn, M. J., E. F. Plow, et al. (2002). "Platelet glycoprotein IIb/IIIa inhibitors: recognition of a two-edged sword?" Circulation 106(3): 379-85.

Rosa, J.-P. and R. P. McEver (1989). "Processing and assembly of the integrin, glycoprotein IIb-IIIa, in HEL cells." J Biol Chem 264: 12596-12603.

Shen, Y., L. Meunier, et al. (2002). "Identification and characterization of a novel endoplasmic reticulum (ER) DnaJ homologue, which stimulates ATPase activity of BiP in vitro and is induced by ER stress." J Biol Chem 277(18): 15947-56.

Tiwari, S., J. E. Italiano, Jr., et al. (2003). "A role for Rab27b in NF-E2-dependent pathways of platelet formation." Blood 102(12): 3970-9.

Topol, E. J., A. M. Lincoff, et al. (2002). "Multi-year follow-up of abciximab therapy in three randomized, placebo-controlled trials of percutaneous coronary revascularization." Am J Med 113(1): 1-6.

Watkins, N. A., A. Gusnanto, et al. (2009). "A HaemAtlas: characterizing gene expression in differentiated human blood cells." Blood 113(19): e1-9.

7

Neutrophil Chemotaxis and Polarization: When Asymmetry Means Movement

Doris Cerecedo

Laboratorio de Hematobiología, Escuela Nacional de Medicina y Homeopatía,
Instituto Politécnico Nacional (IPN), México DF,
México

1. Introduction

Neutrophils (also known as polymorphonuclear leukocytes or PMN), the first line of defense against intruding microorganisms, are produced in the bone marrow from stem cells that in turn proliferate and differentiate into mature neutrophils. They play an important role in host defense and contribute to inflammation-related tissue injuries. During inflammation, neutrophils extravasate across the endothelium that lines the blood vessel wall through a multistep process [1, 2], which includes rolling on and subsequent firm adhesion to endothelial cells.

Neutrophil migration through the vascular endothelial layer into lymphoid or inflamed tissues involves a dynamic regulation of cell adhesion in which new adhesions are formed at the cell's leading edge, [3] while filipodia and lamellipodia are generated as exploratory and motile projections and, coordinately, adhesions are released from the trailing edge [4].

For these events, the supply of adhesion molecules to the site of pseudopodial protrusion must be necessarily replenished in order to enable the cell to move forward. There is evidence that the membrane trafficking pathways that recycle adhesion receptors contribute to cell migration [5], which is crucial for polarization and migration in various cell types [6]. Preferential targeting of proteins to the leading or lagging edge of migrating cells is important for polarity and chemotaxis. Asymmetric distribution of proteins has implications beyond polarity and chemotaxis because these same proteins display characteristic localization patterns when cells undergo morphological changes in general. Several proteins have been identified as contributing to cell polarity organization and subsequent inflammatory-cell migration by regulating membrane trafficking. Ly49Q directs the organization of neutrophil polarization as well as neutrophil migration to inflammation sites by regulating membrane raft functions, reorganizing neutrophils in the presence of inflammatory signals, and maintaining neutrophil homeostasis in the absence of such signals [7]. In addition, regulated exocytosis plays a crucial role in conversion of inactive, circulating neutrophils into fully activated cells capable of chemotaxis, phagocytosis, and bacterial killing [8].

Polarity gives cells morphologically and functionally distinct spatial restriction to leading and/or lagging edges by relocating certain proteins or their activities selectively to the poles. Polarization provides cells with morphological, functional, and sensitivity differences to the chemoattractant, altering the way the cell responds to a gradient. Thus, polarization generates a bipolar mechanosensory state with a dynamic leading edge for acquiring new contacts and signals, a stiff mid-body, and a sticky uropod that is dragged along the substrate and stabilizes the cell position in complex environments [9, 10]. Hence, integration of signals generated in both cellular poles leads to a coordinated movement of the leukocyte.

Chemotaxis is conceptually divided into motility, directional sensing, and polarity; however, chemotaxis typically incorporates these features. Many molecules involved in chemotaxis include both lipids and proteins and are localized on the membrane or in the cortex, specifically at either the leading or the lagging edge of polarized cells.

Freely diffusing chemoattractant or soluble molecular cues, known as Damage-associated molecular patterns (DAMP), are liberated from damaged tissue in high abundance. DAMP include Adenosine triphosphate (ATP), bacterial peptides, heat-shock proteins, chromatin, and galectins [11], providing short-lived or pulsatile directional information, in addition to longer-lived cues provided by constitutive or induced tissue-bound chemoattractants [11]. Beyond adhesive migration arrest, local reduction of promigratory signals is achieved by down-modulation of chemoattractant receptors, receptor desensitization, and ligand competition, whereas termination of chemoattractant activity occurs through uptake by neutralizing chemoattractant receptors and/or proteolytic degradation. After ligation, chemoattractant receptors become internalized and are either recycled to the leading edge or stored in vesicles in the uropod, thus limiting the availability of both the chemoattractant and its receptor [12]. The end result is a cascade of activation and adhesion events designed to uptake leukocytes along vessel walls, activate these for them to make stable adhesions, allow them to locomote along the endothelial surface, and to transmigrate across endothelial junctions and through the subendothelial basal lamina, guiding them onto the damage site (Figure 1) [13].

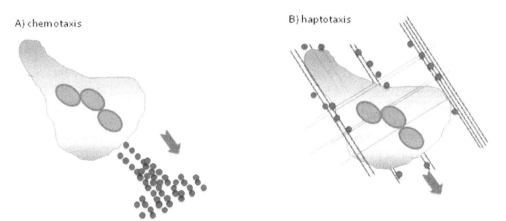

Fig. 1. Type chemotaxis in neutrophils. A) Chemotaxis triggered by soluble diffusing compounds leading to formation of the leading edge. B) Directed-mediated migration toward chemoattractants trapped on tissue structures.

2. Trafficking requirements

Trafficking leukocytes often reduce their migration speed, pause, and polarize toward the bound cell or the tissue structure to execute crucial functions including phagocytosis, cell-to-cell signaling, activation, and the release of cytokines or toxic factors toward an encountered cell.

At least three basic kinetic states govern leukocyte positioning in tissues, including fast migration (5 to 25 µm/min), slow and often locally confined movement (2 to 5 µm), and adhesive arrest, and these rapidly interconvert. Based on these kinetic states, leukocyte accumulation in tissues occurs by means of at least three distinct mechanisms: 1) local engagement of adhesion receptors causes individual leukocytes to stick and become immobilized at a specific spot; 2) degradation of promigratory signals causes cell populations to slow down or stop movement, and 3) loss of exit signals confines cells to a local microenvironment despite ongoing migration [14].

Complete migration arrest is mediated by activation of adhesion receptors on the moving cell followed by attachment to counter-receptors on other cells or on Endothelial cell migration (ECM) structures, leading to an immobilized cell. Within seconds, adhesion overrides ongoing promigratory signals; this is followed by cytoskeletal polarization toward the bound cell or the ECM structure [15].

3. Ensuring tightened adhesion

Endothelial cells (EC) are the critical substrate for leukocyte attachment and motility within the vascular lumen via adhesion molecules such as integrin, ligands whose expression is enhanced on activated ECs, which in turn react to molecules generated during infection and inflammation such as Tumor necrosis factor alpha (TNF- α), interleukin 1β (IL-1 β), and interleukin 17 (IL-17). Expression of these molecules can be further regulated through the cross-talk between EC and leucocytes; binding of PSGL-1 to P-selectin and E-selectin establishes the initial contact between neutrophils and activated ECs. Interaction of EC adhesion molecules (ICAM-1 and VCAM-1) with leukocyte ligands triggers the formation of docking structures or transmigrating cups [16, 17], which embrace adherent leucocytes [18]. Additionally, formation of pro-adhesive sites termed "endothelial adhesive platforms" (EAP) is determined by the existence of pre-formed, tetraspanin-enriched microdomains such as CD9, CD151, and CD81 [19].

Adherent leukocytes may transmigrate at the point of initial arrest, but sometimes rather locomote laterally to preferred sites of Transendothelial cell migration (TECM) [20, 21]; *in vitro* and *in vivo* luminal crawling is dependent on β2 integrins and its blockade appears to increase the incidence of trans- as opposed to paracellular cell migration [21]. The junctional adhesion molecule A (JAM-A), an adhesion molecule expressed on both EC and leukocytes [22], regulate integrin internalization and re-cycling [23].

There are other molecules and mechanisms that have been recently implicated in leukocyte motility; for example, it has been demonstrated both *in vivo* and *in vitro* that platelets enhance neutrophil TECM in inflammation, which is consistent with a mechanistic role for PSGL-1 for this response [24].

4. Neutrophil mobilization

Leukocyte interactions with the endothelial surface trigger cellular and sub-cellular events that initiate and/or facilitate leukocyte passage through the endothelium by interaction of docking structures with cytoskeleton via adaptor proteins such as vinculin, paxilin, and Ezrin, radixin, and moesin (ERM) proteins [18, 25], although Guanosine triphosphate (GTP)ases (RhoG and RhoA) induce actin polymerization leading to the formation of small membrane protrusions called apical cups or docking structures.

Once firm adhesion is established, two routes can be taken for transendothelial migration: the transcellular road, whereby neutrophils penetrate the individual EC, or the paracellular road, by which neutrophils squeeze between EC Figure 2.

A number of molecules at EC junctions actively facilitate leukocyte transmigration via a paracellular route such as Platelet endothelial adhesion molecular-1 (PECAM-1), Intracellular adhesion molecule-2 (ICAM-2), CD99, Endothelial cell-selective adhesion molecules (ESAM), and junctional adhesion molecules (JAM) [22, 26] and, according to *in vivo* and *in vitro* evidence, a sequence of events has been suggested that regulate neutrophil transmigration to EC walls and that include the following: (i) ICAM-1 and ICAM-2 on the luminal surface of EC and within the junction may provide a haptotactic gradient to guide neutrophils to EC junctions via their β2 partners (LFA-1 and MAC-1) [27]; (ii) once within junctions, endothelial-cell JAM-A (through interaction, possibly with LFA-1) [28], facilitates completion of neutrophil passage through the EC layer, and (iii) within the EC junction, homophilic interactions between endothelial and leukocyte PECAM-1 stimulates neutrophils to express the key leukocyte laminin receptor, integrin α6β1, on their surface, which facilitates neutrophil passage through the vascular basement membrane [29-31]. It is also noteworthy that signals from ICAM-1 activate Src and Pyk-2 tyrosine kinases, which phosphorylate VE-Cadherin, destabilizing its bonds and loosening endothelial cell-cell junctions [32].

The transcellular route is taken by some 20% of neutrophils and has been observed in a broad range of tissues including bone marrow, thymus, lymph nodes, pancreas, and the blood brain barrier [33]. Apparently, there is clear evidence for the formation of a transcellular pore requiring membrane fusion and displacement of cytoplasmic organelles during transcellular migration. Vesicular vacuolar organelles (VVO) are enriched at pore-formation sites, apparently providing additional membrane to the area and facilitating the fusion of apical and basal membranes in a process dependent on SNARE-containing membrane fusion complexes [34], and there is increasing evidence for a role for caveolin-1 in determining transendothelial migration route [35].

Carman et al. (2008) [34] have identified *in vitro* and *in vivo* the existence of protrusive podosomes on the basal side of crawling lymphocytes ; these protrusive podosomes appear to identify the cell's thinner peripheral areas rather than the perinuclear region in order to identify a pore formation-permissive site. These dynamic investigatory podosomes can then extend to form invasive podosomes, resembling invadopodia of metastatic tumor cells, which extend down into the EC, bringing the apical and basal membranes into close apposition.

5. Mobilization beyond the endothelium

Beyond the endothelium, migrating cells face two further barriers; the pericyte sheath, and the tough venular Basement membrane (BM) [36, 37]. Neutrophils have the ability to migrate through the pericyte sheath via both para- [38] and transcellular pathways

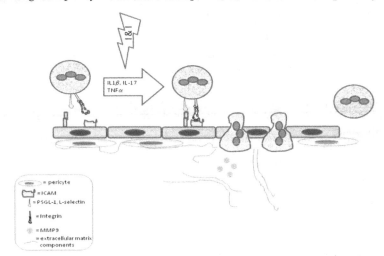

Fig. 2. Hypothetical sequence of events during neutrophil transmigration. Neutrophils are tethered by P- and E-selectin on endothelial cells and PSGL, L-selectin, and CD44 on neutrophils simultaneously participate in neutrophil rolling and activation. Endothelium activation by stimuli such as IL-1β, IL17, TNF-α promote transmigration dependent of molecules such as PECAM-1, ICAM-1, and JAM-A, thus unzipping the tight junctions and restoring themselves while TNF- α promote transmigration via ESAM. Neutrophils take trans- or paracellular routes. Postendothelial cleavage of structural proteins occurs by means of secreted or membrane-anchored matrix metalloproteases (MMPs). Abbreviations: Basement membrane (BM), Endothelial cells (EC), Platelet endothelial cell adhesion molecule (PECAM-1), Intracellular adhesion molecule-1 (ICAM-1), Endothelial cell-selective adhesion molecule (ESAM), Tumor necrosis factor- α (TNF-α) [39].

On the other hand, leukocyte penetration of the vascular BM depends on the vascular bed. Additionally, it has recently been shown that the venular BM contains pre-formed regions with low expression of certain BM components, denominated Low expression regions (LER), which are preferentially utilized by transmigrating neutrophils and monocytes [29, 40]. Alignment of these regions with gaps between adjacent pericytes suggests a key role for these cells in vascular BM generation *in vivo*. Vascular BM architecture depends on the migration of neutrophils, but not monocytes, through the LER remodeling these regions and increasing their size [41, 42], suggesting the involvement of proteases in this response.

6. Neutrophil polarization and migration structures

Neutrophils present in the blood are able to tissue-injury or infection signals by adhering to vascular endothelial cells, then transmigrating across the endothelium through the basement membrane and homing into sites of infection or inflammation.

The following four steps mediate the multiple cycles of attachment and detachment generating neutrophil forward movement during migration: the leading edge protrudes one or several pseudopods by actin flow; protruding membrane and surface receptors interact with the substrate; actomyosin-mediated contraction of the cell body occurs in mid-region, thus the rear of the cell moves forward. Neutrophil migration moves at up to 30 μm/min, lacks strong adhesive interactions to the tissue, and commonly preserves tissue integrity [9].

Receptors such as β2 integrins in neutrophils show discrete relocation toward the tips of ruffles [43]. The mid-region of amoeboid cells contains the nucleus and a relatively immobile cell region that maintains the front-rear axis. The trailing edge contains the highly glycosylated surface receptors CD43 and CD44, adhesion receptors including intercellular adhesion molecule (ICAM)-1, ICAM-3, β1 integrins, and Ezrin-radixin-moesin adaptor proteins (ERM), as well as GM-1-type cholesterol-rich microdomains [44]. The uropod mediates cell–matrix and cell–cell interactions during migration and has a putative anchoring function [45]. The uropod extends rearward from the nucleus and contains the microtubule-organizing center and rearward-polarized microtubules, the Golgi, and abundant actin-binding ERM proteins. In association with microtubules, mitochondria localize to the rear of the cell that, presumably, due to local ATP delivery to the region of ATP-dependent actomyosin contraction, is required for proper polarization, uropod retraction, and migration [10, 46].

7. Polarization of cytoskeletal and signaling scaffolds

In neutrophils, polarization and migration to chemoattractant gradients such as chemokines and cytokines, lipid mediators, bacterial factors, and Extracellular matrix (ECM) degradation products including collagen, fibronectin, and elastin fragments [47, 48], is known as chemotaxis. After chemokines and chemoattractants bind to the extracellular domains of their cognate G protein-coupled receptor (GPCRs) pseudo- and lamellipodia protrusion are induced. In leukocytes, the majority of GPCRs transmit through the α subunit of Giα. These GPCR include the following: the fMLP (N-formyl-Met-Leu-Phe) receptor and the C5a receptor; chemokine receptors including CCR7, CXCR4, CXCR5, and CCR3; the leukotriene B4 receptor BLT1; sphingosine-1-phosphate receptors 1–4 (S1P1–4), and Lysophosphatidic acid (LPA) receptors 1–3 [49]. All these GPCR mediate promigratory signals but also enhance cell activation. A key GPCR-mediated pathway is signaling through the Phosphatidylinositol-3-kinase (PI(3)K), which contains the p110γ catalytic subunit). PI(3)K-γ is recruited into the inner leaflet of the plasma membrane by the G protein βγ subunit, where it becomes activated and subsequently phosphorylates Phosphatidylinositol phosphates (PIP) and other effectors [50]. PIP serve as docking sites for pleckstrin-homology domain-containing proteins, notably Akt (also known as protein kinase B), which is implicated in inducing actin polymerization and pseudopod protrusion by phosphorylating downstream effectors [51] such as the actin-binding protein girdin [52]. A second pathway linked with PI(3)K activation is induced by ζ-chain-associated receptors, including T cell receptors (TCRs) and receptors FC (FcRs). These receptors signal through tyrosine kinases Lck and Zap-70 to class Ia PI(3)Ks (consisting of p110δ) and activate downstream Akt, as well as the GTPases Rac and Cdc42 [53]. A third, PI(3)K-independent pathway induced by the fMLP receptor in neutrophils leads to the activation of p38 mitogen-associated protein kinase and downstream Rac activation [54, 55]. Ultimately, Rac induces actin polymerization through WAVE (Scar) and Arp2/3. WAVE, a member of the WASP family of actin-binding proteins, mediates actin filament formation [56], while Arp2/3 causes sideward branching of actin filaments. Together, these activities generate interconnected, branched networks [57]. Thus, promigratory signals received at the leading edge generate local Rac activation and actin network protrusion, pushing the plasma membrane outward. Preferential receptor-sensitivity mechanisms at the leading edge are likely diverse and may include local signal- amplification mechanisms [58] and exclusion of counter-regulatory proteins. The mid-region generates actomyosin-based stiffness and contractility, limits lateral protrusions, and thereby maintains a stable, bipolar cortex. The cytoskeletal motor protein myosin II, located in the central and rear regions of leukocytes, promotes actin-filament contraction and limits lateral protrusions. Myosin II cross-links actin filaments in parallel, forming the contractile shell required to hold the extending cell together and propelling the cell nucleus, the most rigid part of the cell, forward [59].

8. Leukocyte movement in different environments and initial migration

Neutrophils are able to migrate along or through 2- or 3- dimensional (2-D or 3-D) surfaces. 2-D Surfaces, such as inner vessel walls, peritoneum, and pleura, require integrin-mediated attachment known as haptokinesis and polarized adhesion through binding of integrins α4β1 and LFA-1 (αLβ2) to their counterparts (VCAM-1 and ICAM-1)(Figure 3A). In contrast, migration in 3-D, ECM environments, which are composed mainly of cellular (lymph node) or fibrillar ECM components, is integrin-independent and cells use weakly adhesive-to-nonadhesive interaction and traction mechanisms that are mediated by actin flow along the confining ECM scaffold structure, contributing to shape change and squeezing [9, 44, 60] (Figure 3B). It is likely that neutrophils adapt to tissue geometry and follow paths of least resistance, a process known as contact guidance (Figure 2).

For passage, the first postendothelial tissue structure and barrier to cells undergoing diapedesis, locally confined cleavage of the structural proteins laminin-10 and type IV collagen, occurs by secreted or membrane-anchored Matrix metalloproteases (MMPs) and serine proteases [61, 62]. Cell-body deformation is coupled with cytoplasmic propulsion and streaming through preexisting or newly formed pores; the deformation and constriction capability of leukocytes is considerable, especially for neutrophils [63].

Interestingly, a recent study showed the existence of venule-wall regions in which laminin-10, collagen IV, and nidogen-2 expression is considerably diminished; neutrophil transmigration enlarges the size of these regions, and their protein content is further reduced, an effect that appears to involve neutrophil-derived serine proteases [40]. Location of proteases at the leukocyte cell surface takes place through two different mechanisms: either by endogenous expression as transmembrane proteins or by binding of extracellular proteases to integral membrane receptors. Integrins are shown to act as anchoring receptors for several proteases including MMPs; such interactions have been detected in caveolae, invadopodia, and at the leading edge of migrating cells, where directed proteolytic activity is required [64]. In this regard, pro-MMP-2 and pro-MMP-9 are bound to αLβ2 and αMβ2 on the surface of activated leukemic cells, and inhibition of these complexes blocks β2 integrin-dependent leukocyte migration [65]. Pro-MMP-9– αMβ2 complexes are primarily localized into intracellular granules of resting neutrophils, but after cellular activation, they are relocalized to the cell surface [66]. Neutrophils secrete laminin, suggesting that leukocyte-derived matrix proteins might also contribute to the transmigration process [67].

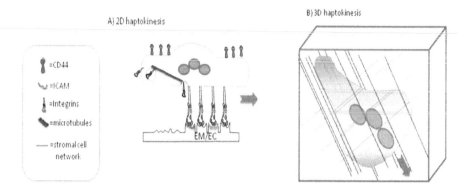

Fig. 3. Type-substrate interaction with neutrophils. A) Two-dimensional integrin-mediated neutrophil migration. *In vivo* 2-D haptokinetic migration is present during crawling on Endothelial cell (EC) or through Extracellular matrix (EM). B) Three-dimensional integrin-independent neutrophil migration. *In vivo*, this occurs through organized tissue structures.

9. Role of cytoskeleton in regulating integrin adhesiveness

Integrins are a superfamily of heterodimeric cell-surface receptors that are found in a broad range of animal species [68]; their main role, as their name implies, is to integrate the cell cytoskeleton with adhesion points of extracellular matrix and cell-surface ligands in order to mediate essential cellular processes such as cell-cell and cell-extracellular matrix interactions, polarization in response to extracellular cues, cell migration, differentiation, survival, and cell-pathogen interactions [69].

In vertebrates, 19 different integrin α subunits and eight different integrin β subunits have been reported, in combination forming about 25 αβ heterodimers [70]. The majority of α/β-subunit combinations can be organized into three fundamental groups based on subunit type (β1, β2, and β3, or αv chains, on the extracellular matrix protein-type recognized, or on the specific adhesion motifs [71] (Table 1).

β1 integrins form the first and largest group of integrins and are ubiquitously distributed in nucleated cells as well as in platelets. β1 Integrins are expressed in bone marrow-derived cells (except for neutrophils), in certain tumor cells, and in muscle development. A second major group of integrins shares either the β3 or the αv subunit (Table 1) and recognizes different ligands from a broad gamma of cell and tissue sources. Integrins with the αv subunit may form dimers with at least five different β chains, including the β1 chain. Subunits αv and β3 recognize Arg-Gly-Asp (RGD) domains present in extracellular matrix proteins.

The third group of integrins shares the β2 integrin chain, whose expression is restricted to leukocytes [72] (Table 1). Receptors such as α4β2, also known as the LFA-1 integrin, determine the capability of leukocytes in endothelial epithelium transmigration and recognize members of the Intercellular adhesion molecule (ICAM) family of adhesion proteins. In contrast, expression of αMβ2 is restricted to monocytes, macrophages, and granulocytes; it recognizes

	Ligands	Motifs	Distribution
β1 integrin			
α1β1	*Co1,Lm*	ND	*EC, SMC, TC, Monos*
α2β1	*Col, Fn, Lm, Echovirus 1*	*DGEA*	*Plt, EC, Fb, SMC, TC, EPC*
α3β1	*Col, Epiligrin, Fn, Lm, Invasin*	*RGD*	*EC, TC, EPC, Fb*
α4β1	Fn, Invasin, VCAM-1	EILDV (Fn) QIDSPL(VCAM-1)	TC, Monos, Eos, LC, ER
α5β1	Fn, Invasin	RGD	Fb, EC, Monos, TC, Plt
α6β1	Lm, Invasin	ND	Plts, TC, EC, EPC
α7β1	Lm	ND	Myocytes
α8β1		ND	*SMC*
α9β1	Col, Lm, Tenascin	RGD	EPC, Myocytes
αϖβ1	Fn,Vn	RGD	Fb
αv and β3 integrins			
αvβ1	Fn, Vn	RGD	Fb
αvβ5	Vn, HIV Tat, Adenovirus	RGD	EC, EPC, Fb, Tumors
αvβ6	Fn, Tenascin	RGD	
αvβ3	Vn	RGD	Melanoma
αvβ3	Col, Fib, Fn, Lm Opn, Pn, TSP, Vn	RGD	EC, FB, Monos, SMC, OC
	vWf, HIV Tat, Tenascin, Adenovirus		Plt, Tumors
αIIbβ3	Col, Fib, Fn, TSP, Vn, vWf, *Borrelia*	KQAGDV	Plt, Mega
αRβ3	Fib, Fn, Vn, vWf	RGD	PMN
β2 integrin			
αLβ2	ICAMs (1-3)	ND	TC, BC, LGL, Monos, PMN, Eos
αMβ2	Fib, Fn, Factor X, ICAM-1, iC3b		PMN, Monos, Macros, LGL
αχβ2	Fib, iC3b	GPRP	Monos, Macros, PMN
αΔβ2		ND	TC. Macros
Other integrins			
α6β4	Lm	ND	EC, EPC, Schwann cells
α4β7	Fn, MAdCAM, VCAM-1	EILDV (Fn)	Gut homing, TC
αEβ7	E-Cadherin	ND	Epithelial TC

Table 1. Classification of integrins according to ligand motifs and distribution.
Abbreviations: BC = B cells; Col = Collagen; EC = Endothelial cells; Eos = Eosinophils; EPC = Epithelial cells; Fb = Fibroblasts; Fib = Fibrinogen; Fn = Fibronectin; iC3b = inactivated component of complement; Lm = Laminin; LGL = Large granular lymphocytes; Macros = Macrophages; Mega = Megakaryocytes; Monos = Monocytes; OPN = Osteopontin; Plt = Platelets; PMN = Neutrophils or Polymorphonuclear leukocytes; SMC = Smooth muscle cells; TC = T cells; TSP = Thrombospondin; Vn = Vitronectin; vWf = von Willebrand disease. (Modified from [71]).

fibrinogen and inactivated C3b, playing an important role in the phagocytosis of opsonized particles and bacteria [73]. The fourth group of integrins includes three integrins (α6β4, α4β7, and αEβ7); these integrins recognize extracellular matrix components as well as adhesion molecules of the Immunoglobulin superfamily (IgSF). Common integrins expressed on leukocytes and their counterparts are summarized in Table 1.

Association of extended forms of integrins with the cortical cytoskeleton is required to integrate mechanical forces from shear flow and F-actin and to undergo ligand-induced strengthening at endothelial contacts. Key differences between α4 and β2 integrins regarding their increase in cytoskeleton-mediated avidity may occur. The α4 integrins can bind paxillin upon dephosphorylation of Ser988 in their cytoplasmic domain at the sides and rear pole of the cell, whereas PKA-mediated phosphorylation of these integrins is confined to the cell's leading edge. Paxillin regulates α4 integrin function (tethering and firm adhesion) [74], enhancing their migration rate and reducing their spreading, and paxillin–α4 interaction downregulates the formation of focal adhesions, stress fibers, and lamellipodia by triggering activation of different tyrosine kinases, such as Focal adhesion kinase (FAK), Pyk2, Src, and Abl [75, 76]. The α4–paxillin complex inhibits stable lamellipodia by recruiting an ADP-ribosylation factor (Arf)-GTPase-activating protein that decreases Arf activity, thereby inhibiting Rac, and limiting lamellipodia formation to the cell front [77]. Recently, it was discovered that integrins can induce PIP5K1C-90 polarization independently of chemoattractants. This integrin-induced PIP5K1C-90 polarization works together with chemoattractant signaling in regulating neutrophil polarization and directionality *in vitro* and infiltration *in vivo* [78].

It has been described that LFA-1 and Mac-1 may use adapter molecules talin, α-actinin, filamin, and 14-3-3 to anchor to the actin cytoskeleton properly [79, 80]. Regarding subcellular localization, LFA-1 pattern ranges from low- in the lamellipodia to high expression in the uropod. However, it has been reported that high-affinity clustered LFA-1 is restricted to a mid-cell zone, termed the "focal zone", different from focal adhesions and focal contacts. In addition, talin, properly activated by phosphorylation or by phosphatidylinositol-4,5-bisphosphate (PIP2), is essential for formation and stability of the focal zone and for LFA-1-dependent migration [81].

Locomotion can be regulated by integrins because the signals involved in integrin-mediated leukocyte firm adhesion to endothelium are subsequently attenuated to allow leukocyte migration toward an appropriate transmigration site. β2 integrins appear to promote direct locomotion, success in correct positioning at the endothelial junction, and effective diapedesis [82, 83]. Upon interaction with their ligands, integrins activate distinct myosin-contractility effectors, actin-remodeling GTPases, and molecules involved in microtubule-network regulation at motile leukocyte leading and trailing edges [84]. During cell polarization, Cdc42, Myosin light chain kinase (MLCK), Rac, RapL, Rap1, mDia, myosin-IIA, and chemokine receptors are redistributed to the cellular front, participating in exploratory filopodia formation and in lamellipodia extension. In contrast, Rho- and Rho-associated kinase (ROCK) (both involved in trailing- edge retraction), the Microtubule-organizing center (MTOC), and adhesion receptors ICAM-1, ICAM-3, CD44, and CD43 move toward the rear pole [85].

Recently, dystrophin protein-adhesion complex proteins such as short dystrophins, utrophins, and the dystrophin-associated protein complex (α-dystroglycan, α–syntrophin and α–dystrobrevins) form part of actin-based structures such as lamellipodia and uropod, in which their polarized distribution is evident and their feasible role in chemotaxis and migration is strongly suggested [86].

Other proteins with differential distribution appear in Figure 4 and the list is increasing.

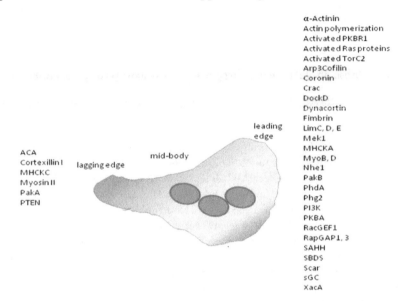

Fig. 4. Neutrophil regions observed after triggered activation and differential protein distribution. Adapted from [87].

10. Conclusions

For exiting the vasculature, leukocytes follow a consecutive sequence of events that starts with the first contact of free-flowing neutrophil to the vascular endothelium followed by leukocyte rolling along the vessel wall. Both events are mediated by specialized receptor ligand pairs consisting of a member of the selectin family of adhesion molecules and specific carbohydrate determinants on selectin ligands. During rolling, leukocytes are in intimate contact with the vascular endothelium, enabling endothelial-bound chemokines to interact with their respective chemokine receptors on the neutrophil surface. Upon binding to the receptor, chemokine receptor-mediated signaling events trigger the activation of β2 integrins. Activated integrins subsequently interact with endothelium-expressed ligands, which lead to a reduction in leukocyte rolling velocity and eventually, to mediate stable adhesion and migration across the blood vessel wall. Following neutrophil spreading and intravascular crawling along the endothelium, tethered neutrophils reach the correct spot for exiting into tissue. Upon neutrophil stimulation, actin, which is one of the major components of the cytoskeleton in neutrophils, is reorganized through reversible cycles of polymerization and depolymerization, thereby comprising the driving motor for the formation of lamellipodia and pseudopodia during migration and phagocytosis. Activated neutrophils become polarized with a contracted tail (uropod) in the rear and F-actin-rich protrusions at the front and start crawling. Actin and the proteins regulating actin polymerization are key players in the establishment of morphological and functional cell polarity. Actin polymerization and membrane ruffling comprise the first events leading to the establishment of chemoattractant-stimulated neutrophil polarization.

Morphological changes imply cytoskeleton redistribution triggered by certain activated pathways which are spatiotemporally coordinated.

Undesrtanding the molecular and cellular interactions that regulate neutrophil transmigration could be of great value to design novel therapeutic strategies directed to promote or suppress an inflammatory response, which may be of potential benefit under physiological or pathological circumstances.

11. References

[1] Luo BH, Carman CV, and Springer TA. Structural basis of integrin regulation and signaling. Annu Rev Immunol. 2007; 25:619-47.

[2] Rose DM, Alon R, and Ginsberg MH. Integrin modulation and signaling in leukocyte adhesion and migration. Immunol Rev. 2007; 218:126-34.

[3] Alcaide P, Auerbach S, and Luscinskas FW. Neutrophil recruitment under shear flow: it's all about endothelial cell rings and gaps. Microcirculation. 2009; 16:43-57.

[4] Woodfin A, Voisin MB, Beyrau M, Colom B, Caille D, Diapouli FM, Nash GB, Chavakis T, Albelda SM, Rainger GE, Meda P, Imhof BA, and Nourshargh S. The junctional adhesion molecule JAM-C regulates polarized transendothelial migration of neutrophils in vivo. Nat Immunol. 2011; 12:761-9.

[5] Veale KJ, Offenhauser C, and Murray RZ. The role of the recycling endosome in regulating lamellipodia formation and macrophage migration. Commun Integr Biol. 2011; 4:44-7.

[6] Pierini LM, Eddy RJ, Fuortes M, Seveau S, Casulo C, and Maxfield FR. Membrane lipid organization is critical for human neutrophil polarization. J Biol Chem. 2003; 278:10831-41.

[7] Sasawatari S, Yoshizaki M, Taya C, Tazawa A, Furuyama-Tanaka K, Yonekawa H, Dohi T, Makrigiannis AP, Sasazuki T, Inaba K, and Toyama-Sorimachi N. The Ly49Q receptor plays a crucial role in neutrophil polarization and migration by regulating raft trafficking. Immunity. 2010; 32:200-13.

[8] Faurschou M and Borregaard N. Neutrophil granules and secretory vesicles in inflammation. Microbes Infect. 2003; 5:1317-27.

[9] Wolf K, Muller R, Borgmann S, Brocker EB, and Friedl P. Amoeboid shape change and contact guidance: T-lymphocyte crawling through fibrillar collagen is independent of matrix remodeling by MMPs and other proteases. Blood. 2003; 102:3262-9.

[10] Friedl P and Brocker EB. The biology of cell locomotion within three-dimensional extracellular matrix. Cell Mol Life Sci. 2000; 57:41-64.

[11] Kono H and Rock KL. How dying cells alert the immune system to danger. Nat Rev Immunol. 2008; 8:279-89.

[12] Servant G, Weiner OD, Neptune ER, Sedat JW, and Bourne HR. Dynamics of a chemoattractant receptor in living neutrophils during chemotaxis. Mol Biol Cell. 1999; 10:1163-78.

[13] Muller WA. Mechanisms of leukocyte transendothelial migration. Annu Rev Pathol. 2011; 6:323-44.

[14] Friedl P and Weigelin B. Interstitial leukocyte migration and immune function. Nat Immunol. 2008; 9:960-9.

[15] Gunzer M, Weishaupt C, Hillmer A, Basoglu Y, Friedl P, Dittmar KE, Kolanus W, Varga G, and Grabbe S. A spectrum of biophysical interaction modes between T cells and different antigen-presenting cells during priming in 3-D collagen and in vivo. Blood. 2004; 104:2801-9.

[16] Carman CV and Springer TA. A transmigratory cup in leukocyte diapedesis both through individual vascular endothelial cells and between them. J Cell Biol. 2004; 167:377-88.

[17] Barreiro O, Yanez-Mo M, Serrador JM, Montoya MC, Vicente-Manzanares M, Tejedor R, Furthmayr H, and Sanchez-Madrid F. Dynamic interaction of VCAM-1 and ICAM-1 with moesin and ezrin in a novel endothelial docking structure for adherent leukocytes. J Cell Biol. 2002; 157:1233-45.

[18] Barreiro O, de la Fuente H, Mittelbrunn M, and Sanchez-Madrid F. Functional insights on the polarized redistribution of leukocyte integrins and their ligands during leukocyte migration and immune interactions. Immunol Rev. 2007; 218:147-64.

[19] Barreiro O, Zamai M, Yanez-Mo M, Tejera E, Lopez-Romero P, Monk PN, Gratton E, Caiolfa VR, and Sanchez-Madrid F. Endothelial adhesion receptors are recruited to adherent leukocytes by inclusion in preformed tetraspanin nanoplatforms. J Cell Biol. 2008; 183:527-42.

[20] Schenkel AR, Mamdouh Z, and Muller WA. Locomotion of monocytes on endothelium is a critical step during extravasation. Nat Immunol. 2004; 5:393-400.

[21] Phillipson M, Heit B, Colarusso P, Liu L, Ballantyne CM, and Kubes P. Intraluminal crawling of neutrophils to emigration sites: a molecularly distinct process from adhesion in the recruitment cascade. J Exp Med. 2006; 203:2569-75.

[22] Ley K, Laudanna C, Cybulsky MI, and Nourshargh S. Getting to the site of inflammation: the leukocyte adhesion cascade updated. Nat Rev Immunol. 2007; 7:678-89.

[23] Cera MR, Fabbri M, Molendini C, Corada M, Orsenigo F, Rehberg M, Reichel CA, Krombach F, Pardi R, and Dejana E. JAM-A promotes neutrophil chemotaxis by controlling integrin internalization and recycling. J Cell Sci. 2009; 122:268-77.

[24] Lam FW, Burns AR, Smith CW, and Rumbaut RE. Platelets enhance neutrophil transendothelial migration via P-selectin glycoprotein ligand-1. Am J Physiol Heart Circ Physiol. 2011; 300:H468-75.

[25] Wittchen ES. Endothelial signaling in paracellular and transcellular leukocyte transmigration. Front Biosci. 2009; 14:2522-45.

[26] Dejana E. Endothelial cell-cell junctions: happy together. Nat Rev Mol Cell Biol. 2004; 5:261-70.

[27] van Buul JD, van Rijssel J, van Alphen FP, van Stalborch AM, Mul EP, and Hordijk PL. ICAM-1 clustering on endothelial cells recruits VCAM-1. J Biomed Biotechnol. 2010:120328.

[28] Wojcikiewicz EP, Koenen RR, Fraemohs L, Minkiewicz J, Azad H, Weber C, and Moy VT. LFA-1 binding destabilizes the JAM-A homophilic interaction during leukocyte transmigration. Biophys J. 2009; 96:285-93.

[29] Voisin MB, Woodfin A, and Nourshargh S. Monocytes and neutrophils exhibit both distinct and common mechanisms in penetrating the vascular basement membrane in vivo. Arterioscler Thromb Vasc Biol. 2009; 29:1193-9.

[30] Woodfin A, Voisin MB, Imhof BA, Dejana E, Engelhardt B, and Nourshargh S. Endothelial cell activation leads to neutrophil transmigration as supported by the sequential roles of ICAM-2, JAM-A, and PECAM-1. Blood. 2009; 113:6246-57.

[31] Dangerfield J, Larbi KY, Huang MT, Dewar A, and Nourshargh S. PECAM-1 (CD31) homophilic interaction up-regulates alpha6beta1 on transmigrated neutrophils in vivo and plays a functional role in the ability of alpha6 integrins to mediate leukocyte migration through the perivascular basement membrane. J Exp Med. 2002; 196:1201-11.

[32] van Buul JD and Hordijk PL. Endothelial signalling by Ig-like cell adhesion molecules. Transfus Clin Biol. 2008; 15:3-6.

[33] Carman CV. Mechanisms for transcellular diapedesis: probing and pathfinding by 'invadosome-like protrusions'. J Cell Sci. 2009; 122:3025-35.

[34] Carman CV, Sage PT, Sciuto TE, de la Fuente MA, Geha RS, Ochs HD, Dvorak HF, Dvorak AM, and Springer TA. Transcellular diapedesis is initiated by invasive podosomes. Immunity. 2007; 26:784-97.

[35] Marmon S, Hinchey J, Oh P, Cammer M, de Almeida CJ, Gunther L, Raine CS, and Lisanti MP. Caveolin-1 expression determines the route of neutrophil extravasation through skin microvasculature. Am J Pathol. 2009; 174:684-92.

[36] Hirschi KK and D'Amore PA. Pericytes in the microvasculature. Cardiovasc Res. 1996; 32:687-98.

[37] Rowe RG and Weiss SJ. Breaching the basement membrane: who, when and how? Trends Cell Biol. 2008; 18:560-74.

[38] Voisin MB, Probstl D, and Nourshargh S. Venular basement membranes ubiquitously express matrix protein low-expression regions: characterization in multiple tissues and remodeling during inflammation. Am J Pathol. 2010; 176:482-95.

[39] Feng D, Nagy JA, Pyne K, Dvorak HF, and Dvorak AM. Neutrophils emigrate from venules by a transendothelial cell pathway in response to FMLP. J Exp Med. 1998; 187:903-15.

[40] Wang S, Voisin MB, Larbi KY, Dangerfield J, Scheiermann C, Tran M, Maxwell PH, Sorokin L, and Nourshargh S. Venular basement membranes contain specific matrix protein low expression regions that act as exit points for emigrating neutrophils. J Exp Med. 2006; 203:1519-32.

[41] Mamdouh Z, Kreitzer GE, and Muller WA. Leukocyte transmigration requires kinesin-mediated microtubule-dependent membrane trafficking from the lateral border recycling compartment. J Exp Med. 2008; 205:951-66.

[42] Reichel CA, Rehberg M, Lerchenberger M, Berberich N, Bihari P, Khandoga AG, Zahler S, and Krombach F. Ccl2 and Ccl3 mediate neutrophil recruitment via induction of protein synthesis and generation of lipid mediators. Arterioscler Thromb Vasc Biol. 2009; 29:1787-93.

[43] Fernandez-Segura E, Garcia JM, and Campos A. Topographic distribution of CD18 integrin on human neutrophils as related to shape changes and movement induced by chemotactic peptide and phorbol esters. Cell Immunol. 1996; 171:120-5.

[44] Friedl P, Entschladen F, Conrad C, Niggemann B, and Zanker KS. CD4+ T lymphocytes migrating in three-dimensional collagen lattices lack focal adhesions and utilize beta1 integrin-independent strategies for polarization, interaction with collagen fibers and locomotion. Eur J Immunol. 1998; 28:2331-43.

[45] Fais S and Malorni W. Leukocyte uropod formation and membrane/cytoskeleton linkage in immune interactions. J Leukoc Biol. 2003; 73:556-63.

[46] Campello S, Lacalle RA, Bettella M, Manes S, Scorrano L, and Viola A. Orchestration of lymphocyte chemotaxis by mitochondrial dynamics. J Exp Med. 2006; 203:2879-86.

[47] Laskin DL, Kimura T, Sakakibara S, Riley DJ, and Berg RA. Chemotactic activity of collagen-like polypeptides for human peripheral blood neutrophils. J Leukoc Biol. 1986; 39:255-66.

[48] Senior RM, Gresham HD, Griffin GL, Brown EJ, and Chung AE. Entactin stimulates neutrophil adhesion and chemotaxis through interactions between its Arg-Gly-Asp (RGD) domain and the leukocyte response integrin. J Clin Invest. 1992; 90:2251-7.

[49] Thelen M and Stein JV. How chemokines invite leukocytes to dance. Nat Immunol. 2008; 9:953-9.

[50] Marone R, Cmiljanovic V, Giese B, and Wymann MP. Targeting phosphoinositide 3-kinase: moving towards therapy. Biochim Biophys Acta. 2008; 1784:159-85.

[51] Stambolic V and Woodgett JR. Functional distinctions of protein kinase B/Akt isoforms defined by their influence on cell migration. Trends Cell Biol. 2006; 16:461-6.

[52] Enomoto A, Murakami H, Asai N, Morone N, Watanabe T, Kawai K, Murakumo Y, Usukura J, Kaibuchi K, and Takahashi M. Akt/PKB regulates actin organization and cell motility via Girdin/APE. Dev Cell. 2005; 9:389-402.

[53] Rommel C, Camps M, and Ji H. PI3K delta and PI3K gamma: partners in crime in inflammation in rheumatoid arthritis and beyond? Nat Rev Immunol. 2007; 7:191-201.

[54] Heit B, Robbins SM, Downey CM, Guan Z, Colarusso P, Miller BJ, Jirik FR, and Kubes P. PTEN functions to 'prioritize' chemotactic cues and prevent 'distraction' in migrating neutrophils. Nat Immunol. 2008; 9:743-52.

[55] Billadeau DD. PTEN gives neutrophils direction. Nat Immunol. 2008; 9:716-8.

[56] Ibarra N, Pollitt A, and Insall RH. Regulation of actin assembly by SCAR/WAVE proteins. Biochem Soc Trans. 2005; 33:1243-6.

[57] Machesky LM, Mullins RD, Higgs HN, Kaiser DA, Blanchoin L, May RC, Hall ME, and Pollard TD. Scar, a WASp-related protein, activates nucleation of actin filaments by the Arp2/3 complex. Proc Natl Acad Sci U S A. 1999; 96:3739-44.

[58] Charest PG and Firtel RA. Feedback signaling controls leading-edge formation during chemotaxis. Curr Opin Genet Dev. 2006; 16:339-47.

[59] Bendix PM, Koenderink GH, Cuvelier D, Dogic Z, Koeleman BN, Brieher WM, Field CM, Mahadevan L, and Weitz DA. A quantitative analysis of contractility in active cytoskeletal protein networks. Biophys J. 2008; 94:3126-36.

[60] Lammermann T, Bader BL, Monkley SJ, Worbs T, Wedlich-Soldner R, Hirsch K, Keller M, Forster R, Critchley DR, Fassler R, and Sixt M. Rapid leukocyte migration by integrin-independent flowing and squeezing. Nature. 2008; 453:51-5.

[61] Monaco S, Sparano V, Gioia M, Sbardella D, Di Pierro D, Marini S, and Coletta M. Enzymatic processing of collagen IV by MMP-2 (gelatinase A) affects neutrophil migration and it is modulated by extracatalytic domains. Protein Sci. 2006; 15:2805-15.

[62] Delclaux C, Delacourt C, D'Ortho MP, Boyer V, Lafuma C, and Harf A. Role of gelatinase B and elastase in human polymorphonuclear neutrophil migration across basement membrane. Am J Respir Cell Mol Biol. 1996; 14:288-95.

[63] Yap B and Kamm RD. Cytoskeletal remodeling and cellular activation during deformation of neutrophils into narrow channels. J Appl Physiol. 2005; 99:2323-30.

[64] Smart EJ, Graf GA, McNiven MA, Sessa WC, Engelman JA, Scherer PE, Okamoto T, and Lisanti MP. Caveolins, liquid-ordered domains, and signal transduction. Mol Cell Biol. 1999; 19:7289-304.

[65] Stefanidakis M and Koivunen E. Cell-surface association between matrix metalloproteinases and integrins: role of the complexes in leukocyte migration and cancer progression. Blood. 2006; 108:1441-50.

[66] Stefanidakis M, Ruohtula T, Borregaard N, Gahmberg CG, and Koivunen E. Intracellular and cell surface localization of a complex between alphaMbeta2 integrin and promatrix metalloproteinase-9 progelatinase in neutrophils. J Immunol. 2004; 172:7060-8.

[67] Wondimu Z, Geberhiwot T, Ingerpuu S, Juronen E, Xie X, Lindbom L, Doi M, Kortesmaa J, Thyboll J, Tryggvason K, Fadeel B, and Patarroyo M. An endothelial laminin isoform, laminin 8 (alpha4beta1gamma1), is secreted by blood neutrophils, promotes neutrophil migration and extravasation, and protects neutrophils from apoptosis. Blood. 2004; 104:1859-66.

[68] Humphries MJ. Integrin structure. Biochem Soc Trans. 2000; 28:311-39.

[69] Hynes RO. Integrins: bidirectional, allosteric signaling machines. Cell. 2002; 110:673-87.

[70] Shimaoka M, Takagi J, and Springer TA. Conformational regulation of integrin structure and function. Annu Rev Biophys Biomol Struct. 2002; 31:485-516.

[71] Gille J and Swerlick RA. Integrins: role in cell adhesion and communication. Ann N Y Acad Sci. 1996; 797:93-106.

[72] Springer TA. Adhesion receptors of the immune system. Nature. 1990; 346:425-34.

[73] Tuffery-Giraud S, Saquet C, Chambert S, Echenne B, Marie Cuisset J, Rivier F, Cossee M, Philippe C, Monnier N, Bieth E, Recan D, Antoinette Voelckel M, Perelman S, Lambert JC, Malcolm S, and Claustres M. The role of muscle biopsy in analysis of the dystrophin gene in Duchenne muscular dystrophy: experience of a national referral centre. Neuromuscul Disord. 2004; 14:650-8.

[74] Han J, Rose DM, Woodside DG, Goldfinger LE, and Ginsberg MH. Integrin alpha 4 beta 1-dependent T cell migration requires both phosphorylation and dephosphorylation of the alpha 4 cytoplasmic domain to regulate the reversible binding of paxillin. J Biol Chem. 2003; 278:34845-53.

[75] Rose DM, Liu S, Woodside DG, Han J, Schlaepfer DD, and Ginsberg MH. Paxillin binding to the alpha 4 integrin subunit stimulates LFA-1 (integrin alpha L beta 2)-dependent T cell migration by augmenting the activation of focal adhesion kinase/proline-rich tyrosine kinase-2. J Immunol. 2003; 170:5912-8.

[76] Cohen-Hillel E, Mintz R, Meshel T, Garty BZ, and Ben-Baruch A. Cell migration to the chemokine CXCL8: paxillin is activated and regulates adhesion and cell motility. Cell Mol Life Sci. 2009; 66:884-99.

[77] Nishiya N, Kiosses WB, Han J, and Ginsberg MH. An alpha4 integrin-paxillin-Arf-GAP complex restricts Rac activation to the leading edge of migrating cells. Nat Cell Biol. 2005; 7:343-52.

[78] Xu W, Wang P, Petri B, Zhang Y, Tang W, Sun L, Kress H, Mann T, Shi Y, Kubes P, and Wu D. Integrin-induced PIP5K1C kinase polarization regulates neutrophil polarization, directionality, and in vivo infiltration. Immunity. 2010; 33:340-50.

[79] Fagerholm SC, Hilden TJ, Nurmi SM, and Gahmberg CG. Specific integrin alpha and beta chain phosphorylations regulate LFA-1 activation through affinity-dependent and -independent mechanisms. J Cell Biol. 2005; 171:705-15.

[80] Pavalko FM and LaRoche SM. Activation of human neutrophils induces an interaction between the integrin beta 2-subunit (CD18) and the actin binding protein alpha-actinin. J Immunol. 1993; 151:3795-807.

[81] Smith A, Carrasco YR, Stanley P, Kieffer N, Batista FD, and Hogg N. A talin-dependent LFA-1 focal zone is formed by rapidly migrating T lymphocytes. J Cell Biol. 2005; 170:141-51.

[82] Springer TA. Traffic signals for lymphocyte recirculation and leukocyte emigration: the multistep paradigm. Cell. 1994; 76:301-14.

[83] Laudanna C, Kim JY, Constantin G, and Butcher E. Rapid leukocyte integrin activation by chemokines. Immunol Rev. 2002; 186:37-46.

[84] Chrzanowska-Wodnicka M and Burridge K. Rho-stimulated contractility drives the formation of stress fibers and focal adhesions. J Cell Biol. 1996; 133:1403-15.

[85] Vicente-Manzanares M and Sanchez-Madrid F. Role of the cytoskeleton during leukocyte responses. Nat Rev Immunol. 2004; 4:110-22.

[86] Cerecedo D, Cisneros B, Gomez P, and Galvan IJ. Distribution of dystrophin- and utrophin-associated protein complexes during activation of human neutrophils. Exp Hematol. 2010; 38:618-628 e3.

[87] Swaney KF, Huang CH, and Devreotes PN. Eukaryotic chemotaxis: a network of signaling pathways controls motility, directional sensing, and polarity. Annu Rev Biophys. 2010; 39:265-89.

8

Intravascular Leukocyte Chemotaxis: The Rules of Attraction

Sara Massena and Mia Phillipson
Department of Medical Cell Biology, Integrative Physiology
Uppsala University
Sweden

1. Introduction

The security system of the body against pathogenic invaders includes leukocytes that efficiently scan the organism. Leukocytes within the vasculature utilize the comprehensive circulatory system to examine the blood vessels of the entire body for signs of *e.g.* bacteria displayed on vascular endothelial cells. Upon infection, a successful immune response is dependent on prompt recruitment of leukocytes from the bloodstream to the afflicted site where they exert their effector functions. A critical aspect of leukocyte recruitment out of vasculature is the chemotactic gradient that guides leukocytes over the blood vessel wall, and further through the extracellular matrix towards the affected site. Leukocyte recruitment is a strictly regulated cascade of events involving different molecular mechanisms. To rapidly and efficiently reach their target, specific interactions between circulating leukocytes and vascular endothelium orchestrates leukocyte activation and guides them already within blood vessels to optimal transmigration sites at endothelial *loci* close to the source of inflammation.

Despite the obvious need for effective leukocyte recruitment to eradicate bacteria and to maintain tissue homeostasis, amplified and dysregulated recruitment of leukocytes is a key factor in diverse disorders including autoimmune diseases and sepsis. For many of these conditions, therapeutic options are limited and unspecific. Understanding the triggering signals, involved molecules and underlying mechanisms by which the body enhances, controls and limits immune responses is therefore critical for the development of novel therapeutic interventions.

In this chapter we summarize leukocyte recruitment during inflammation, highlighting a recent finding, namely intravascular leukocyte chemotaxis.

2. Leukocyte recruitment and chemotaxis

Over the last years, research groups have been dedicating their efforts to delineate the cellular and molecular mechanisms behind leukocyte recruitment using a wide range of *in vivo* imaging techniques (*e.g.* fluorescence intravital microscopy, spinning disk confocal, as well as two-photon confocal microscopy). These techniques, together with genetically altered mice (transgenic or knockout) combined with fluorescently labeled proteins and antibodies, allow detailed examination of leukocyte-endothelial cell interactions, adhesion molecule expression and chemokine distribution. Thereby, an expanded and more detailed version of the leukocyte recruitment cascade was established.

Leukocyte recruitment can be described as a sequential process having at least five distinct events, as depicted in **Figure 1**, induced by upregulation of endothelial adhesion molecules and molecular guidance signals (chemotactic stimuli).

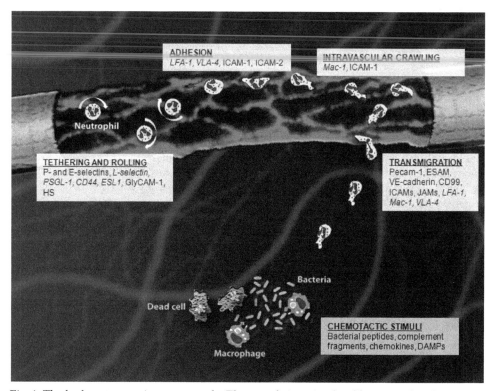

Fig. 1. The leukocyte recruitment cascade. The vessels is stained red by monoclonal antibodies to CD31 conjugated to Alexa Fluor 555, and cartoon neutrophils are added to the phtograph. The white boxes contain involved adhesion molecules, where the ones expressed by neutrophils are written in italics. Illustration adapted with permission from Phillipson M, Kubes P, *Nature Medicine*, 2011.

2.1 Leukocyte tethering and rolling

In order to leave the vasculature at the site of infection, leukocytes have to become marginated, leave the center of the blood stream, and decelerate to come in contact with the vascular endothelium. However, due to the force of blood flow in postcapillary venules (shear rate ~150 to 1600 s^{-1}, depending on flow rate and vessel diameter) collisional contact duration between leukocytes and unstimulated endothelium is brief (*i.e.* <25 ms) (Simon S. I., Goldsmith H. L., 2002). Specific interaction mechanisms between leukocytes and activated endothelium under shear flow are therefore required for leukocyte recruitment to inflammatory foci.

In fact, during inflammation, locally released stimuli (*e.g.* bacterial peptides, complement fragments, chemokines, histamine, and damage-associated molecular patterns) activate endothelial cells in the nearby venules to upregulate adhesion molecules on the plasma membrane which will aid leukocyte tethering, slow rolling and adhesion to the endothelium, leading ultimately to leukocyte transmigration into the tissue.

Selectins are a family of long adhesive molecules, extending from the plasma membrane, which facilitate attachment of circulating leukocytes to the endothelium (Patel K. D. *et al.*, 1995; Kansas G.S., 1996). Increased expression of P- and E-selectin (CD62P and CD62E, respectively) on activated venular endothelium induces leukocyte tethering (Kunkel E. J., Ley K., 1996; Petri B. *et al.*, 2008). While P-selectin is stored in Weibel-Palade bodies within the endothelial cells, E-selectin requires *de novo* synthesis. Once tethered, leukocytes can rapidly release and reengage selectin ligand bonds, resulting in a slow rotational movement along the vessel wall termed rolling (Norman M. U., Kubes P., 2005; Kelly M. *et al.*, 2007; Ley K. *et al.*, 2007). Rolling dynamics is optimized by force-regulated transitions from catch bonds to slip bonds[1], which explains the requirement for a shear threshold to support rolling (McEver R. P., Zhu C., 2010). L-selectin (CD62L), constitutively expressed on leukocytes, participates redundantly with P- and E-selecting, and supports both capture and rolling of leukocytes in blood vessels (Kunkel E. J., Ley K., 1996; Petri B. *et al.*, 2008).

Each of the three selectins binds with different affinity to sialylated and fucosylated oligosaccharides including sialyl Lewis[X] (sLe[X]) moieties, which are present on multiple glycolipids and glycoproteins on leukocytes and endothelium (McEver R. P., 2001; Simon S. I., Green C. E., 2005; Kelly M. *et al.*, 2007). The best characterized selectin ligand is PSGL-1 (P-selectin glycoprotein ligand-1), a heavily sialylated mucin present on leukocytes and endothelial cells, which can serve as a ligand to P-, E- and L-selectins although it binds P-selectin with the highest affinity (Kansas G. S., 1996). Besides PSGL-1, other ligands have been identified for E-selectin, *e.g.* sialophorin (leukosialin, CD43), hematopoietic cell E-selectin ligand (HCELL, CD44), and E-selectin ligand-1 (ESL1) (Kelly M. *et al.*, 2007; Ley K. *et al.*, 2007). L-selectin can also bind other ligands *e.g.* glycosylation-dependent cell adhesion molecule-1 (GlyCAM-1), mucosal addresin cell adhesion molecule-1 (MAdCAM-1), podocalyxin (CD34), heparan sulfate (HS) and sulphated glycoprotein-200 (Sgp200) (Wang L. *et al.*, 2005).

Rolling along the endothelium provides leukocytes a great opportunity to interact with and be further activated by chemokines or other inflammatory mediators presented on the luminal endothelium.

2.2 Intravascular chemokine presentation to rolling leukocytes

To initiate activation and recruitment of circulating leukocytes to tissue, tissue-derived chemokines need to be presented to rolling leukocytes at the apical endothelium. Within blood vessels, immobilization of chemokines on the endothelium is essential to avoid that they are washed away from the site of inflammation by the blood flow.

---

[1] *Catch bond:* a bond that prolongs its lifetime in response to tensile force; *Slip bond:* a bond that shortens its lifetime in response to tensile force (McEver R. P., Zhu C., 2010).

Heparan sulfate proteoglycans (HSPGs) are proteins bearing covalently attached complex polysaccharide chains that are negatively charged (heparan sulfate, HS), and are found on cell surfaces of most cell types as well as in the extracellular matrix (Bernfield M. *et al.*, 1999, Parish C., 2005). Chemokines and a variety of positively charged proteins bind to HS through specific and/or electrostatic interactions (Lindhal U., Kjellén L., 1991; Lindhal U., 2007). Indeed, interstitially released chemokines were shown to cross the endothelium and to be presented by luminal HSPGs to leukocytes both *in vitro* (Ihrcke N. S. *et al.*, 1993; Parish C., 2005; Wang L. *et al.*, 2005; Lindhal U., 2007) and *in vivo* (Massena S. *et al.*, 2010). Binding of chemokines to endothelial HSPG may promote molecular encounters between rolling leukocytes and chemokines, and thereby further inducing leukocyte activation. Moreover, endothelial HS acts as a ligand for L-selectin aiding neutrophil slow rolling (Wang L. *et al.*, 2005), which increase the propensity for leukocyte-chemokine encounters.

How chemokines originating from the afflicted site or released by tissue leukocytes reach the luminal side of the endothelium in order to be presented by HS to leukocytes is not completely established. However, electron microscopy studies suggested that chemokines bound to HS are transported through the endothelium by transcytosis (Middleton J. *et al.*, 1997) as endothelium exposed to interleukin-8 (IL-8, CXCL8) contained IL-8 within intracellular caveola, while no chemokines were found at endothelial cell junctions. Nevertheless, under the experimental conditions of this study, it is impossible to tell if the intracellular chemokines are being transported through endothelium towards the apical membrane or if they are on their way to lyzosomes for degradation. In addition, soluble chemokines passing through junctions cannot be detected using electron microscopy, as they would be lost during tissue preparation prior to examination.

Edema formation is one of the cardinal signs of inflammation, and is caused by increased vascular permeability and consequent plasma leakage. The primary cause of increased vascular permeability is leakage of plasma through paracellular gaps (Curry F. E., Adamson R. H., 2010; Lindbom L., Kenne E., 2011), which is regulated by the interplay of adhesive forces between adjacent endothelial cells and counter adhesive forces generated by endothelial actomyosin contraction (Mehta D., Malik A. B., 2006). The physiological importance of this event for leukocyte recruitment is debated. It is well documented that increased vascular permeability in presence of inflammatory mediators is accompanied by increased leukocyte adhesion and diapedesis (Curry F.E., Adamson R. H., 1999; Michel C. C., Curry F. E., 1999). Nevertheless, temporal and spatial uncoupling between these two events has also been described. During inflammation, vascular permeability can increase at a faster rate than leukocyte transmigration (Kim M. H. *et al.*, 2009), suggesting that increased vascular permeability precedes leukocyte recruitment. Further, in aseptic wounds, vascular permeability and leukocyte extravasation were shown to be uncoupled (Curry F.E., Adamson R. H., 1999; Kim M. H. *et al.*, 2009). It is generally believed that increased permeability supports chemokine influx into the vessels and one hypothesis is that the increase in vascular permeability during inflammation grants the paracellular transport of chemokines for rapid presentation to intravascular leukocytes, guiding them out to the afflicted area in the tissue. A recent study using intravital spinning-disk confocal microscopy in anesthetized mice revealed that chemokines added extravascularly became accumulated intra-luminally at endothelial cell junctions (Massena S. *et al.*, 2010). High junctional sequestration of chemokines suggests that chemokines are transported either paracellularly into blood vessels or longitudinally on the apical endothelial cell membrane towards junctions after being transcytosed. Further, this observation might simply reflect high concentrations of HS in junctional regions. However, these findings suggest that increased vascular permeability during inflammation does not necessary account for amplified leukocyte extravasation *per se,* but instead might promote cytokine/chemokine transport and thereby induce leukocyte recruitment.

Endothelial cells display extraordinary phenotypic and functional heterogeneity. Endothelial cell structural features such as shape, thickness, molecular characteristics of apical membrane and junctions, as well as the thickness of the luminal glycocalyx are some of the features, which vary across the vascular tree (Van Den Berg B. M. *et al.,* 2003; Aird W. C., 2007). Heparan sulfate is known to display miscellaneous structural features in various tissues and on different cell types (Lindhal U., Li J. P., 2009), which accounts for binding of proteins in a selective fashion. Differences in proteoglycan composition (altered structure of HS epitopes or sequences, and/or expression pattern of different syndecans) might result in different chemokine binding properties, explaining the observed differences in leukocyte recruitment of different organs upon diverse inflammatory stimuli.

2.3 Leukocyte activation and adhesion to the endothelium

After being stimulated by chemokines sequestered on the endothelium, rolling leukocytes adhere to the endothelium by rapid formation of shear-resistant bindings mediated by specialized leukocyte integrins (Rose D. M. *et al.,* 2007). Integrins are noncovalently associated heterodimeric cell surface adhesion molecules consisting of combinations of α and β-molecules. Leukocytes express at least 10 members of the integrin family belonging to the β_1-, β_2- and β_7-subfamilies (Luo B. H. *et al.,* 2007). Leukocyte adhesion molecules relevant for recruitment belong to the β_1- and β_2-integrin families (Ley K. *et al.,* 2007), of which LFA-1 (Lymphocyte function-associated antigen-1, ITGAL, CD11a/CD18, $\alpha_L\beta_2$), Mac-1 (Macrophage antigen-1, ITGAM, CD11b/CD18, $\alpha_M\beta_2$) and VLA-4 (very late antigen-4, CD49d/CD29, $\alpha_4\beta_1$) are the most studied.

Members of the β_1-subfamily (also called VLA integrins) contain the β_1-subunit associated to one of at least six different α subunits (Hemler M. E., 1990). VLA-4 integrin is amply expressed on peripheral blood B-lymphocytes, T-lymphocytes and monocytes (Hemler M. E., 1990). Peripheral blood neutrophils are believed to generally be devoid of cell surface β_1-integrin structures (Hemler M. E., 1990), even though some reports claim that immature neutrophils expressing surface VLA-4 can also be found in circulation (Lund-Johansen F., Terstappen L. W., 1993; Pillay J. *et al.,* 2010).

Most circulating leukocytes express integrins in a low affinity state (Carman C. V., Springer T. A., 2003). Upon binding of chemokines to G-protein-coupled receptors (GPCRs) expressed on leukocytes, a complex intracellular signaling network is triggered within milliseconds (Shamri R. *et al.,* 2005; Ley K. *et al.,* 2007). This induces integrins to undergo an almost instantaneous change in avidity and ligand affinity (Von Andrian U. H. *et. al.,* 1992; Shamri R. *et al.,* 2005; Hyduk S. J., Cybulsky M. I., 2009). Thus, inside-out signaling after chemokine binding to GPCRs shifts the integrins from a resting to an active conformation (Simon S.I., Goldsmith H. L., 2002; Simon S. I., Green C. E., 2005), which is necessary for binding to its ligands expressed on activated endothelial cells (Ley K. *et al.,* 2007).

Differential leukocyte expression levels of integrins and chemokine receptors as well as receptor affinity for chemokines might account for selective arrest and recruitment of leukocyte subtypes. Additionally, chemokine-triggered signaling networks can regulate distinct integrins in specific leukocyte subtypes, contributing for differential leukocyte recruitment.

2.3.1 Neutrophil adhesion

β_2-integrin dependent neutrophil adhesion is fundamental for effective bacterial clearance. In fact, the genetic disorder leukocyte adhesion deficiency I (LAD I) is characterized by a profound defect in leukocyte recruitment and therefore severe immunodeficiency, due to neutrophils failing to adhere to the activated endothelium since the surface levels of β_2-integrins are dramatically reduced or absent (Bunting M. et al., 2002).

It was recently found that binding of the β_2-integrin LFA-1 to intercellular adhesion molecule-1 (ICAM-1, CD54) expressed by endothelial cells, mediates neutrophil firm adhesion to the vascular endothelium under shear flow (Shamri R. et al., 2005; Phillipson M. et al., 2006; Ley K. et al., 2007; Petri B. et al., 2008). LFA-1 is also able to bind to other immunoglobulin superfamily members, ICAM-2 (CD102) and ICAM-3 (CD50), albeit with lower affinity relative to ICAM-1 (De Fougerolles A. R. et al., 1994), in addition to JAM-A (junction adhesion molecule-A).

However, there is some evidence that neutrophils adhere via other adhesion molecules than LFA-1, or by non-adhesion processes such as physical trapping, described to occur in lung capillaries or liver sinusoids (Doerschuk C. M. et al., 1990; Wong J. et al., 1997; Norman M. U., Kubes P., 2005). Indeed, anti-CD18 treatment did not reduce leukocyte recruitment to the lung of rabbits (Doerschuk C. M. et al., 1990), or in the rat liver (Jaeschke H. et al., 1996). In the liver, neutrophils have been reported to adhere via CD44 interacting with sinusoidal hyaluronan (McDonald B. et al., 2008). Furthermore, under systemic inflammatory conditions, such as sepsis, neutrophils have been suggested to adhere to the endothelium via VLA-4 (Ibbotson G. C. et al., 2001). This integrin was also proposed to be involved in neutrophil adhesion in the lung microvasculature (Ibbotson G. C. et al., 2001).

2.3.2 Monocyte adhesion

In contrast to neutrophil adhesion, β_2-integrins seem to play a moderate role in monocyte arrest, since monocytes both adhere and polarize after blockade of β_2-integrins as well as after blockade of ICAM-1 or ICAM-2 in vitro (Schenkel A. R. et al., 2004). Instead, β_1-integrins seem to play a more substantial role in monocyte adhesion to the endothelium. In fact, recent mouse models showed that monocytes firmly adhered to endothelium by VLA-4 binding to endothelial VCAM-1 (vascular cell adhesion molecule-1, CD106) (Luscinkas F. W. et al., 1994; Meerschaert J., Furie M. B., 1995; Lee T. D. et al., 2003; Ley K. et al., 2007; Soehnlein O. et al., 2009).

2.3.3 Lymphocyte adhesion

During lymphocyte recruitment to peripheral tissues, LFA-1 is the dominant integrin involved in firm adhesion (Dustin M., Springer T. A., 1989; Shamri R. et al., 2005) by binding to its ligand ICAM-1 (Shamri R. *et al.*, 2005). As described for neutrophils, LFA-1 prevails in a low affinity state on most circulating lymphocytes. Stimulation of lymphocyte-GPCRs rapidly shifts LFA-1 integrin to a high avidity state (Carman C. V., Springer T. A., 2003). This high avidity state of LFA-1 on T-lymphocytes is transient, peaking 5 to 10 minutes after receptor stimulation and returns to the low affinity state by 30 min to 2 hours (Dustin M., Springer T. A., 1989).

T-lymphocytes are not only recruited to tissue, they also home to lymph nodes. *In vitro* studies of T-lymphocyte adhesion to the specialized lymph node endothelium (high endothelial venules, HEV), demonstrated that besides LFA-1, VLA-4 is involved in T-cell adhesion (Faveew C. *et al.*, 2000). Adhesion was reduced by 40-50% upon treatment with inhibiting antibodies to either integrin. Interestingly, the effects of VLA-4 and LFA-1 antibodies were additive, giving >90% inhibition of T-lymphocyte adhesion.

2.4 Intravascular chemotactic gradients and leukocyte crawling

Using time-lapse *in vivo* microscopy, adherent neutrophils and monocytes were recently observed to crawl significant distances within the vessels (Phillipson M. *et al.*, 2006; Auffray C. *et al.*, 2007; Phillipson M. *et al.*, 2009). The crawling neutrophils were searching the endothelium for optimal sites for transmigration, since inhibition of crawling significantly delayed neutrophil transmigration (Phillipson M. *et al.*, 2006; Sumagin R. *et al.*, 2010).

2.4.1 Neutrophil crawling

Intravascular crawling of neutrophils is dependent on the leukocyte β_2-integrin Mac-1 and its ligand ICAM-1 on endothelial cells (Phillipson M. *et al.*, 2006; Sumagin R. *et al.*, 2010). Compared to LFA-1, Mac-1 binds a wider spectrum of ligands, including complement fragment iC3b, fibrinogen, fibronectin, laminin, collagen, myeloperoxidase, elastase, JAM-B and –C to name just a few (Simon S. I., Green C. E., 2005; Kelly M. *et al.*, 2007; Luo B. H. *et al.*, 2007) suggesting that this integrin might have other roles apart from intravascular crawling.

Neutrophil crawling on the stimulated endothelium occurs in two distinct stages. In the initial phase directly following neutrophil adhesion, a mechanotactic signal provided by shear stress induces neutrophil crawling perpendicular to blood flow until an endothelial cell junction is encountered (Phillipson M. *et al.*, 2009). This observation has also been made *in vitro* when adherent neutrophils crawled perpendicular to the direction of flow when shear was applied to the system (Phillipson M. *et al.*, 2009). However, as soon as the crawling neutrophils meet the junction, the shear stress signal is ignored and neutrophils instead begin to follow the junction. Considering that endothelial cells are elongated in the direction of flow, perpendicular crawling generates the greatest probability for a neutrophil to find an endothelial junction in the shortest period of time.

More recently, the existence of an intravascular gradient of chemokines (macrophage inflammatory protein-2, CXCL2 [MIP-2]; keratinocyte-derived chemokine, CXCL1 [KC]) originating from the infection or released by tissue leukocytes on endothelial cells has been described (Massena S. *et al.*, 2010). Indeed, this chemotactic gradient is sequestered on endothelial HS and provides directional cues to crawling neutrophils, which follow this gradient to optimal transmigration sites close to the origin of the infection (Massena S. *et al.*,

2010). However, whether haptotactic gradients can be established by all chemokines remains unclear, since different chemokines have diverse affinity to HS (Lindhal U., Kjellén L., 1991; Lindhal U., 2007).

Directional intravascular crawling along a chemotactic gradient expedites neutrophil recruitment, compared to when no chemokine gradient is formed due to homogenous extravascular chemokine concentrations (Massena S. *et al.*, 2010). Disruption of the chemokine gradient is translated into random crawling and inefficient recruitment of neutrophils which ultimately leads to a decreased ability to clear infections, as seen in *Staphylococcus aureus* infected mice with truncated HS chains (overexpressing heparanase, Massena S. *et al.*, 2010).

2.4.2 Monocyte crawling

Intravascular crawling monocytes have been reported *in vivo* (Auffray C. *et al.*, 2007; Sumagin R. *et al.*, 2010), and crawling on endothelium is critical to reach optimal transmigration sites, as demonstrated *in vitro* (Schenkel A. R. *et al.*, 2004).

Whereas the integrin Mac-1 alone is responsible for crawling of neutrophils, LFA-1 and Mac-1 integrins were in some studies reported to play a redundant role in monocyte crawling via binding to ICAM-1 and ICAM-2 (Schenkel A. R. *et al.*, 2004; Sumagin R. *et al.*, 2010). Blockade of each of these molecules led to a pirouette behavior at the adhesion site (Schenkel A. R. *et al.*, 2004). Nevertheless, monocytes were shown to be able to adhere and polarize.

Recently, a distinct role for each of these integrins on monocyte crawling under different endothelial activation states has been described. Monocytes were shown to crawl long distances on resting endothelium in a patrolling behavior (*i.e.* monitoring healthy tissue) in a LFA-1-dependent manner (Auffray C. *et al.*, 2007; Sumagin R. *et al.*, 2010). However, upon inflammatory stimulation, monocyte crawling became Mac-1-dependent and assumed a neutrophil-like crawling pattern, *i.e.* similar crawling distance and confinement ratio (Sumagin R. *et al.*, 2010). These results have been suggested to correspond to differences between two different monocyte populations rather than to a shift in integrin expression upon inflammatory stimulation.

Two monocyte subsets distinguished by their expression levels of selectins, integrins and chemokine receptors have already been characterized in various mammals (Geissman F. *et al.*, 2003; Gordon S., Taylor P. R., 2005). These phenotypic differences encompass distinct effector functions. A monocyte subset termed "resident" (CX_3CR1^{hi} CCR2- Ly6C- in mice; $CD14^{lo}$ CD16+ in humans) is involved in tissue remodeling and wound repair (Gordon S., Taylor P. R., 2005; Auffray C. *et al.*, 2007; Soehnlein O. *et al.*, 2009). In contrast, another monocyte subset denominated "inflammatory" (CX_3CR1^{lo} CCR2+ Ly6C+ in mice; $CD14^{hi}$ CD16- in humans) is specialized in pro-inflammatory activities such as bacterial phagocytosis, secretion of inflammation-promoting cytokines and reactive species as well as proteolytic activity (Gordon S., Taylor P. R., 2005; Auffray C. *et al.*, 2007; Soehnlein O. *et al.*, 2009). Resident monocytes, express high amounts of LFA-1. In contrast, inflammatory monocytes do not express LFA-1, even though no differences were found for Mac-1 between the two monocyte subsets (Auffray C. *et al.*, 2007).

It is possible that the two subsets of circulating monocytes might use different integrins and display different crawling patterns to achieve the different effector functions.

2.4.3 Lymphocyte crawling

In vitro, adherent T-lymphocytes have been reported to crawl over the luminal surface of the endothelium in a LFA-1-dependent manner (Shulman *et al.*, 2009). LFA-1 is also responsible for T-lymphocyte adhesion, but the distribution of the membrane LFA-1 is altered correlating with changes in cell morphology as soon as the T-lymphocyte starts to migrate (Smith A. *et al.*, 2005). LFA-1 turnover at numerous focal points ensures rapid crawling and resistance to detachment by shear forces (Shulman *et al.*, 2009). Low expression levels of LFA-1 were detected at the leading edge of the cell and high expression level in the non-attached uropod at the rear (Smith A. *et al.*, 2005). Interestingly, LFA-1 in the leading edge was not in a high-affinity state, as detected by use of specific antibodies that recognize LFA-1 in different conformational states (Smith A. *et al.*, 2007). Instead LFA-1 in the leading edge was in an intermediate affinity conformation allowing crawling possibly by weaker interactions with ICAM-1.

Published studies have identified intravascular natural killer T-lymphocytes (NKT cells) with possible sentinel functions for the detection of bacteria in the blood (Geissmann F. *et al.*, 2005; Lee T. D. *et al.*, 2010; Thomas S. Y. *et al.*, 2011). These cells are distinguished by their restricted repertoire of T-cell receptor (TCR) variants that recognize lipids and glycolipids presented by CD1d (Kawano T. *et al.*, 1997; Brossay L. *et al.*, 1998). NKT cells primarily reside and wander within the vasculature of the liver and spleen (Geissmann F. *et al.*, 2005; Bendelac A. *et al.*, 2007) but have also been suggested to accumulate in smaller amounts in the vascular compartment of the lung (Thomas S. Y. *et al.*, 2011). The mechanisms underlying adhesion and crawling of NKT cells are still poorly understood. It has been reported that treatment of mice with blocking antibodies to LFA-1 and ICAM-1 induced rapid detachment of adherent NKT cells from sinusoidal endothelium (Thomas S. Y. *et al.*, 2011). In contrast, blocking VLA-4 or VCAM-1 had no effect. Integrin activation typically relies on inside–out signaling after chemokine binding to GPCRs (Ley K. *et al.*, 2007). However, genetic ablation of CXCR6 (the major chemokine receptor expressed on NKT cells) or treatment with an inhibitor of GPCRs, did not induce detachment of NKT cells from liver microvasculature (Geissmann F. *et al.*, 2005; Lee T. D. *et al.*, 2010). Furthermore, previous studies on NKT cells transferred into CD1d-deficient mice suggested that TCR activation was not a prerequisite for NKT cells sinusoidal adhesion (McNab F. W. *et al.*, 2005; Wei D. G. *et al.*, 2005). Crawling was also unimpeded in mice treated with anti-CD1d antibody (Lee T. D. *et al.*, 2010). Interestingly, upon infection with the blood-borne pathogen *Borrelia burgdorferi* (a spirochete injected intravenously through tick bite), NKT cells were reported to slow their crawling and to accumulate in clusters on Kupffer cells in a GPCRs-dependent way (CXCR3, and CD1d) (Lee T. D. *et al.*, 2010). Kupffer cells are specialized ramified macrophages, which line the walls of liver sinusoids and prevent the dissemination of pathogens via the blood by capturing and engulfing them. Kupffer cells can then present glycolipid antigens via CD1d (Lee T. D. *et al.*, 2010). In the absence of Kupffer or NKT cells, dissemination of *Borrelia burgdorferi* occurred, suggesting a role for NKT cells in vascular surveillance for blood-borne pathogens captured by Kupffer cells (Lee T. D. *et al.*, 2010).

2.5 Diapedesis: Trans- and paracellular routes

Leukocyte diapedesis out of vasculature into affected tissue can occur both between neighboring endothelial cells (paracellularly through junctions) and directly through the endothelium (transcellularly) (Feng D. *et al.*, 1998; Shaw S. K. *et al.*, 2001; Carman C. V., Springer T. A., 2004; Engelhardt B., Wolburg H., 2004; Yang L. *et al.*, 2005; Phillipson M. *et al.*, 2006). The route employed most likely depends on inflammatory stimuli, as well as the type of leukocyte and vascular bed.

Diapedesis has been reported to be mediated by numerous endothelial adhesion molecules expressed in high density at endothelial junctions, such as platelet-endothelial cell adhesion molecule 1 (PECAM-1, CD31), CD99, vascular endothelial-cadherins (VE-cadherins), endothelial cell-selective adhesion molecule (ESAM), ICAM-1 and -2 and JAMs (Luscinskas F. W. *et al.*, 2002; Engelhardt B., Wolburg H., 2004; Yang L. *et al.*, 2005; Ley K. *et al.*, 2007; Lou O. *et al.*, 2007; Petri B. *et al.*, 2008; Woodfin A. *et al.*, 2011). Other molecules involved in leukocyte transmigration are integrins expressed on leukocytes (*e.g.* LFA-1, Mac-1, VLA-4) (Ley K. *et al.*, 2007; Petri B. *et al.*, 2008; Woodfin A. *et al.*, 2011). The specific molecules involved in either of the transmigration pathways remains to be identified.

The different molecules appear to mediate leukocyte transmigration in either a stimulus-specific or leukocyte-specific manner. For example PECAM-1, ICAM-2 and JAM-A mediate leukocyte transmigration in response to interleukin-1β (IL-1β) but not to tumor necrosis factor-alpha (TNF-α) (Wang S. *et al.*, 2006; Ley K. *et al.*, 2007). Direct activation of leukocytes by TNF-α, fMLP (N-formyl-methionyl-leucyl-phenylalanine) or leukotriene-B4 (LTB4) appears to bypass the need for these molecules. Studies of activated mouse cremaster muscle and intravital microscopy in mice knocked down for ESAM gene (Ley K. *et al.*, 2007) have shown that ESAM does not show a stimulus-specific role but appears to mediate neutrophil rather than T-lymphocyte transmigration.

Neutrophils have been found to transmigrate predominantly through the paracellular route, *i.e.* between adjacent endothelial cells (Phillipson M. *et al.*, 2006; Woodfin A. *et al.*, 2011). Paracellular transmigration was found to be dependent on the ability for leukocytes to crawl to optimal transmigration sites at the endothelial cell junctions. In Mac-1 deficient mice, due to inhibition of intravascular crawling, transcellular transmigration predominated (Phillipson M. *et al.*, 2006).

Using *in vivo* spinning disk or multi-photon confocal microscopy, profound anatomical changes of the endothelium that facilitated leukocyte extravasation without compromising vascular barrier integrity were observed (Phillipson M. *et al.*, 2008; Petri B. *et al.*, 2011). Docking cup-like structures were formed by endothelial cells (endothelial projections) at the base of the transmigrating neutrophil, which has also been described for T-lymphocytes *in vitro* (Carman C. V., Springer T. A., 2004). The endothelial projections extended towards the top of the neutrophil and eventually formed a dome that surrounded the entire neutrophil, prior to basolateral opening and neutrophil migration further into tissue. If the dome formations were prevented, neutrophil transmigration was delayed (Petri B. *et al.*, 2011), further implicating an active role of endothelium during leukocyte diapedesis, while maintaining the barrier function and vascular permeability.

2.5.1 Migration through the subendothelial basement membrane and pericyte sheet

To overcome the barrier of the blood vessel and finally reach the inflamed tissue, leukocytes also have to transmigrate across the subendothelial basement membrane (BM) surrounding the venular endothelium. This has been shown to occur in areas low in collagen IV, laminin-10 and nidogen-2 (Wang S. *et al.*, 2006). These areas were seen to be closely associated to gaps between pericytes (Wang S. *et al.*, 2006). Interestingly, leukocytes have been observed to initiate transmigration through endothelium at sites superimposing these specific areas. How intravascular crawling leukocytes can detect these areas from the luminal side of the endothelium remains unknown.

2.6 Extravascular crawling

Following leukocyte diapedesis across the vessel wall, further movement in tissue is required in order for the leukocytes to reach the affected site to exert their effector functions. As within the vasculature, leukocyte movement in the tissue is guided by chemotactic gradients leading to the source (Foxman E. F. *et al.*, 1997; Lindbom L., Werr J., 2002). Upon binding to GPCRs on leukocytes, chemoattractants trigger downstream signaling, which translates to cytoskeletal reorganization, polarization and directional locomotion (Friedl P. *et al.*, 2001). Migrating leukocytes thereby adopt a polarized morphology consisting of a leading edge and a tail-like uropod (Friedl P. *et al.*, 2001).

In order to initiate movement, leukocytes have to establish adhesive contacts with the tissue stroma via interactions between the extracellular integrin domains and components of the extracellular matrix (ECM) (Friedl P. *et al.*, 2001; Lindbom L., Werr J., 2002). Stimulation by encountered chemoattractants activates surface integrins and recruits additional integrins from cytoplasmic stores (Diamond M. S., Springer T. A., 1994; Friedl P. *et al.*, 2001). Binding to ECM macromolecules triggers integrin-mediated signals, which regulate further integrin apposition, actin assembly, cell polarity, and migration (Friedl P. *et al.*, 2001).

Accumulating evidence suggests that leukocyte chemotaxis in the ECM is mostly associated with β_1-integrins while a limited role for β_2-integrins is described (Sixt M. *et al.*, 2001). Members of the β_1-family shown to be involved in leukocyte locomotion (Gao J. X., Issekutz A. C., 1997; Werr J. *et al.*, 1998; Sixt M. *et al.*, 2001) show high affinity interactions with proteins of the ECM, including fibronectin, vibronectin, collagen and laminin (Hemler M. E., 1990). Circulating neutrophils are not believed to constitutively express β_1-integrins. However, it has been suggested that upregulation of β_2-integrins by chemotactic stimuli induced an outside-in signaling leading to mobilization of β_1-integrins to the neutrophil surface, in order to prepare recruited neutrophils for subsequent interactions with ECM (Lindbom L., Werr J., 2002). There are also studies demonstrating upregulation of neutrophil surface expression of β_1-integrins in association with emigration from the vasculature (Kubes P. *et al.*, 1995; Werr J. *et al.*, 1998).

Another adhesion molecule involved in extravascular crawling is L-selectin. Indeed, studies using L-selectin-deficient mice revealed no role of L-selectin on leukocyte rolling or adhesion, but transmigration was significantly impaired (Hickey M. J. *et al.*, 2000). Furthermore, leukocytes in L-selectin-deficient mice were unable to respond to directional cues (platelet activating factor [PAF]; KC) in the interstitium (Hickey M. J. *et al.*, 2000). These findings provided strong evidence of an important L-selectin function in leukocyte emigration and extravascular locomotion. Intriguingly, L-selectin expression on emigrated leukocytes is dramatically reduced in comparison to levels on circulating leukocytes (Hickey M. J. *et al.*, 2000). Shedding of L-selectin upon transmigration has been reported both *in vitro* (Smith C. W. *et al.*, 1991; Allport J. R. *et al.*, 1997) and *in vivo* (Jutila M. A. *et al.*, 1989). These results raise the possibility that L-selectin early in the recruitment cascade triggers downstream signals that modulate consecutive transmigration and migration in the interstitium (Hickey M. J. *et al.*, 2000).

Further, integrins bind different components of the tissue stroma and with diverse affinities (Lindbom L., Werr J., 2002). Leukocyte chemotaxis in the tissue is therefore influenced not only by the stimuli encountered but also by the matrix proteins in the tissue.

2.6.1 Prioritazing chemotactic cues

During bacterial infections, the chemotaxing leukocytes are exposed to a cacophony of different chemotactic gradients of diverse origins. Chemoattractants originate from the bacteria themselves (*e.g.* fMLP; lipopolysaccharide [LPS]) or complement fragments bound to bacteria (*e.g.* complement fragment C5a), but also from nearby activated leukocytes and endothelial cells (*e.g.* LTB$_4$; IL-8) (Foxman E. F. *et al.*, 1997; Heit B. *et al.*, 2008; Muller W. A., 2011). A microenvironment where numerous chemoattractants are encountered requires tightly regulated intracellular mechanisms for leukocytes to readily prioritize between the cues, in order for them to effectively reach the target. Thus, to fulfill their missions, leukocytes need to find the bacteria without being distracted by opposing gradients. A hierarchical relationship between chemotactic factors has developed, and "end-target" chemotactic factors like bacterial products *versus* the "intermediate" chemokines released by activated endothelium or tissue leukocytes have been shown to activate separate signaling pathways in neutrophils (p38-mitogen-activated protein kinase [p38MAPK] and phosphoinositide 3-kinase [PI3K], respectively [Campbell J. J. *et al.*, 1997; Heit B. *et al.*, 2002]). In this way, neutrophils are able to sort signals in the noisy environment of inflammation, and respond to chemotactic cues in a hierarchical manner, preferring "end-target" chemoattractant factors like fMLP and C5a over "intermediate" chemokines like IL-8 (Foxman E. F. *et al.*, 1997). This has been suggested to occur through the p38MAPK pathway inhibiting PI3K through relocalization of phosphatase and tensin homologue (PTEN) on the basolateral cell membrane of the polarized moving cell (Heit B. *et al.*, 2008). However, additional parallel scenarios of how chemotacting leukocytes are directed to their goal have been described (PLA2, cGMP and DOCK2/phosphatic acid). Despite the mentioned advances in understanding how leukocytes find their way in tissue, many issues remain to be deciphered considering the very complex nature of the extravascular environment during infection. Leukocytes will not only encounter bacterial chemoattractants and chemokines, but also cytokines, lipids and complement fragments. Cytokines (IL-1β, TNF-α) are released simultaneously during infection and induce chemokine production. Chemokines and cytokines have been shown to act in concert to direct leukocyte delivery and activation, and chemokines of different families have been demonstrated *in vitro* to synergistically enhance influx of both neutrophils and monocytes (Gouwy M. *et al.*, 2008; Kuscher K. *et al.*, 2009). Further, interplay between lipid chemoattractant LTB$_4$, the cytokine IL-1β and the chemokine ligands to first CCR1 and later CXCR2 was shown in a model of arthritogenesis (Chou R. C. *et al.*, 2010). This vividly demonstrates that leukocyte recruitment *in vivo*, in contrast to during *in vitro* settings hardly is the result of release of a single chemokine, and that synergistic as well as opposing effects of involved signaling molecules are to be expected to enhance as well as steer the inflammatory response. This interplay needs to be further clarified and the importance of these observations has to be confirmed *in vivo*, to determine therapeutic targets during different inflammatory conditions.

3. Additional stimuli for leukocyte recruitment

Inflammation is closely linked to hypoxia, and numerous leukocytes are detected at sites of tissue ischemia (Eltzschig H. K., Carmeliet P., 2011). Severe hypoxia causes both apoptosis and necrosis of somatic cells, which results in release of various damage-associated danger signals, like DAMPs (danger associated molecular pattern molecules). DAMPs include molecules originating from the cytosol or the nucleus, such as adenosine triphosphate (ATP), formylated peptides from mitochondria, heat shock proteins, chromatin and galectins, that often undergo denaturation when leaving the intracellular milieu, where after they become pro-inflammatory (Kono H., Rock K. L., 2008). Even though most of them are not considered directly chemotactic, they induce leukocyte recruitment by activating tissue macrophages and nearby endothelial cells to secrete pro-inflammatory cytokines (*e.g.* IL-1β) and chemokines (*e.g.* IL-8), in addition to upregulating expression of adhesion molecules on endothelial cells (Muller W. A., 2011). However, fomylated peptides originating from mitochondria were recently found to recruit neutrophils via activation of the fMLP receptor formyl-peptide receptor-1 (McDonald B. *et al.*, 2010; Zhang Q. *et al.*, 2010).

During hypoxia and cell injury, recruited neutrophils are believed to contribute to wound healing processes by clearing the area of debris through phagocytosis. In addition to phagocytosis, leukocytes have recently been acknowledged for their role in angiogenesis and tissue remodeling both during health and disease. Neutrophils produce and store within their granules pro-angiogenic molecules such as VEGF-A (vascular endothelial growth factor-A, [Gaudry M. *et al.*, 1997]) and MMP-9 (matrix metalloproteinase-9, [Ardi V. C. *et al.*, 2007]). VEGF is a key player in blood vessel formation and has a direct chemotactic effect on endothelial cells, while the pro-angiogenic function of MMP-9 is attributed to its ability to digest extra cellular matrix (ECM), which pave way for new vessels as well as release and thereby activate ECM-bound VEGF and other growth factors. The neutrophils are in fact the only cells in the body that release MMP-9 free of its endogenous inhibitor TIMP (tissue inhibitor of metalloproteinase), and are therefore capable of deliver highly active MMP-9 to sites of angiogenesis (Ardi V. C. *et al.*, 2007). The pro-angiogenic capacity of neutrophils has been demonstrated in a corneal injury model, where the number of infiltrated neutrophils positively correlated to angiogenesis and VEGF levels (Gong Y., Koh D. R., 2010). Neutrophil depletion significantly impaired tissue healing in this model, as well as the release of VEGF. Further, neutrophils recruited to islets of Langerhans transplanted to striated muscle were recently shown to be crucial for revascularization to occur, as transplantation of islets to neutropenic mice resulted in complete inhibition of islets revascularization (Christoffersson G. *et al.*, 2010). Neutrophils were shown to accumulate at sites for islet engraftment and were specifically localized at the newly formed vessels, as demonstrated in **Figure 2**.

Monocytes have also been shown to have pro-angiogenic properties. For instance, tissue healing following myocardial infarction requires sequential mobilization of the two

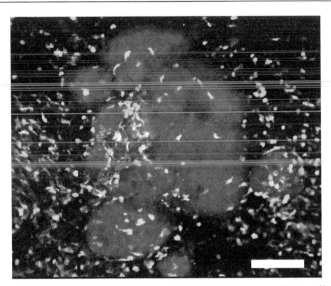

Fig. 2. Isolated pancreatic islets (blue) transplanted to muscle causes Gr1+ cell (green) accumulation (courtesy of G. Christoffersson). Blood vessels are stained with anti-CD31 (red). Scale bar equals 100 μm.

described monocyte subsets which exhibit opposing phenotypes (Nahrendorf M. et al., 2007). Recruited "inflammatory" monocytes exhibit proteolytic activity and inflammatory functions, whereas monocytes of the "resident" subtype contribute to angiogenesis and have attenuated inflammatory properties (Nahrendorf M. et al., 2007).

In the field of tumor biology, it is known that the ability of tumors to create an immunomodulating microenvironment to escape cytotoxic immune cells and to allow for angiogenesis is central for tumor growth. Different factors have been shown to skew tumor-associated leukocytes including neutrophils and macrophages from a pro-inflammatory, anti-tumorigenic to a pro-tumorigenic, pro-angiogenic phenotype (Fridlender Z. G. et al., 2009; Hanahan D., Weinberg R. A., 2011; Rolny C. et al., 2011). Indeed, the angiogenic switch in islet dysplasia and tumors in the RIP1-Tag2 transgenic mouse model of pancreatic cancer was mediated by tumor-infiltrated MMP-9 expressing neutrophils (Nozawa H. et al., 2006).

The identity of these pro-angiogenic leukocytes is currently being investigated, and whether circulating subpopulations with pro-angiogenic and anti-inflammatory properties exist, or if they attain their phenotype giving the stimuli, are under debate. Myeloid-derived suppressor cells (MDSCs) are a heterogenic population that increases in numbers in the spleen and bone marrow of tumor bearing mice, and consists of monocyte and neutrophil subsets with potent ability of suppressing immune functions such as T-lymphocyte activation (Bronte V. et al., 2000). In mice, they express CD11b and Gr-1, where the GR-1hi CD11b+ corresponds to immature and mature neutrophil subpopulations while the Gr-1int CD11b+ to the monocyte subset (Peranzoni E. et al., 2010; Youn J. I., Gabrilovich D. I., 2010). How other surface markers differ from the classical pro-inflammatory neutrophils or monocytes are not completely established, but the roles of neutrophils during restitution and angiogenesis described above might indeed involve the neutrophil subset of MDSC.

Further characterization of the identities of leukocytes involved in tissue restitution and angiogenesis, and even more importantly their functions during these situations, is of great relevance.

4. Therapeutic interventions

A variety of disorders are associated with leukocyte activation and infiltration. Asthma (Fanta C. H., 2009; Broide D. H. *et al.*, 2011; Minnicozzi M. *et al.*, 2011); emphysema (Martinez F. J. *et al.*, 2011); atherosclerosis (Ross R., 1999; Hansson G., 2005); inflammatory bowel disease (Khor B. *et al.*, 2011); rheumatoid arthritis (Olsen N. J., Stein C. M., 2004; O'Dell J. R., 2004; Scott D. L., Kingsley G. H., 2006); multiple sclerosis (Frohman E. M. *et al.*, 2006); sepsis (Hotchkiss R. S., Karl I. E., 2003); and allograft rejection after transplantation (Savasta M., Lentini S., 2011; Arias M. *et al.*, 2011), are just some examples of this broad spectrum. Although many details remain to be delineated, the consensus is that the over-exuberant, maladaptive and/or uncontrolled inflammation is in the pathogenesis of these conditions and leads to tissue injury.

Over the past few years, pharmacotherapeutic advances have been made, with most therapeutic options focusing on means to prevent leukocyte activation and recruitment. Anti-adhesion therapies directed against different adhesion molecules have been evaluated. However, despite positive data from animal studies, many of the integrin antagonists have failed in clinical trials or are associated with severe side effects (Rutgeerts P. *et al.*, 2009; Fontoura P., 2010; Del Zoppo G. J., 2010).

A new approach for reducing leukocyte recruitment to tissue was recently described in mice (Maiguel D. *et al.*, 2011). This study was based upon a nearly 20-year-old observation for eosinophils, which, in response to activating antibodies trapping VLA-4-integrin in a high-avidity state, were able to adhere but not migrate (Kuijpers T. W. *et al.*, 1993). Accordingly, the recent study screened for selective small-molecule Mac-1 agonists, named leukadherins. These agonists caused increased intravascular adhesion, but not transmigration of neutrophils, resulting in reduced leukocyte recruitment in experimental models of acute peritonitis and nephritis. Integrin clustering or outside-in signaling were not induced by binding of the agonist, which might account for the lack of detectable vascular injury, even though the effects on tissue blood flow by the increased number of intravascular adherent neutrophils remains to be studied. These observations are all very intriguing, even though further experimental evaluation of this course of action is required.

5. Conclusion

Leukocyte recruitment is a hallmark event in acute and chronic inflammation. Tightly regulated activation of circulating leukocytes and intravascular leukocyte guidance by the establishment of chemokine gradients within blood vessels is fundamental for leukocytes to efficiently transmigrate to the inflamed tissue, where they finally exert their effector functions. Specific interactions between transmigrating leukocytes and the activated vascular endothelium orchestrate profound anatomical changes of the endothelium which facilitate leukocyte extravasation while maintaining the barrier function and vascular permeability. Targeting intravascular leukocyte chemotaxis and the gating property of the endothelium would limit leukocyte transmigration and/ or vascular permeability during detrimental inflammation. Understanding the underlying mechanisms behind these processes might therefore contribute for the development of novel therapeutic interventions.

6. Acknowledgements

The authors would like to acknowledge Gustaf Christoffersson who kindly supplied the image presented as Figure 2.

This work was supported by grants from the Swedish Medical Research Council, the Royal Swedish Academy of Sciences, Magnus Bergvalls Foundation, the Swedish Society for Medical Research, the Swedish Diabetes Foundation, Lars Hiertas Foundation, Harald and Greta Jeanssons Foundation, Åke Wibergs Foundation, and the Wallenberg Foundation.

7. References

Aird W. C. Phenotypic heterogeneity of the endothelium: II. Representative vascular beds. Circ. Res. (2007); 100 (2): 174-190.

Allport J. R., Ding H. T., Ager A., Steeber D. A., Tedder T. F., Luscinskas F. W. L-selectin shedding does not regulate human neutrophil attachment, rolling, or transmigration across human vascular endothelium *in vitro*. J. Immunol. (1997); 158 (9): 4365-4372.

Ardi V. C., Kupriyanova T. A., Deryugina E. I., Quingly J. P. Human neutrophils uniquely release TIMP-free MMP-9 to provide a potent catalytic stimulator of angiogenesis. Proc. Natl. Acad. Sci. U. S. A. (2007); 104 (51): 20262-20267.

Arias M., Serón D., Moreso F., Bestard O., Praga M. Chronic renal allograft damage: existing challenges. Transplantation (2011); 91 (9 Suppl): S4-S5.

Auffray C., Fogg D., Garfa M., Elain G., Join-Lambert O., Kayal S., Sarnacki S., Cumano A., Lauvau G., Geissmann F. Monitoring blood vessels and tissues by a population of monocytes with patrolling behavior. Science (2007); 317 (5838): 666-670.

Bendelac A., Savage P. B., Teyton L. The biology of NKT cells. Annu. Rev. Immunol. (2007); 25: 297-336.

Bernfield M., Götte M., Park P. W., Reizes O., Fitzgerald M. L., Lincecum J., Zako M. Functions of cell surface heparan sulfate proteoglycans. Annu. Rev. Biochem. (1999); 68: 729-777.

Broide D. H., Finkelman F. Bochner B. S., Rothenberg M. E. Advances in mechanisms of asthma, and immunology in 2010. J. Allergy Clin. Immunol. (2011); 127 (3): 689-695.

Bronte V., Apolloni E., Cabrelle A., Ronca R., Serafini P., Zamboni P., Restifo N. P., Zanovello P. Identification of a CD11b(+)/Gr-1(+)/CD31(+) myeloid progenitor capable of activating or suppressing CD8(+) T cells. Blood (2000); 96 (12): 3838-3846.

Brossay L., Chioda M., Burdin N., Koezuka Y., Casorati G., Dellabona P., Kronenberg M. CD1d-mediated recognition of an alpha-galactosylceramide by natural killer T cells is highly conserved through mammalian evolution. J. Exp. Med. (1998); 188 (8): 1521-1528.

Bunting M., Harris E. S., McIntyre T. M., Prescott S. M., Zimmerman G. A. Leukocyte adhesion deficiency syndromes: adhesion and tethering defects involving beta 2 integrins and selectin ligands. Curr. Opin. Hematol. (2002); 9 (1): 30-35.

Campbell J. J., Foxman E. F., Butcher E. C. Chemoattractant receptor cross talk as a regulatory mechanism in leukocyte adhesion and migration. Eur. J. Immunol. (1997); 27 (10): 2571-2578.

Carman C. V., Springer T.A. Integrin avidity regulation: are changes in affinity and conformation underemphasized? Curr. Opin. Cell Biol. (2003); 15 (5): 547-556.

Carman C. V., Springer T.A. A transmigratory cup in leukocyte diapedesis both through individual vascular endothelial cells and between them. J. Cell Biol. (2004); 167 (2): 377-388.

Chou R. C., Kim N. D., Sadik C. D., Seung E., Lan Y., Byrne M. H., Haribabu B., Iwakura Y., Luster A. D. Lipid-cytokine-chemokine cascade drives neutrophil recruitment in a murine model of inflammatory arthritis. Immunity (2010); 33 (2): 266-278.

Christoffersson G., Henriksnäs J., Johansson L., Rolny C., Ahlström H., Caballero-Corbalan J., Segersvärd R., Permert J., Korsgren O., Carlsson P. O., Phillipson M. Clinical and experimental pancreatic islet transplantation to striated muscle: establishment of a vascular system similar to that in native islets. Diabetes (2010); 59 (10): 2569-2578.

Curry F. R., Adamson R. H. Transendothelial pathways in venular microvessels exposed to agents which increase permeability: the gaps in our knowledge. Microcirculation (1999); 6(1): 3-5.

Curry F. R., Adamson R. H. Vascular permeability modulation at the cell, microvessel, or whole organ level: towards closing gaps in our knowledge. Cardiovasc. Res. (2010); 87 (2): 218-229.

De Fougerolles A. R., Qin X., Springer T. A. Characterization of the function of intercellular adhesion molecule (ICAM)-3 and comparison with ICAM-1 and ICAM-2 in immune responses. J. Exp. Med. (1994); 179 (2): 619-629.

Del Zoppo G. J. Acute anti-inflammatory approaches to ischemic stroke. Ann. N. Y. Acad. Sci. (2010); 1207: 143-148.

Diamond M. S., Springer T. A. The dynamic regulation of integrin adhesiveness. Curr. Biol. (1994); 4 (6): 506-517.

Doerschuk C. M., Winn R. K., Coxson H. O., Harlan J. M. CD18-dependent and independent mechanisms of neutrophil emigration in the pulmonary and systemic microcirculation of rabbits. J. Immunol. (1990); 144 (6): 2327-2333.

Dustin M. L., Springer T. A. T-cell receptor cross-linking transiently stimulates adhesiveness through LFA-1. Nature (1989); 341 (6243): 619-624.

Eltzschig H. K., Carmeliet P. Hypoxia and inflammation. N. Engl. J. Med. (2011); 364 (7); 656-665.

Engelhardt B., Wolburg H. Mini-review: Transendothelial migration of leukocytes: through the front door or around the sides of the house? Eur. J. Immunol. (2004); 34 (11): 2955-2963.

Fanta C. H. Asthma. N. Engl. J. Med. (2009); 360 (10): 1002-1014.

Faveew C., Di Mauro M. E., Price A. A., Ager A. Roles of alpha(4) integrins/ VCAM-1 and LFA-1/ ICAM-1 in the binding and transendothelial migration of T lymphocytes and T lymphoblasts across high endothelial venules. Int. Immunol. (2000); 12 (3): 241-251.

Feng D., Nagy J. A., Pyne K., Dvorak H. F., Dvorak A. M. Neutrophils emigrate from venules by transendothelial cell pathway in response to FMLP. J. Exp. Med. (1998); 187 (6): 903-915.

Friedl P., Borgmann S., Bröcker E. B. Amoeboid leukocyte crawling through extracellular matrix: lessons from the Dictyostelium paradigm of cell movement. J. Leukoc. Biol. (2001); 70 (4): 491-509.

Frohman E. M., Racke M. K., Raine C. S. Multiple Sclerosis – The plaque and its pathogenesis. N. Engl. J. Med. (2006); 354 (9): 942-955.

Fontoura P. Monoclonal antibody therapy in multiple sclerosis: Paradigm shifts and emerging challenges. MAbs. (2010); 2 (6): 670-681.

Foxman E. F., Campbell J. J., Butcher E. C. Multistep navigation and the combinatorial control of leukocyte chemotaxis. J. Cell Biol. (1997); 139 (5): 1349-1360.

Fridlender Z. G., Sun J., Kim S., Kapoor V., Cheng G., Ling L., Worthen G. S., Albelda S. M. Polarization of tumor-associated neutrophil phenotype by TGF-beta: "N1" *versus* "N2" TAN. Cancer Cell (2009); 16 (3): 183-194.

Gao J. X., Issekutz A. C. The beta 1 integrin, very late activation antigen-4 on human neutrophils can contribute to neutrophil migration through connective tissue fibroblast barriers. Immunology (1997); 90 (3): 448-454.

Gaudry M., Brégerie O., Andrieu V., El Benna J., Pocidalo M. A., Hakim J. Intracellular pool of vascular endothelial growth factor in human neutrophils. Blood (1997); 90 (10): 4153-4161.

Gouwy M., Struyf S., Noppen S., Schutyser E., Springael J. Y., Parmentier M., Proost P., Van Damme J. Synergy between coproduced CC and CXC chemokines in monocyte chemotaxis through receptor-mediated events. Mol. Pharmacol. (2008); 74 (2): 485-495.

Geissmann F., Cameron T. O., Sidobre S., Manlongat N., Kronenberg M., Briskin M. J., Dustin M. L., Littman D. R. Intravascular immune surveillance by CXCR6+ NKT cells patrolling liver sinusoids. PLoS Biol. (2005); 3 (4): e113.

Geissmann F., Jung S., Littman D. R. Blood monocytes consist of two principal subsets with distinct migratory properties. Immunity (2003); 19 (1): 71-82.

Gong Y., Koh D. R. Neutrophils promote inflammatory angiogenesis via release of preformed VEGF in an *in vivo* corneal model. Cell Tissue Res. (2010); 339 (2): 437-448.

Gordon S., Taylor P. R. Monocyte and macrophage heterogeneity. Nat. Rev. Immunol. (2005); 5 (12): 953-964.

Hanahan D., Weinberg R. A. Hallmarks of cancer: the next generation. Cell (2011); 144 (5): 646-674.

Hansson G. K. Inflammation, Atherosclerosis, and Coronary Artery Disease. N. Engl. J. Med. (2005); 352 (16): 1685-1695.

Heit B., Robbins S. M., Downey C. M., Guan Z., Colarusso P., Miller B. J., Jirik F. R., Kubes P. PTEN functions to 'prioritize' chemotactic cues and prevent 'distraction' in migrating neutrophils. Nat. Immunol. (2008); 9: 716-718.

Heit B., Tavener S., Raharjo E., Kubes P. An intracellular signaling hierarchy determines direction of migration in opposing chemotactic gradients. J. Cell. Biol. (2002); 159 (1): 91-102.

Hemler M. E. VLA proteins in the integrin family: structures, functions, and their role on leukocytes. Annu. Rev. Immunol. (1990); 8: 365-400.

Hickey M. J., Forster M., Mitchell D., Kaur J., De Caigny C., Kubes P. L-selectin facilitates emigration and extravascular locomotion of leukocytes during acute inflammatory responses *in vivo*. J. Immunol. (2000); 165 (12): 7164-7170.

Hotchkiss R. S., Karl I. E. The Pathophysiology and Treatment of Sepsis. N. Engl. J. Med. (2003); 348 (2): 138-150.

Hyduk S. J., Cybulsky M. I. Role of alpha4beta1 integrins in chemokine-induced monocyte arreest under conditions of shear stress. Microcirculation (2009); 16 (1): 17-30.

Ibbotson G. C., Doig C., Kaur J., Gill V., Ostrovsky L., Fairhead T., Kubes P. Functional alpha4-integrin: a newly identified pathway of neutrophil recruitment in critically septic patients. Nat. Med. (2001); 7 (4): 465-470.

Ihrcke N. S., Wrenshall L. E., Lindman B. J., Platt J. L. Role of heparan sulfate in immune system-blood vessel interactions. Immunol. Today (1993); 14: 500-505.

Jaeschke H., Farhood A., Fisher M. A., Smith C. W. Sequestration of neutrophils in the hepatic vasculature during endotoxemia is independent of beta 2 integrins and intercellular adhesion molecule-1. Shock (1996); 6 (5): 351-356.

Jutila M. A., Rott L., Berg E. L., Butcher E. C. Function and regulation of the neutrophil MEL-14 antigen *in vivo*: comparison with LFA-1 and MAC-1. J. Immunol. (1989); 143 (10): 3318-3324.

Kansas G. S. Selectins and their ligands: current concepts and controversies. Blood (1996); 88 (9): 3259-3287.

Kawano T., Cui J., Koezuka Y., Toura I., Kaneko Y., Motoki K., Ueno H., Nakagawa R., Sato H., Kondo E., Koseki H., Taniguchi M. CD1d-restricted and TCR-mediated activation of valpha14 NKT cells by glycosylceramides. Science (1997); 278 (5343): 1626-1629.

Kelly M., Hwang J. M., Kubes P. Modulating leukocyte recruitment in inflammation. J. Allergy Clin. Immmunol. (2007); 120 (1): 3-10.

Kenne E., Lindbom L. Imaging inflammatory plasma leakage *in vivo*. Thromb. Haemost. (2011); 105 (5): 783-789.

Kim M. H., Curry F. R., Simon S. I. Dynamics of neutrophil extravasation and vascular permeability are uncoupled during aseptic cutaneous wounding. Am. J. Physiol. Cell Physiol. (2009); 296 (4): C848-856.

Kono H., Rock K. L. How dying cells alert the immune system to danger. Nat. Rev. Immunol. (2008); 8 (4): 279-289.

Kubes P., Niu X. F., Smith C. W., Kehrli M. E. Jr., Reinhardt P. H., Woodman R. C. A novel β_1-dependent adhesion pathway on neutrophils: a mechanism invoked by dihydrocytochalasin B or endothelial transmigration. FASEB J. (1995); 9 (11): 1103-1111.

Kuijpers T. W., Mul E. P., Blom M., Kovach N. L., Gaeta F. C., Tollefson V., Elices M. J., Harlan J. M. Freezing adhesion molecules in a state of high-avidity binding blocks eosinophil migration. J. Exp. Med. (1993); 178 (1): 279-284.

Kunkel E. J., Ley K. Distinct phenotype of E-selectin-deficient mice. E-selectin is required for slow rolling *in vivo*. Circ. Res. (1996); 79 (6); 1196-1204.

Kuscher K., Danelon G., Paoletti S., Stefano L., Schiraldi M., Petkovic V., Locati M., Gerber B. O., Uguccioni M. Synergy-inducing chemokines enhance CCR2 ligand activities on monocytes. Eur. J. Immunol. (2009); 39 (4): 1118-1128.

Lee T. D., Gonzalez M. L., Kumar P., Grammas P., Pereira H. A. CAP37, a neutrophil-derived inflammatory mediator, augments leukocyte adhesion to endothelial monolayers. Microvasc. Res. (2003); 66 (1): 38-48.

Ley K., Laudanna C., Cybulsky M. I., Nourshargh S. Getting to the site of inflammation: the leukocyte adhesion cascade updated. Nat. Rev. Immunol. (2007); 7 (9): 678-689.

Lindbom L., Werr J. Integrin-dependent neutrophil migration in extravascular tissue. Semin. Immunol. (2002); 14 (2): 115-121.

Lindhal U. Heparan sulfate-protein interactions: a concept for drug design? Thromb. Haemost. (2007); 98 (1): 109-115.

Lindhal U., Kjellén L. Heparin or heparan sulfate: what is the difference? Thromb. Haemost. (1991); 66 (1): 44-48.

Lindahl U., Li J. P. Interactions between heparan sulfate and proteins-design and functional implications. Int. Rev. Cell Mol. Biol. (2009); 276: 105-159.

Lou O., Alcaide P., Luscinskas F. W., Muller W. A. CD99 is a key mediator of the transendothelial migration of neutrohils. J. Immunol. (2007); 178 (2): 1136-1143.

Lund-Johansen F., Terstappen L. W. Differential surface expression of cell adhesion molecules during granulocyte maturation. J. Leukoc. Biol. (1993); 54 (1): 47-55.

Luo B. H., Carman C. V., Springer T. A. Structural basis of integrin regulation and signaling. Annu. Rev. Immunol (2007); 25: 619-647.

Luscinskas F. W., Kansas G. S., Ding H., Pizcueta P., Schleiffenbaum B. E., Tedder T. F., Gimbrone M. A. Jr. Monocyte rolling, arrest and spreading on IL-4-activated vascular endothelium under flow is mediated via sequential action of L-selectin, beta 1-integrins, and beta 2-integrins. J. Cell Biol. (1994); 125 (6): 1417-1427.

Luscinskas F. W., Ma S., Nusrat A., Parkos C. A., Shaw S. K. Leukocyte transendothelial migration: a junctional affair. Semin. Immunol. (2002); 14 (2): 105-113.

Maiguel D., Faridi M. H., Wei C., Kuwano Y., Balla K. M., Hernandez D., Barth C. J., Lugo G., Donnelly M., Nayer A., Moita L. F., Schürer S., Traver D., Ruiz P., Vazquez-Padron R. I., Ley K., Reiser J., Gupta V. Small Molecule-Mediated Activation of the Integrin CD11b/CD18 Reduces Inflammatory Disease. Sci. Signal. (2011); 4 (189): ra57.

Martinez F. J., Donohue J. F., Rennard S. I. The future of chronic obstructive pulmonary disease treatment – difficulties of and barriers to drug development. Lancet (2011); 378: 1027-1037.

Massena S., Christoffersson G., Hjertström E., Zcharia E., Vlodavsky I., Ausmees N., Rolny C., Li J. P., Phillipson M. A chemotactic gradient sequestered on endothelial heparan sulfate induces directional intraluminal crawling of neutrophils. Blood (2010); 116 (11): 1924-1931.

McDonald B., McAvoy E. F., Lam F., Gill V., de la Motte C., Savani R. C., Kubes P. Interaction of CD44 and hyaluronan is the dominant mechanism for neutrophil sequestration in inflamed liver sinusoids. J. Exp. Med. (2008); 205 (4): 915-927.

McDonald B., Pittman K., Menezes G. B., Hirota S. A., Slaba I., Waterhouse C. C., Beck P. L., Muruve D. A., Kubes P. Intravascular danger signals guide neutrophils to sites of sterile inflammation. Science (2010); 330 (6002): 362-366.

McEver R. P. Adhesive interactions of leukocytes, platelets, and the vessel wall during hemostasis and inflammation. Thromb. Haemost. (2001); 86 (3): 746-756.

McEver R. P., Zhu C. Rolling Cell Adhesion. Annu. Rev. Cell Dev. Biol. (2010); 26: 363-396.

McNab F. W., Berzins S. P., Pellicci D. G., Kyparissoudis K., Field K., Smyth M. J., Godfrey D. I. The influence of CD1d in postselection NKT cell maturation and homeostasis. J. Immunol. (2005); 175 (6): 3762-3768.

Meerschaert J., Furie M. B. The adhesion molecules used by monocytes for migration across the endothelium include CD11a/CD18, CD11b/CD18, and VLA-4 on monocytes and ICAM-1, VCAM-1, and other ligands on endothelium. J. Immunol (1995); 154 (8): 4099-4112.

Mehta D., Malik A. B. Signaling mechanisms regulating endothelial permeability. Physiol. Rev. (2006); 86 (1): 279-367.

Michel C. C., Curry F. E. Microvascular permeability. Physiol. Rev. (1999); 79 (3): 703-761.

Middleton J., Neil S., Wintle J., Clark-Lewis I., Moore H., Lam C., Auer M., Hub E., Rot A. Transcytosis and surface presentation of IL-8 by venular endothelial cells. Cell (1997); 91: 385-395.

Minnicozzi M., Sawyer R. T., Fenton M. J. Innate immunity in allergic disease. Immunol Rev. (2011); 242 (1): 106-127.

Muller W. A. Sorting the signals from the signals in the noisy environment of inflammation. Sci. Signal. (2011); 4 (170): pe23.

Nahrendorf M., Swirski F. K., Aikawa E., Stangenberg L., Wurdinger T., Figueiredo J. L., Libby P., Weissleder R., Pittet M. J..The healing myocardium sequentially mobilizes two monocyte subsets with divergent and complementary functions. J. Exp. Med. (2007); 204 (12): 3037-3047.

Norman M. U., Kubes P. Therapeutic intervention in inflammatory diseases: a time and place for anti-adhesion therapy. Microcirculation (2005); 12 (1): 91-98.

Nozawa H., Chiu C., Hanahan D. Infiltrating neutrophils mediate the initial angiogenic switch in a mouse model of multistage carcinogenesis. PNAS (2006); 103 (33): 12493-12498.

O'Dell J. R. Therapeutic targets for rheumatoid arthritis. N. Engl. J. Med. (2004); 350 (25): 2591-2602.

Olsen N. J., Stein C. M. New drugs for rheumatoid arthritis. N. Engl. J. Med. (2004); 350 (21): 2167-2179.

Parish C. Heparan sulfate and inflammation. Nat. Immunol. (2005); 6 (9): 861-862.

Patel K. D., Nollert M. U., McEver R. P. P-selectin must extend a sufficient length from the plasma membrane to mediate rolling of neutrophils. J. Cell. Biol. (1995); 131: 1893-1902.

Peranzoni E., Zilio S., Marigo I., Dolcetti L., Zanovello P., Mandruzzato S., Bronte V. Myeloid-derived suppressor cell heterogeneity and subset definition. Curr. Opin. Immunol. (2010); 22 (2): 238-244.

Petri B., Kaur J., Long E. M., Li H., Parsons S. A., Butz S., Phillipson M., Vestweber D., Patel K. D., Robbins S. M., Kubes P. Blood (2011); 117 (3): 942-952.

Petri B., Phillipson M., Kubes P. The physiology of leukocyte recruitment: an *in vivo* perspective. J. Immunol. (2008); 180 (10): 6439-6446.

Phillipson M., Heit B., Colarusso P., Liu L., Ballantyne C. M., Kubes P. Intraluminal crawling of neutrophils to emigration sites: a molecularly distinct process from adhesion in the recruitment cascade. J. Exp. Med. (2006); 203 (12): 2569-2575.

Phillipson M., Heit B., Parsons S. A., Petri B., Mullaly S. C., Colarusso P., Gower R. M., Neely G., Simon S. I., Kubes P. Vav1 is essential for mechanotactic crawling and migration of neutrophils out of the inflamed microvasculature. J. Immunol. (2009); 182 (11): 6870-6878.

Phillipson M., Kaur J., Colarusso P., Ballantyne C. M., Kubes P. Endothelial domes encapsulate adherent neutrophils and minimize increases in vascular permeability in paracellular and transcellular emigration. PLoS One (2008); 3: e1649.

Phillipson M., Kubes P. The neutrophil in vascular inflammation. Nat. Med. (2011); 17 (11): 1381-1390.

Pillay J., Ramakers B. P., Kamp V. M., Loi A. L., Lam S. W., Hietbrink F., Leenen L. P., Tool A. T. Pickkers P., Koenderman L. Functional heterogeneity and differential priming of circulating neutrophils in human experimental endotoxemia. J. Leukoc. Biol. (2010); 88 (1): 211-220.

Rolny C., Mazzone M., Tugues S., Laoui D., Johansson I., Coulon C., Squadrito M. L., Segura I., Li X., Knevels E., Costa S., Vinckier S., Dresselaer T., Åkerud P., De Mol M., Salomäki H., Phillipson M., Wyns S., Larsson E., Buysschaert I., Botling J., Himmelreich U., Van Ginderachter J. A., De Palma M., Dewerchin M., Claesson-Welsh L., Carmeliet P. HRG inhibits tumor growth and metastasis by inducing macrophage polarization and vessel normalization through downregulation of PlGF. Cancer Cell (2011); 19 (1): 31-44.

Rose D. M., Alon R., Ginsberg M. H. Integrin modulation and signaling in leukocyte adhesion and migration. Immunol. Rev. (2007); 218: 126-134.

Ross R. Atherosclerosis – An Inflammatory Disease. N. Engl. J. Med. (1999); 340 (2): 115-126.

Rutgeerts P.,Vermeire S., Van Assche G. Biological therapies for inflammatory bowel diseases. Gastroenterology (2009); 136 (4): 1182-1197.

Savasta M., Lentini S. Immunology insights into cardiac allograft rejection. Rev. Cardiovasc. Med. (2011); 12 (2): e68-76.

Schenkel A. R., Mamdouh Z., Muller W. A. Locomotion of monocytes on endothelium is a critical step during extravasation. Nat. Immunol. (2004); 5: 393-400.

Scott D. L., Kingsley G. H. Tumor necrosis factor inhibitors for rheumatoid arthritis. N. Engl. J. Med. (2006); 355 (7): 704-712.

Shamri R., Grabovsky V., Gauguet J. M., Feigelson S., Manevich E., Kolanus W., Robinson M. K., Stauton D. E., Andrian U. H., Alon R. Lymphocyte arrest requires instantaneous induction of an extended LFA-1 conformation mediated by endothelium-bound chemokines. Nat. Immunol. (2005); 6 (5): 497-506.

Shaw S. K., Bamba P. S., Perkins B. N., Luscinskas F. W. Real-time imaging of vascular endothelial-cadherin during leukocyte transmigration across endothelium. J. Immunol. (2001); 164 (4): 2323-2330.

Shulman Z., Shinder V., Klein E., Grabovsky V., Yeger O., Geron E., Montresor A., Bolomini-Vittori M., Feigelson S. W., Kirchhausen T., Laudanna C., Shakhar G., Alon R. Lymphocyte crawling and transendothelial migration require chemokine triggering of high-affinity LFA-1 integrin. Immunity (2009); 30 (3): 384-396.

Simon S. I., Goldsmith H. L. Leukocyte adhesion dynamics under in shear flow. Ann. Biomed. Eng. (2002); 30 (3): 315-332.

Simon S. I., Green C. E. Molecular mechanisms and dynamics of leukocyte recruitment during inflammation. Annu. Rev. Biomed. Eng. (2005); 7: 151-185.

Sixt M., Hallmann R., Wendler O., Scharffetter-Kochanek K., Sorokin L. M. Cell adhesion and migration properties of beta 2-integrin negative polymorphonuclear granulocytes on defined extracellular matrix molecules. Relevance for leukocyte extravasation. J. Biol. Chem. (2001); 276 (22): 18878-18887.

Smith A., Carrasco Y. R., Stanley P., Kieffer N., Batista F. D., Hogg N. A talin-dependent LFA-1 focal zone is formed by rapidly migrating T lymphocytes. J. Cell. Biol. (2005); 170 (1): 141-151.

Smith A., Stanley P., Jones K., Svensson L., McDowall A., Hogg N. The role of the integrin LFA-1 in T-lymphocyte migration. Immunol. Rev. (2007); 218: 135-146.

Smith C. W., Kishimoto T. K., Abbassi O., Hughes B., Rothlein R., McIntire L. V., Butcher E., Anderson D. C. Chemotactic factors regulate lectin adhesion molecule 1 (LECAM-1)-dependent neutrophil adhesion to cytokine-stimulated endothelial cells *in vitro*. J. Clin. Invest. (1991); 87 (2): 609-618.

Soehnlein O., Lindbom L., Weber C. Mechanisms underlying neutrophil-mediated monocyte recruitment. Blood (2009); 114 (21): 4613-4623.

Sumagin R., Prizant H., Lomakina E., Waugh R. E., Sarelius I. H. LFA-1 and Mac-1 define characteristically different intraluminal crawling and emigration patterns for monocytes and neutrophils in situ. J. Immunol. (2010); 185 (11): 7057-7066.

Van Den Berg B. M., Vink H., Spaan J. A. The endothelial glycocalyx protects against myocardial edema. Circ. Res. (2003); 92 (6): 592-594.

Von Andrian U. H., Hansell P., Chambers J. D., Berger E. M., Torres Filho I., Butcher E. C., Arfors K. E. L-selectin function is required for beta-2-integrin-mediated neutrophil adhesion at physiological shear rates *in vivo*. Am. J. Physiol. (1992); 263: H1034-1044.

Wang L., Fuster M., Sriramarao P., Esko J. D. Endothelial heparan sulfate deficiency impairs L-selectin- and chemokine-mediated neutrophil trafficking during inflammatory responses. Nat. Immunol. (2005); 6: 902-910.

Wang S., Voisin M. B., Larbi K. Y., Dangerfield J., Scheiermann C., Tran M., Maxwell P. H., Sorokin L., Nourshargh S. Venular basement membranes contain specific matrix protein low expression regions that act as exit points for emigrating neutrophils. J. Exp. Med. (2006); 203 (6): 1519-1532.

Wei D. G., Lee H., Park S. H., Beaudoin L., Teyton L., Lehuen A., Bendelac A. Expansion and long-range differentiation of the NKT cell lineage in mice expressing CD1d exclusively on cortical thymocytes. J. Exp. Med. (2005); 202 (2): 239-248.

Werr J., Xie X., Hedqvist P., Ruoslahti E., Lindbom L. Beta1 integrins are critically involved in neutrophil locomotion in extravascular tissue *In vivo*. J. Exp. Med. (1998); 187 (12): 2091-2096.

Wong J., Johnston B., Lee S. S., Bullard D. C., Smith C. W., Beaudet A. L., Kubes P. A minimal role for selectins in the recruitment of leukocytes into the inflamed liver microvasculature. J. Clin. Invest. (1997); 99 (11): 2782-2790.

Woodfin A., Voisin M. B., Beyrau M., Colom B., Caille D., Diapouli F. M., Nash G. B., Chevakis T., Albelda S. M., Rainger G. E., Meda P., Imhof B. A., Nourshargh S. The junctional adhesion molecule JAM-C regulates polarized transendothelial migration of neutrophils *in vivo*. Nat. Immunol. (2011); 12 (8): 761-769.

Yang L., Froio R. M., Sciuto T. E., Dvorak A. M., Alon R., Luscinskas F. W. ICAM-1 regulates neutrophil adhesion and transcellular migration of TNF-alpha-activated vascular endothelium under flow. Blood (2005); 106 (2): 584-592.

Youn J. I., Gabrilovich D. I. The biology of myeloid-derived suppressor cells: the blessing and the curse of morphological and functional heterogeneity. Eur. J. Immunol. (2010); 40 (11): 2969-2975.

Zhang Q., Raoof M., Chen Y., Sumi Y., Sursal T., Junger W., Brohi K., Itagaki K., Hauser C. J. Circulating mitochondrial DAMPs cause inflammatory responses to injury. Nature (2010); 464 (7285): 104-107.

9

SATB1: Key Regulator of T Cell Development and Differentiation

Kamalvishnu P. Gottimukkala, Mithila Burute and Sanjeev Galande

Indian Institute of Science Education and Research
Sai Trinity, Garware Circle, Pashan, Pune
India

1. Introduction

Vertebrates have evolved a lymphocyte based adaptive immune system which specifically recognises antigens (Pancer and Cooper, 2006). The lymphoid progenitor cells migrate to the thymus a primary lymphoid organ for the development of T cells (Yang et al., 2010; Zlotoff and Bhandoola, 2011). Progenitor cells undergo a stringent selection process which leads to the development of T cells which have a T cell receptor that specifically reacts with the foreign antigens and not with the self antigens. The pre-T cells further differentiate into many subpopulations in the thymus or the peripheral organs, which perform different functions and are responsible for the adaptive immune responses. The maturation and development of T cells is typically defined by the expression of specific cell surface receptors. The early immature thymocytes that do not express either CD4 or CD8 are called double negative (DN) thymocytes. At these stage the cells undergo the rearrangement of T cell receptor (TCR) β chain. Subsequently, these cells express both CD4$^+$ CD8$^+$ and are referred to as the double positive (DP) cells. During this stage, the rearrangement of the α chain of TCR happens and the cells express the complete T cell receptor (Kreslavsky et al., 2010). The DP thymocytes undergo proliferation and depending on the strength of TCR signaling further develop into either CD4$^+$ or CD8$^+$ single positive (SP) T cells via repression of the gene encoding the other receptor.

The mature T cells migrate to the periphery wherein they encounter the antigens and develop into effector cells. The differentiation of naïve cells into the effector cells depends on the signaling pathways, the pathogen or the cytokines secreted by the antigen presenting cells (APCs). Naïve CD4 T cells mature into various subpopulations which secrete characterisic effector cytokines that define the functions of T cells. Based on the cytokines produced the CD4 T cells are distinguished into multiple subtypes such as T_H1, T_H2, T_H17, induced regulatory T cells (iTregs), Tfh and T_H9 (Zhu et al., 2010). Table 1 provides general overview of various lineages of CD4$^+$ T cells with their key factors and cytokines secreted. The first functionally distinct subpopulations of CD4$^+$ T cells were identified and described as the T_H1/T_H2 paradigm by Mosmann and Coffman, (Mosmann et al., 1986; Mosmann & Coffman, 1987) followed by delineation of the roles of T_H1 and T_H2 cells in cell-mediated and humoral immunity respectively. IL-12 signaling via STAT-4 results in the development of T_H1 cells. IL-4 signaling in conjunction with STAT-6 skews the cells towards T_H2

phenotype. Another major subtype of CD4+ T cells that has gained considerable importance in recent years is T$_H$17 which produce IL-6 and IL-17. The transcription factors STAT-3 and RORγt act as master regulators for T$_H$17 differentiation (Park et al., 2005; Dong et al., 2008). Major function of T$_H$ cells is to help B cells to develop antigen-specific antibody response. A subset of T$_H$ cells enter into germinal center and interact with developing B cells and assist them for class-switching. This subset of cells is known as Follicular Helper T cells (Tfh). The Tfh cells secrete IL-4 or IFNγ depending upon their priming (King et al., 2008). Naïve peripheral CD4+ T cells can be induced to give rise to iTreg cells which require FOXP3 transcription factor. These cells are shown to be involved in suppressor function of immune system and for maintainance of tolerance to self-antigens (DiPaolo et al., 2007). T$_H$9 is another recently discovered type of CD4+ T cells which produce IL-9 and whose function is not clearly understood. However it is proposed that these cells might be involved in confering immunity against helminth infection (Staudt et al., 2010).

Subset of CD4+ T cells	Important Transcription factors	Hallmark cytokines secreted by cells	Function (Described in)
T$_H$1	STAT-4, T-bet	IFN-γ	Cell mediated Immunity (Mosmann & Coffman, 1987)
T$_H$2	STAT-6, SATB1, GATA-3	IL-5, IL-4, IL-13	Humoral Immunity (Mosmann & Coffman, 1987)
Treg	FOXP3		Maintainance of tolerance (Sakaguchi et al., 2008)
T$_H$17	STAT-3, ROR γt	IL-17A, IL-17F	Inflammation, autoimmunity (Hirota et al., 2011)
Tfh	Bcl-6	IL-21	Mediate help and class switching in B cells in germinal centers (Kitano et al., 2011)
T$_H$9	IRF-4	IL-9	Immunity against helminth infection, most important cell type responsible for the pathogenesis of Asthma (Staudt et al., 2010)

Table 1. **Functional subtypes of CD4+ T lineage.** Various characterized subtypes of CD4+ T cells are listed with their reported essential factors required for lineage determination, key cytokine secreted and function of these cells. For details see text.

2. SATB1 and its role in transcriptional regulation of multiple genes

The cell signaling pathways which initiate the differentiation process ultimately lead to expression of a specific transcription factor. The key transcription factors are important for the expression of specific cytokine gene and maintenance of the phenotype. SATB1 is a T cell enriched transcription factor that regulates large number of genes involved in T cell development and is also required for the maintainance of higher-order chromatin architecture (Alvarez et al., 2000; Kumar et al., 2006; Cai et al., 2003; Cai et al., 2006, Kumar et al., 2007). Ablation of SATB1 causes dysregulation of genes required for the development of T cells and the development is stalled at the DP stage (Alvarez et al., 2000). Thymocytes from SATB1 knockout mice revealed ectopic expression of genes such as *IL-2R* and *IL-7R*. SATB1 is known to regulate genes by selectively tethering their regulatory regions and via formation of a characteristic cage-like structure around the heterochromatic regions in Thymocytes (Cai et al., 2004), presumably demarcating the active and inactive domains (Galande et al., 2007). SATB1 also acts as a docking site for chromatin remodeling/modifying factors such as ISWI, ASF1 and NURD complex containing HDAC1, leading to the repression of genes (Yasui et al., 2000). Post-translational modifications of SATB1 such as acetylation and phosphorylation act as molecular switches regulating its ability to govern gene expression. The PDZ-like domain of SATB1 undergoes phosphorylation by PKC and acetylation by PCAF acetyltransferase in signal-dependent manner (Kumar et al., 2006). Acetylation of SATB1 negatively influences the DNA binding activity of SATB1 whereas phosphorylated form of SATB1 is shown to bind tightly to the *Il-2* promoter and repress *Il-2*. Interaction of SATB1 with the CtBP1 corepressor via its N-terminal PDZ-like domain represses transcription. Upon inhibition of Wnt signaling by LiCl treatment SATB1 is acetylated, loses its interaction with CtBP1 and thus leads to activation of *Il-2* (Purbey et al., 2009). Further, SATB1 is also known to regulate chromatin loop domain organization ('loopscape') in a cell type-specific manner. In Jurkat T cells, SATB1 organizes the MHC class I locus into a 'loopscape' comprising six loops. However, CHO cells which express comparatively less SATB1 exhibit a different 'loopscape' of the MHC locus. Intersstingly, overexpression of SATB1 in CHO cells rendered the 'loopscape' similar to that in Jurkat cells underscoring the importantance of SATB1 in cell-type specific higher-order chromatin organization (Kumar et al., 2007; Galande et al., 2007). In T_H2 cells, SATB1 organizes the loop domain architecture of the T_H2 cytokine locus and governs the coordinated expression of *IL-4*, *IL-5* and *IL-13* and thus regulate T_H2 differentiation (Cai et al., 2006). Thus, SATB1 has emerged as an important factor orchestrating gene expression by modulating the higher-order chromatin architecture in a cell-type specific and signal-dependent manner.

Number of studies in the past few years have demonstrated the role of SATB1 in cancer. It has been shown that siRNA-mediated knockdown of SATB1 in higly aggressive breast cancer cells reversed the tumorogenic capability of cells and also inhibited the tumor growth (Han et al., 2008). Downregulation of SATB1 in cancerous cells resulted in alteration in the expression of about thousand genes. Furthermore, overexpression of SATB1 in a non-aggressive tumor cell line resulted in augmenting the tumorigenic and metastatic capacity of these cells indicating its direct role in coordinated regulation of multiple genes. SATB1 presumably reprogrammes gene expression by inducing specific epigenetic modifications at target gene loci, leading to upregulation of metastasis-associated genes and simultaneously causing downregulation of tumor suppressor genes (Han et al., 2008). These studies point to a coordinated mechanism of tumor progression.

3. SATB1 in T cell development and differentiation

3.1 Overview of T cell development

T cells arise from the hematopoietic stem cell precursors that migrate to the thymus. Early stage T cell precursors (ETPs) that migrate to the thymus lose the capability to give rise to B cells, however they have the propensity to develop into lineages other than T cells such as macrophages, dendritic cells and NKT cells (Yui et al., 2010). The ETPs also called DN1 phenotypically are CD4-, CD8-, CD3-, CD25-, CD44+ cells. These cells undergo extensive proliferation and are not yet completely committed to T lineage (Rothenberg et al., 2010). The next stage of development is characterized by upregulation of CD25 and is called DN2 stage at which cells are CD4-, CD8-, CD3-, CD25+, CD44+. Further, CD44 is downregulated and such cells are referred to as DN3 stage (CD4-, CD8-, CD3-, CD25+, CD44-) and at this stage they are committed to the T cell lineage. The DN3 cells stop dividing and undergo rearrangement of TCRβ chain. Successful assembly of the β chain facilitates the movement of cells and this process is known as β-selection (Michie & Zuniga-Pflucker, 2002). Subsequently, these cells downregulate both CD25 (IL-2Rα) and CD44, the stage is called DN4 and these are fully committed towards T lineage and start proliferation. Following the successful rearrangement of αβ TCR, thymocytes start expressing CD4 and CD8 coreceptors on the cell surface. The DP thymocytes undergo a stringent selection process, where the TCRs that cannot bind to self antigens undergo death by neglect, whereas those which bind to self MHC with intermediate affinity undergo positive selection (Marrack & Kappler, 1997). Further, these thymocytes either develop into CD4+ or CD8+ SP thymocytes dependent on the TCR signals and the expression of specific transcription factor(s) (Singer et al., 2008). In the periphery, the mature T cells differentiate into effector T cells depending on the antigen encountered and cytokine signals.

3.2 Role of SATB1 in thymocyte development

SATB1 knockout mice exhibit a severe defect in T cell development. SATB1-null mice have disproportionately small thymi and spleens as compared to the wild-type mice. At the cellular level, these mice exhibit multiple defects in T-cell development. The population of immature CD3-,CD4-,CD8- triple negative (TN) thymocytes is greatly reduced. Most strikingly, the thymocyte development is blocked at the double positive stage and the CD4+ or CD8+ SP thymocytes fail to develop (Alvarez et al., 2000). Ablation of SATB1 also results in dysregulation of multiple genes such as Il-2R and Il-7R involved in T cell development and differentiation (Alvarez et al., 2000). Within the thymus majority of the DP thymocytes are eliminated via apoptosis during positive and negative selection process (Surh & Sprent, 1994). Dexamethasone-induced apoptosis of thymocytes resulted in rapid dissociation of SATB1 from chromatin. Furthermore, SATB1 is specifically cleaved by caspase-6 after the aspartate residue at position 254 which led to the identification of the PDZ-like domain in the N-terminal region of SATB1. In vitro analysis revealed that caspase-6 cleavage also abolished the DNA-binding ability of SATB1 (Galande et al., 2001). The cleavage of SATB1 during T cell apoptosis might be required for the initiation of DNA fragmentation. In SATB1- null mice peripheral CD4+ T cells fail to respond to activation stimulus and undergo apoptosis demonstrating indispensible role of SATB1 during proper T cell development (Alvarez et al., 2000). Comparison of the wild-type mice with the SATB1-/- mice indicated that repression of Il-2R gene was caused specifically by recruitment of histone deacetylases by SATB1 (Yasui et al., 2002). Immunostaining of SATB1 in mouse thymocytes revealed that it forms a unique cage-like structure differentiating euchromatin from heterochromatin (Cai et al., 2003; Notani et al., 2010). In thymocytes, SATB1 is also known to cooperate with other regulatory factors such as β-catenin and CtBP-1 in signal-dependent manner and regulate gene expression (Purbey et al., 2009; Notani et al., 2010). SATB1-binding site-driven reporter assays revealed that SATB1:β-catenin interaction regulates the expression of Wnt target genes in TCF-independent manner (Notani et al., 2010). The recruitment of β-catenin to SATB1 target genes is preceded by deacetylation of SATB1 upon Wnt/β-catenin signaling in thymocytes and CD4+ T cells. SATB1 directly binds to cis regulatory elements at the CD8 enhancer and required for the CD8 SP thymocyte development from the DP thymocytes (Yao et al., 2010). Thus, SATB1 which is highly expressed in thymocytes acts as a global regulator in their development.

3.3 Role of SATB1 in T_H2 differentiation

CD4+ SP thymocytes from the thymus migrate to peripheral lymphoid organs, where they encounter antigen presented by the antigens presenting cells (APCs) and further differentiate into T helper (T_H) effector phenotypes. T_H1 population is involved in cellular immunity wherein they assist macrophages and cytotoxic T cells (Tc) for clearance of infected cells while T_H2 cells help B cells in generating humoral response by increasing production of neutralising antibodies against the pathogen (Zhu and Paul, 2008). T_H2 population is characterized by the effector cytokines it secretes viz., IL-5, IL-13 and IL-4. Strikingly, SATB1 which is known to have a important role during thymocyte development is upregulated during T_H2 differentiation (Lund et al., 2005; Notani et al., 2010). SATB1 was shown to regulate the expression of T_H2 cytokines by remodeling the chromatin in an actively transcribed loop form (Cai et al., 2006). T cell activation along with IL-4 cytokine stimulus showed that SATB1 forms higher-order chromatin structure of the 200 Kb T_H2 cytokine locus and regulates *Il-5*, *Il-13* and *Il-4*. SATB1 induces expression of these cytokines by recruiting chromatin modifying enzyme Brg1 and RNA Pol II converting the locus into transcriptionally active region (Cai et al., 2006). Furthermore, induction of SATB1 expression in CD4+ cells during T_H2 differentiation is STAT-6 dependent (Lund et al., 2005 and Ahlfors et al., 2010). Transcriptome profiling of differentiating CD4+ cells into T_H1/ T_H2 subtypes revealed that SATB1 is involved in regulation of over 300 genes indicating its crucial role during T_H cell differentiation (Ahlfors et al., 2010).

An important insight into the role of SATB1 in T_H differentiation was obtained when the gene expression profiles of various subsets of T_H cells were compared with the TCR-activated CD4+ T cells, a condition referred to as T_H0. To ascertain whether SATB1 regulated genes are involved in T_H cell differentiation, Ahlfors et al., (2010) silenced expression of SATB1 using siRNAs in T_H cells. Their studies revealed that expression of multiple genes was altered upon SATB1 knockdown in T_H1, T_H2 and T_H0 population. The RNA expression profile revealed that in differentiating CD4+ T cells, expression of 319 genes was altered. Out of these, 70 genes were selectively affected in T_H2 population while 43 genes had altered expression in T_H1 population. Thus total of 40% (43+14+43=127) genes showed altered expression upon cytokine treatment suggesting SATB1 targets were partly specific to T_H subsets. Notably, 48% of SATB1 target genes were regulated by IL-4. Furthermore, TCR stimulation alone regulated one third of SATB1 targets and only 18% of SATB1 target genes were not regulated by TCR or combination of T_H1/T_H2 polarizing cytokines. The gene expression profiling clearly indicated that SATB1 is likely to play an essential role in the development or function of various T_H subtypes (Ahlfors et al., 2010). Another important contribution of this study was the finding that IL-5 which is predominantly secreted by T_H2 cells is repressed by SATB1 during early stages of polarization. The repression of *Il-5* promoter by SATB1 was during brought about by recruiting HDAC1 corepressor to the *Il-5* locus (Figure 1). Later the course of differentiation, the competition between binding of SATB1 and GATA-3 results in binding of GATA-3 to the *Il-5* promoter which derepresses *Il-5* locus and IL-5 is produced (Ahlfors et al., 2010). IL-5 plays important role in differentiation and activation of eosinophils and dysregulation of *Il-5* results into eosinophila (Mosmann & Coffman 1987; Campbell et al., 1988; Sanderson, 1988). Hence regulation of IL-5 is not only important in proper T_H differentiation but also in understanding its role in diseases such as eosinophila.

T_H2 differentiation is also regulated by the downstream transcription factors like GATA-3 and STAT-6. GATA-3 is a transcription factor predominantly expressed in T cells and brain (Oosterwegel et al., 1992). GATA-3 has been shown to play an important role in thymocyte development and also during T_H2 differentiation (Ho et al., 2010). The essential role of GATA-3 was demonstrated by creating mice lacking GATA-3 expression. GATA-3-deficient CD4+ T cells cannot differentiate into T_H2 phenotype and they produce IFNγ under T_H2 polarizing conditions (Zhu J et. al., 2004). IL-4-STAT6 signaling pathway is known to cause the upregulation of GATA-3 in T_H2 differentiating cells. However, a recent report provided an alternative view by demonstrating that CD4+ T cells can differentiate to T_H2 phenotype in absence of STAT6 via notch signaling although with a reduced efficiency (Amsen et al., 2004). In this review we have focused on the newly dicovered mechanism for regulation of GATA-3 expression by SATB1 in Wnt-dependent manner.

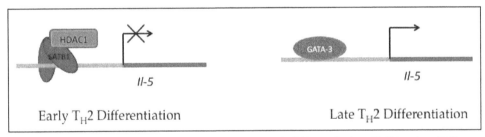

Early T_H2 Differentiation   Late T_H2 Differentiation

Fig. 1. **SATB1 mediated regulation of *Il-5* during T_H2 differentiation.** IL-5 is a late T_H2 cytokine. SATB1 directly binds to *Il-5* promoter and inhibits its expression by recruiting HDAC repressor complex. During allergic conditions GATA-3 displaces SATB1 bound to the *Il-5* promoter and upregulates IL-5 cytokine expression (Ahlfors et al., 2010).

3.4 SATB1 as a mediator of Wnt signaling

Recently, a new role for SATB1 has been discovered as a mediator of Wnt-signaling pathway during T_H differentiation (Notani et al., 2010). Wnt signaling is one of the well studied and highly conserved pathways responsible for various developmental processes and cell fate decisions (Logan and Nusse, 2004). β-catenin is the key transducer of canonical Wnt signaling cascade which upon Wnt signaling is stabilized in the cytoplasm, then translocates to the nucleus and interacts with T cell factor (TCF) family transcriptional factors. Asociation of β-catenin with the TCF family proteins alters the expression of Wnt-responsive genes (Logan and Nusse, 2004). SATB1 brings about T_H2 cell differentiation via Wnt signaling by recruiting β-catenin to its genomic targets (Notani et al., 2010). This study demonstrated that SATB1 represses target genes in undifferentiated cells. Upon Wnt signalling in the polarized cells, SATB1 interacts with β-catenin, recruits it to *Gata-3* promoter and derepresses it leading to T_H2 commitment (Figure 2). Several SATB1 regulated genes are activated by SATB1:β-catenin complex in Wnt-dependent manner. Post-translational modifications of SATB1 act as molecular switches regulating its DNA-binding activity and ability to interact with multiple partner proteins (Kumar et al., 2006). Upon Wnt signaling SATB1 is deacetylated and directly interacts with β-catenin through its PDZ-like domain. The physical interaction between SATB1 and β-catenin is required for T_H2 differentiation. The two prominent factors TCF and SATB1 compete for β-catenin interaction. SATB1 competitively recruits β-catenin and hence also affects the transcription of TCF regulated genes. However, TCF and SATB1 do not interact with each other suggesting that they have non-overlapping effects (Notani et al., 2010). Thus, these two mediators of Wnt signaling presumably bind to their genomic targets independent of each other. LEF/TCF family proteins were the only known β-catenin partners for number of years. Another β-catenin partner known to be involved in pituitary gland development and lineage determination is the homeodomain protein Prop-1 (Olson et al., 2006). The report by Notani et al. (2010), demonstrated that homeodomain-containing transcription regulator SATB1 is also a β-catenin-binding factor and is involved in T_H2 differentiation.

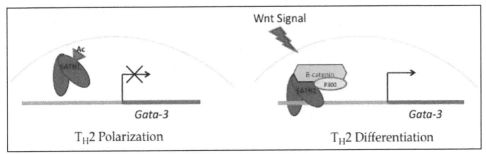

Fig. 2. **SATB1: β-catenin complex regulates *Gata-3* expression during T_H2 differentiation.** Upon Wnt signaling β-catenin translocates into the nucleus. SATB1 interacts with β-catenin and regulates multiple genes. GATA-3 is known to be a master regulator of T_H2 differentiation. In differentiating T_H2 cells, SATB1: β-catenin complex binds to the *Gata-3* promoter and upregulates Gata-3 expression by recruiting the p300 activator complex. SATB1: β-catenin complex regulates *Gata-3* expression in Wnt-dependent manner and thus regulates T_H2 differentiation (Notani et al., 2010).

Role of transcription factor GATA-3 in T_H2 polarization by upregulating IL-4 secretion and inhibiting IFN-γ expression is very well established (Avni et al., 2002; Spilianakis et al., 2004). SATB1 positively regulates GATA-3 expression in T_H2 cells by recruiting p300 acetyltransferase and β-catenin to *Gata-3* promoter upon Wnt signal (Figure 2). The role of Wnt signaling in T_H2 cell differentiation was further demonstrated by using DKK1, an inhibitor of Wnt signaling. Upon DKK1 treatment in T_H cells, GATA-3 expression was suppressed and also T_H2 cytokines were downregulated. Quantitative transcript profiling revealed that expression of GATA-3 was suppressed upon Dkk1 treatment in T_H2 subset, suggesting that Wnt signaling is necessary for the upregulation of GATA-3 during differentiation of T_H2 cells. Overexpression and siRNA mediated silencing of SATB1 and β-catenin provided the conclusive evidence for their direct roles in the differentiation of CD4+ cells. Upon siRNA-mediated silencing of SATB1 the expression of GATA-3 was downregulated in T_H2 cells. Overexpression of SATB1 led to a significant increase in the expression of GATA-3 in T_H2, suggesting that SATB1 positively regulates GATA-3 expression (Notani et al., 2010). In summary, Wnt signaling is essential for T_H2 differentiation whereby SATB1 upregulates GATA-3 expression which further enhances IL-4 secretion. CD4+ T cells are receptive to Wnt signals because they produce different Wnts themselves (Notani et al., 2010). The differential sensitivity of T_H cell subtypes to Wnt signaling could be due to the fact that the downstream processes such as stabilization of β-catenin occur prominently in the T_H2 subtype and not T_H1 (Notani et al., 2010). Thus, these evidences clearly argue in favor of requirement of SATB1 and Wnt/β-catenin signaling during T_H cell differentiation.

GATA3 facilitates chromatin remodeling of T_H2 cytokine locus leading to conversion of the *Il4–Il5–Il13* locus to an open conformation, allowing transcription of this locus by transcription factors involved in T_H2-cell differentiation (Avni et al., 2002). The associated specific epigenetic changes include histone modifications upon binding of GATA-3 to its DNA targets were found to be mainly H3K4 and H3K27 methylation (Wei et al., 2011). Another chromatin protein CTCF binds to T_H2 cytokine locus and assists GATA-3 and SATB1 mediated T_H2 commitment (Almeida et al., 2009). Thus, collectively the three regulators namely SATB1, GATA-3 and CTCF could be responsible for orchestrating the coordinated regulation of T_H cell differentiation.

A model for regulation of T_H2 differentiation by SATB1 is illustrated in Figure 3. T_H0 cell is activated and polarized by TCR docking and IL-4 cytokine respectively. In the absence of

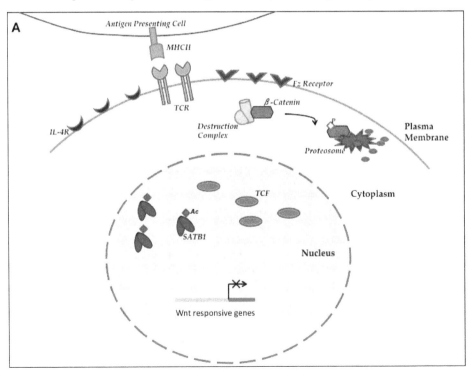

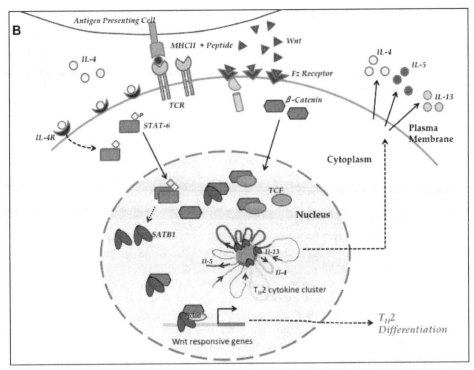

Fig. 3. Model depicting the early events occurring upon Wnt signaling in polarized T_H2 cell and role of SATB1 in this process. In the complex paradigm of T_H2 polarization model there have been several studies suggesting role(s) of different mechanisms and it is now evident that SATB1 plays a major role during this process of T_H2 commitment. **A,** In naïve cells when IL-4 signalling is absent, expression of SATB1 is low and GATA-3 is not upregulated. **B,** Under T_H2 conditions, when a peptide antigen is presented by an antigen presenting cell (APC) to the TCR on T cell surface and IL-4 secreted by the APCs causes the activation of Jak Kinases which phosphorylate STAT-6, which in turn upregulates SATB1 and GATA-3. SATB1 interacts with β-catenin which is translocated to the nucleus in Wnt-dependent manner and this complex regulates *Gata-3* expression. STAT-6, SATB1 and GATA-3 coordinatively regulate *Il-4* expression which is a characteristic cytokine of T_H2 differentiation. However, the role of STAT-6 in regulation of SATB1 as depicted here is speculative.

Wnt signaling, β-catenin is phosporylated by destruction complex and targeted for degradation to proteosomal complex. SATB1 is acetylated and has low DNA-binding affinity in the absence of Wnt signal. Also, in the absence of nuclear β-catenin TCF does not regulate Wnt responsive genes and hence their transcription is suppressed (Figure 3A). Upon Wnt signaling, the destruction complex that sequesters β-catenin does not form and β-catenin is stabilized, which then translocates to nucleus. SATB1 is deacetylated upon Wnt signaling and it then competes with TCF for interaction with β-catenin. Deacetylated SATB1 recruits β-catenin to genomic targets and regulates Wnt-responsive genes resulting into T_H2 differentiation (Notani et al., 2010). SATB1 also binds to T_H2 cytokine locus and upregulates transcription of *Il-4*, *Il-5* and *Il-13* resulting into T_H2 commitment (Figure 3B).

4. Regulation of SATB1 via STAT-6

Signal transducer and activator of transcription (STATs) are important in various biological processes such as development, programed cell death, organogenesis, cell growth regulation and adaptive immunity (Horvath, 2000). Upon appropriate cytokine signaling STAT molecules are phosphorylated by Janus kinases and they form homodimers. The phosphorylated STATs translocate to the nucleus and affect the transcription of their target genes (Schindler and Darnell, 1995). Cytokine signaling mediates the activation of specific STAT molecules and plays an important role during T helper cell differentiation. During the T_H differentiation STAT-4 and STAT-6 play seminal roles during T_H1 and T_H2 differentiation process respectively. IL-12 signaling initiates from binding of IL-12 to the IL-12 receptor, which further associates with protein tyrosine kinases and Jak2. The Jak2 kinase specifically causes the phosphorylation of STAT-4 (Waltford et al., 2004). STAT-4 causes the expression of Interferon γ and transcription factor Tbet during T_H1 differentiation (Thieu et al., 2008, Robertson et al., 2005). IL-4 secreted by the APCs engages to the IL-4 receptor on CD4+ T cells which then recruits Jak 3 kinases and causes the activation of STAT-6 (Witthuhn et al., 1994). STAT-6 regulates the expression of IL-4 and GATA-3 during the T_H2 differentiation (Zhu and Paul, 2008). The knockout models of STAT-4 and STAT-6 have revealed that T cells cannot differentiate into their respective effector phenotypes (Wuster et al., 2000). Genome-wide analysis of occupancy of STAT factors have shown that they preferentially bind to the promoters and intergenic regions in the genome. STAT proteins have a palindromic GAA consensus binding site. STAT molecules generally colocalize with the active histone marks, and it is shown that both proteins SAT4 and SAT6 colocalize with H3K4 trimethylation marks in the genome (Wei et al., 2010). Gene expression studies along with elucidation of the epigenetic marks at key loci using STAT knockout mice have revealed that STAT are important for the maintenance of epigenetic marks on such genes and thus regulation of gene expression.

STAT-6 knockdown caused the downregulation of CRTH2 expression in cells polarised to T_H2 phenotype (Elo et al., 2010). Another study also demonstrated that STAT-6 knockdown resulted in downregulation of SATB1 expression at both RNA and protein level (Ahlfors et al., 2010). Microarray-based gene expression profiling data from different groups using mouse and human models depicted similar results showing downregulation of SATB1 (Wei et al., 2010; Elo et al., 2010). Bsed on these finding, we hypothesize that STAT-6 may directly bind to the SATB1 promoter and mediate activating epigenetic histone modifications leading to the upregulation of SATB1 during T_H2 differentiation. SATB1 in turn causes positive regulation of *Il-4* expression.

Interestingly, two recent studies have implicated Foxp3 in the regulation of SATB1 (Beyer et al. 2011; McInnes et al., 2011). Foxp3 tumor suppressor regulates SATB1 expression in breast epithelial cells and downregulates its expression in miRNA-dependent manner (McInnes et al., 2011). Repression of SATB1 has been also identified as a crucial mechanism for the phenotype and function of T(reg) cells. Foxp3 acts as a transcriptional repressor for the SATB1 locus and indirectly suppresses it through the induction of microRNAs that bound the SATB1 3' untranslated region (Beyer et al., 2011). Thus, elucidation of such regulatory loops will be important steps towards understanding the regulation and in vivo functions of SATB1.

5. Loss of SATB1 function: Sézary syndrome

Adaptive immune response raised against pathogen includes clonal expansion of antigen-specific T cells which are then cleared from the system mainly by activation-induced cell death (AICD), a type of apoptosis (Krammer et al., 2007). Sézary syndrome which is a variant of cutaneous T cell lymphoma results by clonal accumulation of mature T cells originating from skin (Willemze et al., 2005). This accumulation of cells occurs as a result of resistance of cells to AICD (Klemke et al., 2006). The pathogenesis of Sézary Syndrome (SS) is still not very clear. A recent study by Wang et al. (2011) revealed that the deficiency of SATB1 leads to SS. Sézary cells obtained from patients are CD4+ CD7- mature memory T cells and show a T_H2 cytokine profile with loss of expression of CD7. Transcription profiling of the Sézary cells from patients and Hut78 (Sézary-derived cell line) revealed that SATB1 was drastically downregulated in these cells as compared to non-Sézary control cells such as Jurkat T cells. Additionally, immunofluorescence staining showed a lowered nuclear localization of SATB1 in of primary Sézary cells as well as in Hut98 cells (Wang et al., 2011). Retroviral transduction mediated restoration of SATB1 in Hut98 cells increased apoptosis in these cells within 4 days without changing their proliferation rate. Subsequently, it was demonstrated that the SATB1 restored cells were sensitized to AICD. The transcriptome analysis of these SATB1 restored cells showed remarkable up-regulation of FASL/CD95L which is a death receptor ligand. Further, 32 out of total 153 (12%) dysregulated genes in Sézary cells were normalized upon SATB1 restoration in these cells (Wang et al., 2011). The increased AICD in SATB1 restored Sézary cells was shown to be induced by FASL via caspase 8-dependent pathway. These studies strongly suggested that SATB1 plays a very important role in pathogenesis of Sézary syndrome and it plays a vital role in regulation of homeostasis of T cells. Sézary cells are known not to respond to radiation therapy as these cells do not have increased proliferation but rather possess resistance to apoptosis. Currently the therapies for SS include upregulation of FASL to sensitize these cells for apoptosis. Restoration of SATB1 in Sézary cells could be a promising new strategy for the treatment of Sézary syndrome. The SS cells would also serve as a knockout model for studying role of SATB1 in human T cell functions.

6. Conclusions

In the field of T cell biology, T_H differentiation is itself a complex phenomenon, one reason being that T_H cell fate is not pre-decided during development in thymus, it is primarily executed upon the encounter of undifferentiated T cell with the antigen in the peripheral immune system. Hence T_H cell polarization leading to final differentiation is a multi-cascade process with several epigenetic changes invoked in response to various signals. In this Chapter we focused on role of SATB1 which is an important global regulator involved in T cell development, maturation and differentiation. We elaborated on the role of SATB1 during T_H cell differentiation which is an important pool of cells for humoral as well as cell mediated immunity. To summarize the findings of various studies, it can be concluded that SATB1 plays an important role at the very early stages of T_H cell differentiation. The studies discussed here suggest that SATB1 represses the chromatin in undifferentiated cells by recruiting repressors to the gene loci. Upon early events of cell polarization such as TCR signal and cytokine secretion by cells, SATB1 immediately responds to even lower level of cytokine signal such as IL-4 by changing the chromatin 'loopscape' of specific loci in T_H2

cells which culminates into synthesis of downstream transcription factors required for further differentiation such as GATA-3. Wnt signaling acts as a booster for the differentiation signal in these cells which brings about changes in chromatin organization via SATB1 as a mediator of Wnt signaling and promotes GATA-3 transcription. In the later stages of differentiation, T_H subtype specific factors such as GATA-3 take over and competitively overcome the SATB1 mediated repression of T_H2 cytokines and in turn upregulate the T_H2 signature cytokines such as IL-5. Thus, SATB1 presumably acts as a regulatory switch at the very early stages of cell polarization and differentiation by repressing various cell type specific genes, however it specifically responds to polarization signal by changing its acetylation status. The indispensible role of SATB1 in T_H cell differentiation is exemplified by diseases such as Eosinophila and Sézary syndrome, the later manifests as a result of SATB1 deficiency.

7. Future perspectives

The role of SATB1 in differentiation of CD4[+] T cells has come into the limelight as described in this review. However, the role of SATB1 during earlier events such as thymocyte maturation are not studied in detail and requires further investigation. Since SATB1 is known to regulate genes such as *Thpok* which are important for the lineage commitment process, it is essential to evaluate whether SATB1 plays a direct role during the thymocyte lineage commitment. Findings from recent studies have highlighted the requirement for delineation of molecular mechanisms governing the expression of SATB1 during the process of thymocyte maturation. In the CD4[+] T cells, it would be important to study the regulation of SATB1 which might be regulated by an IL-4:STAT6-dependent mechanism as seen during the differentiation of T_H2 cells. It would be also interesting to investigate whether SATB1 plays any role(s) in the differentiation of the other subtypes of CD4[+] T cells. Studies elucidating role of miRNAs in the regulation of SATB1 in these various subtypes of T cells would also shed light on the signaling pathways and associated mechanisms regulating the development and differentiation of various subtypes of T cells.

8. Acknowledgements

Work was supported by grants from the Centre of Excellence in Epigenetics program of the Department of Biotechnology, Government of India and IISER Pune. KG is supported by fellowship from the Council of Scientific and Industrial Research, India.

9. References

Ahlfors A, Limaye A, Elo LL, Tuomela S, Burute M, Notani D, Gottimukkala K, Rasool O, Galande S & Lahesmaa R. (2010) SATB1 dictates expression of multiple genes including IL-5 involved in human T helper cell differentiation. *Blood.* 116:1443-1453.
Almeida C, Heath H, Krpic S, Dingjan G, Hamburg J, Bergen I, Nbelen S, Sleutels F, Grosveld F, Galjart N & Hendriks R (2009) Critical role for the transcription regulator CCCTC-Binding factor in the control of Th2 cytokine expression. *J. Immunol.* 182:999-1010.

Alvarez JD, Yasui DH, Niida H, Joh T, Loh DY & Kohwi-Shigematsu T. (2000) The MAR-binding protein SATB1 orchestrates temporal and spatial expression of multiple genes during T-cell development. *Genes Dev.* 14:521-535.

Amsen D, Blander JM, Lee GR, Tanigaki K, Honjo T & Flavell RA. (2004) Instruction of distinct CD4 T helper cell fates by different notch ligands on antigen-presenting cells. Cell. 117:515-526.

Avni O, Lee D, Macian F, Szabo SJ, Glimcher LH & Rao A. (2002) T(H) cell differentiation is accompanied by dynamic changes in histone acetylation of cytokine genes. *Nature Immunol.* 3:643-651

Beyer M, Thabet Y, Müller RU, Sadlon T, Classen S, Lahl K, Basu S, Zhou X, Bailey-Bucktrout SL, Krebs W, Schönfeld EA, Böttcher J, Golovina T, Mayer CT, Hofmann A, Sommer D, Debey-Pascher S, Endl E, Limmer A, Hippen KL, Blazar BR, Balderas R, Quast T, Waha A, Mayer G, Famulok M, Knolle PA, Wickenhauser C, Kolanus W, Schermer B, Bluestone JA, Barry SC, Sparwasser T, Riley JL & Schultze JL. (2011) Repression of the genome organizer SATB1 in regulatory T cells is required for suppressive function and inhibition of effector differentiation. *Nat Immunol.* 12:898-907.

Cai S, Han HJ & Kohwi-Shigematsu T. (2003) Tissue-specific nuclear architecture and gene expression regulated by SATB1. *Nat Genet.* 34:42-51.

Cai S, Lee CC & Kohwi-Shigematsu T. (2006) SATB1 packages densely looped, transcriptionally active chromatin for coordinated expression of cytokine genes. *Nat Genet.* 38:1278:1288.

Campbell HD, Tucker WQ, Hort Y, Martinson ME, Mayo G, Clutterbuck EJ, Sanderson CJ & Young IG. (1987) Molecular cloning, nucleotide sequence, and expression of the gene encoding human eosinophil differentiation factor (interleukin 5). *Proc Natl Acad Sci U S A.* 84:6629–6633.

DiPaolo RJ, Brinster C, Davidson TS, Andersson J, Glass D, Shevach EM. (2007) Autoantigen-specific TGFbeta-induced Foxp3+ regulatory T cells prevent autoimmunity by inhibiting dendritic cells from activating autoreactive T cells. *J Immunol.* 179:4685-4693.

Dong C. (2008) TH17 cells in development: an updated view of their molecular identity and genetic programming. *Nat Rev Immunol.* 8:337-348.

Elo LL, Järvenpää H, Tuomela S, Raghav S, Ahlfors H, Laurila K, Gupta B, Lund RJ, Tahvanainen J, Hawkins RD, Oresic M, Lähdesmäki H, Rasool O, Rao KV, Aittokallio T & Lahesmaa R. (2010) Genome-wide profiling of interleukin-4 and STAT6 transcription factor regulation of human Th2 cell programming. *Immunity.* 32:852-862.

Galande S, Dickinson LA, Mian IS, Sikorska M & Kohwi-Shigematsu T. (2001) SATB1 cleavage by caspase 6 disrupts PDZ domain-mediated dimerization, causing detachment from chromatin early in T-cell apoptosis. *Mol Cell Biol.* 21:5591-5604.

Galande S, Purbey PK, Notani D & Kumar PP. (2007) The third dimension of gene regulation: organization of dynamic chromatin loopscape by SATB1. *Curr Opin Genet Dev.* 17:408-414.

Han HJ, Russo J, Kohwi Y, Kohwi-Shigematsu T. (2008) SATB1 reprogrammes gene expression to promote breast tumour growth and metastasis. Nature. 452:187-93.

Hirota K, Duarte JH, Veldhoen M, Hornsby E, Li Y, Cua DJ, Ahlfors H, Wilhelm C, Tolaini M, Menzel U, Garefalaki A, Potocnik AJ & Stockinger B. (2011) Fate mapping of IL-17 producing T cells in inflammatory responses. *Nat Immunol.* 12:255-263.

Ho IC, Tai TS, Pai SY. (2009) GATA3 and the T-cell lineage: essential functions before and after T-helper-2-cell differentiation. *Nat Rev Immunol.* 9:125-135.

Horvath CM. (2000) STAT proteins and transcriptional responses to extracellular signals. *Trends Biochem Sci.* 10:496-502.

King C, Tangye SG, Mackay CR. (2008) T follicular helper (TFH) cells in normal and dysregulated immune responses. *Annu Rev Immunol.* 26:741-766.

Kitano M, Moriyama S, Ando Y, Hikida M, Mori Y, Kurosaki T & Okada T. (2011) Bcl6 protein expression shapes pre-germinal center B cell dynamics and follicular helper T cell heterogeneity. *Immunity.* 34:961-972.

Klemke CD, Brenner D, Weiss EM, Schmidt M, Leverkus M, Gülow K & Krammer PH. (2009) Lack of T-cell receptor-induced signaling is crucial for CD95 ligand up-regulation and protects cutaneous T-cell lymphoma cells from activation-induced cell death. *Cancer Res.* 69:4175-4183.

Krammer PH, Arnold R & Lavrik IN. (2007) Life and death in peripheral T cells. *Nat Rev Immunol.* 7:532-542.

Kreslavsky T, Gleimer M, Garbe AI & Von Boehmer H. (2010) αβ versus γδ fate choice: counting the T-cell lineages at the branch point. *Immunol Rev.* 238:169-181.

Kumar PP, Bischof O, Purbey PK, Notani D, Urlaub H, Dejean A & Galande S. (2007) Functional interaction between PML and SATB1 regulates chromatin-loop architecture and transcription of the MHC class I locus. *Nat Cell Biol.* 9:45-56.

Logan CY & Nusse R (2004) The Wnt signaling pathway in development and disease. *Annu Rev Cell Dev Biol.* 20: 781-810.

Lund R, Aittokallio T, Nevalainen O & Lahesmaa R. (2003) Identification of novel genes regulated by IL-12, IL-4 or TGF-β during the early polarization of CD4+ lymphocytes. *J Immunol.* 171:5428-5336.

Lund R, Ahlfors H, Kainonen E, Lahesmaa AM, Dixon C & Lahesmaa R. (2005) Identification of genes involved in the initiation of human Th1 or Th2 cell commitment. *Eur J Immunol.* 35: 3307-3319.

Marrack P & Kappler J. (1997) Positive selection of thymocytes bearing alpha beta T cell receptors. *Curr Opin Immunol.* 9:250-255.

McInnes N, Sadlon TJ, Brown CY, Pederson S, Beyer M, Schultze JL, McColl S, Goodall GJ, Barry SC. (2011) FOXP3 and FOXP3-regulated microRNAs suppress SATB1 in breast cancer cells. Oncogene. doi: 10.1038/onc.2011.293.

Michie AM & Zúñiga-Pflücker JC. (2002) Regulation of thymocyte differentiation: pre-TCR signals and beta-selection. *Semin Immunol.* 14:311-323.

Mosmann TR & Coffman RL. (1987) TH1 and TH2 cells: different patterns of lymphokine secretion lead to different functional properties. *Annu Rev Immunol.* 7:145–173.

Mosmann TR, Cherwinski H, Bond MW, Giedlin MA & Coffman RL. (1986) Two types of murine helper T cell clone. I. Definition according to profiles of lymphokine activities and secreted proteins. *J. Immunol.* 136:2348–574.

Notani D, Gottimukkala KP, Jayani RS, Limaye AS, Damle MV, Mehta S, Purbey PK, Joseph J & Galande S. (2010) Global regulator SATB1 recruits beta-catenin and regulates T(H)2 differentiation in Wnt-dependent manner. *PLoS Biol.* 8(1):e1000296.

Oosterwegel M, Timmerman J, Leiden J & Clevers H. (1992) Expression of GATA-3 during lymphocyte differentiation and mouse embryogenesis. *Dev Immunol.* 3:1-11.

Pancer Z & Cooper MD. (2006) The evolution of adaptive immunity. *Annu Rev Immunol.* 24:497-518.

Pavan Kumar P, Purbey PK, Sinha CK, Notani D, Limaye A, Jayani RS & Galande S. (2006) Phosphorylation of SATB1, a global gene regulator, acts as amolecular switch regulating its transcriptional activity in vivo. *Mol cell.* 22:231-243.

Pavan Kumar P, Purbey PK, Sinha CK, Notani D, Limaye A, Jayani RS, Galande S. (2006) Phosphorylation of SATB1, a global gene regulator, acts as a molecular switch regulating its transcriptional activity in vivo. *Mol Cell.* 22:231-243.

Purbey PK, Singh S, Notani D, Kumar PP, Limaye AS & Galande S. (2009) Acetylation-dependent interaction of SATB1 and CtBP1 mediates transcriptional repression by SATB1. *Mol Cell Biol.* 29:1321-1337.

Rappl G, Muche JM, Abken H & et al. (2001) CD4+CD7- T cells compose the dominant T-cell clone in the peripheral blood of patients with Sezary syndrome. *J Am Acad Dermatol.* 44:456-461.

Robertson MJ, Chang HC, Pelloso D & Kaplan MH (2005) Impaired interferon-gamma production as a consequence of STAT4 deficiency after autologous hematopoietic stem cell transplantation for lymphoma. *Blood.* 106:963-970.

Rothenberg EV, Zhang J & Li L. (2010) Multilayered specification of the T-cell lineage fate. *Immunol Rev.* 238:150-168.

Sakaguchi S, Yamaguchi T, Nomura T & Ono M. (2008) Regulatory T cells and immune tolerance. *Cell.* 133:775-787.

Sanderson CJ. (1988) Interleukin-5: an eosinophil growth and activation factor. *Dev Biol Stand.*69:23–29.

Schindler C & Darnell JE Jr. (1995) Transcriptional responses to polypeptide ligands: the JAK-STAT pathway. *Annu Rev Biochem.* 64:621-651.

Singer A, Adoro S & Park JH. (2008) Lineage fate and intense debate: myths, models and mechanisms of CD4- versus CD8-lineage choice. *Nat Rev Immunol.* 8:788-801.

Singer A. (2002) New prespectives on a developmental dilemma: the kinetic signaling model and the importance of signal duration for the CD4/CD8 lineage decision. *Curr Opin Immunol.* 14:207-215.

Sokolowska-Wojdylo M, Wenzel J, Gaffal E, Steitz J, Roszkiewicz J, Bieber T &Tüting T. (2005) Absence of CD26 expression onskin-homing CLA+ CD4+ T lymphocytes in peripheral blood is a highly sensitive marker for early diagnosis and therapeutic monitoring of patients with Sezary syndrome. *Clin Exp Dermatol.* 30:702-706.

Staudt V, Bothur E, Klein M, Lingnau K, Reuter S, Grebe N, Gerlitzki B, Hoffmann M, Ulges A, Taube C, Dehzad N, Becker M, Stassen M, Steinborn A, Lohoff M, Schild H, Schmitt E & Bopp T. (2010) Interferon-regulatory factor 4 is essential for the developmental program of T helper 9 cells. *Immunity.* 33:192-202.

Surh CD & Sprent J. (1994) T-cell apoptosis detected in situ during positive and negative selection in the thymus. *Nature.* 372:100-103.

Thieu VT, Yu Q, Chang HC, Yeh N, Nguyen ET, Sehra S & Kaplan MH. (2008) Signal transducer and activator of transcription 4 is required for the transcription factor T-bet to promote T helper 1 cell-fate determination. *Immunity.* 29: 679-670.

Wang Y, Su M, Zhou LL, Tu P, Zhang X, Jiang X, Zhou Y. (2011) Deficiency of SATB1 expression in Sezary cells causes apoptosis resistance by regulating FasL/CD95L transcription. *Blood.* 117: 3826-3835.

Watford WT, Hissong BD, Bream JH, Kanno Y, Muul L & O'Shea JJ. (2004) Signaling by IL-12 and IL-23 and the immunoregulatory roles of STAT4. *Immunol Rev.* 202:139-156.

Wei L, Vahedi G, Sun HW, Watford WT, Takatori H, Ramos HL, Takahashi H, Liang J, Gutierrez-Cruz G, Zang C, Peng W, O'Shea JJ & Kanno Y. (2010) Discrete roles of STAT4 and STAT6 transcription factors in tuning epigenetic modifications and transcription during T helper cell differentiation. *Immunity.* 32:840-851.

Willemze R, Jaffe ES, Burg G, Cerroni L, Berti E, Swerdlow SH, Ralfkiaer E, Chimenti S, Diaz-Perez JL, Duncan LM, Grange F, Harris NL, Kempf W, Kerl H, Kurrer M, Knobler R, Pimpinelli N, Sander C, Santucci M, Sterry W, Vermeer MH, Wechsler J, Whittaker S & Meijer CJ. (2005) WHO-EORTC classification for cutaneous lymphomas. *Blood.* 105:3768-3785.

Witthuhn BA, Silvennoinen O, Miura O, Lai KS, Cwik C, Liu ET & Ihle JN. (1994) Involvement of the Jak-3 Janus kinase in signaling by interleukins 2 and 4 in lymphoid and myeloid cells. *Nature.* 370: 153–157.

Yang Q, Jeremiah Bell J & Bhandoola A. (2010) T-cell lineage determination. *Immunol Rev.* 238:12-22.

Yao X, Nie H, Rojas IC, Harriss JV, Maika SD, Gottlieb PD, Rathbun G & Tucker PW. (2010) The L2a element is a mouse CD8 silencer that interacts with MAR-binding proteins SATB1 and CDP. *Mol Immunol.* 48:153-163.

Yasui D, Miyano M, Cai S, Varga-Weisz P & Kohwi-Shigematsu T. (2002) SATB1 targets chromatin remodelling to regulate genes over long distances. *Nature.* 419:641-645.

Yu D, Rao S, Tsai LM, Lee SK, He Y, Sutcliffe EL, Srivastava M, Linterman M, Zheng L, Simpson N, Ellyard JI, Parish IA, Ma CS, Li QJ, Parish CR, Mackay CR & Vinuesa CG. (2009) The transcriptional repressor Bcl-6 directs T follicular helper cell lineage commitment. *Immunity.* 31:457-468.

Yui MA, Feng N & Rothenberg EV. (2010) Fine-scale staging of T cell lineage commitment in adult mouse thymus. *J Immunol.* 185:284-293.

Zhu J & Paul WE. (2008) CD4 T cells: fates, functions and faults. *Blood.* 112:1557-1569

Zhu J, Min B, Hu-Li J, Watson CJ, Grinberg A, Wang Q, Killeen N, Urban JF Jr, Guo L & Paul WE. (2004) Conditional deletion of Gata3 shows its essential function in T_H1-T_H2 responses. *Nat Immunol.* 5:1157-1165.

Zhu J, Yamane H & Paul WE. (2010) Differentiation of effector CD4 T cell populations. *Annu Rev Immunol.* 28:445-489.

Zlotoff DA & Bhandoola A. (2011) Hematopoietic progenitor migration to the adult thymus. *Ann N Y Acad Sci.* 1217:122-138.

10

Membrane Trafficking and Endothelial-Cell Dynamics During Angiogenesis

Ajit Tiwari, Jae-Joon Jung, Shivangi M. Inamdar and Amit Choudhury
Department of Anatomy and Cell Biology, University of Iowa, Iowa City
USA

1. Introduction

The formation of new blood vessels, or neovascularization, involves multiple processes, including cell proliferation and migration, cell-cell and cell-matrix adhesion, and tube morphogenesis. Neovascularization can occur through one of two events: vasculogenesis, the *de novo* formation of blood vessels from angioblasts; or angiogenesis, the extension of new vessels from a pre-existing vasculature. Among these, angiogenesis in particular is relevant throughout life; its dysregulation has been causally related to several disorders that involve malignancy, inflammation, and ischemia. Angiogenesis is thought to depend on a set of signaling proteins – including certain kinases, integrins and vascular endothelial growth factor receptor-2 (VEGFR2) – that are enriched in specific plasma membrane domains. Both physiological and pathological angiogenesis rely on intracellular trafficking, a process that governs signaling by such proteins, as well as cell motility.

In this chapter, we discuss our current understanding of angiogenesis from the perspective of trafficking of the membrane components that are responsible for endothelial-cell (EC) dynamics.

2. Angiogenesis: Mechanism and importance

The vascular system carries out a variety of functions vital to vertebrates. It delivers oxygen and nutrients to tissues and organs. It is required for waste disposal, including the detoxification of toxic metabolites in the liver and their excretion through kidney. It is needed for the onset of immune responses against pathogens, since it transports immune cells to the site of infection and/or inflammation. Finally, its constituent vessels produce instructive signals for organogenesis.

Blood vessels are the main component of the vascular system and comprise: an EC monolayer that lines the vessel lumen, vascular smooth muscle cells that surround the EC monolayer, and a basement membrane that covers the vascular tube (**Figure 1**). The larger vessels, arteries and veins are stabilized by a thick layer of vascular smooth muscle cells, whereas the medium-sized vessels are supported by mural cells, for example pericytes (Gerhardt and Betsholtz, 2003).

The vascular system is among the earliest organ systems to develop in embryos; it first emerges when haemangioblast progenitors proliferate, migrate and differentiate into

ECs and form a primitive vascular plexus. The formation of new blood vessels, or neovascularization, then occurs either through vasculogenesis or angiogenesis, as mentioned above.

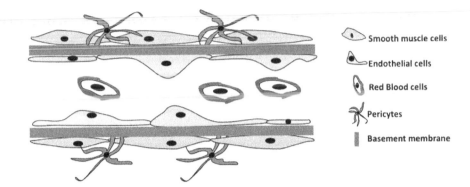

Fig. 1. Schematic representation of a mature blood vessel. Endothelial cells at the luminal side line tubular blood vessel. The smooth muscle cells and the pericytes that remain in contact with the endothelial cell lining through the basement membrane strengthen this tubular structure.

2.1 Vasculogenesis

Vasculogenesis, defined as *de novo* formation of blood vessels from precursor cells, starts with differentiation of precursor cells (angioblasts) into ECs and a primitive vascular network. In the first phase of vasculogenesis (during gastrulation), the splanchnic mesoderm gives rise to hemangioblasts, which are presumed to be the common progenitors of ECs and blood cells (Baron, 2001; Choi, 2002), and subsequently the outer cells of the blood island differentiate into angioblasts. In the second phase, angioblasts differentiate into ECs. In the third and final phase, the ECs participate in tube formation, giving rise to the primitive vascular plexus (**Figure 2**). Growth factor, fibroblast growth factor 2 (FGF2) generates hemangioblasts from the mesoderm, whereas vascular endothelial growth factor (VEGF) and its receptor, VEGFR, cooperate in hemangioblast generation and tube formation, and Angiopoietin-1 (Ang-1) regulates the connection between ECs and pericytes (Hiratsuka, 2011).

2.2 Angiogenesis

Angiogenesis, the establishment of new vessels from a pre-existing vasculature, starts with stimulation of ECs that line the luminal surface of blood vessels. The process of angiogenesis can be classified into two types: "sprouting" and "nonsprouting" (Risau, 1997). Sprouting angiogenesis refers to a process that entails proteolytic degradation of the extracellular matrix, the migration and proliferation of cells, the formation of a lumen, and maturation of ECs into functional capillaries. Specifically, ECs in pre-existing vessels respond to activation by a stimulatory molecule supplied by neighboring cells (e.g. VEGF), by producing a protease that degrades the surrounding basement membrane, to facilitate EC migration towards stimulatory signal. The sprout is comprised of a growth-arrested leading tip cell and proliferating stalk cells (Gerhardt et al., 2003). The tips cells are migratory and extend long filopodia that guide the sprouts towards the stimulus. Subsequently, the sprout anastomoses with other newly formed vessels to allow circulation. The basement membrane reassembles pericytes and gets recruited to newly formed vessels (**Figure 2**). Sprouting angiogenesis occurs during yolk sac and embryo development, and later during brain development (Scappaticci, 2002). Non-sprouting angiogenesis is a process that occurs by invagination involving EC proliferation within a vessel, and results in an enlarged lumen that can be split by transcapillary or by the fusion and splitting of capillaries. Non-sprouting angiogenesis occurs mainly during development of the lung and heart (Scappaticci, 2002). Both sprouting and non-sprouting angiogenesis contribute to vessel formation in the adult, via a process known as "adult vasculogenesis". This process is thought to rely on endothelial progenitor cells (EPCs) that originate from the bone marrow. While circulating in the blood, EPCs are incorporated into vessels at the site of angiogenesis (Caplice and Doyle, 2005).

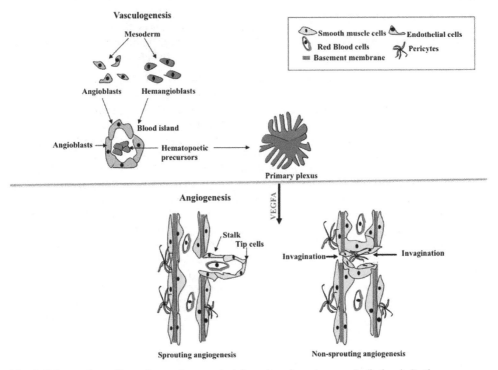

Fig. 2. Schematic outline of vasculogenesis (above) and angiogenesis (below). Both sprouting and non-sprouting mechanism of angiogenesis are shown.

2.3 Pathological angiogenesis

The process of angiogenesis is highly regulated in healthy adults and occurs only rarely, for example during ovulation and the endometrial growth that is central to the menstrual cycle. Angiogenesis is also required for wound healing, and ceases once this process is completed.

Since vessels nourish nearly every organ of the body the strict limitation of angiogenesis to such contexts is essential; deviation from normal vessel growth – in either direction – leads to fatal disease. Excess angiogenesis is characteristic of conditions such as retinopathy, rheumatoid arthritis, psoriasis and tumor growth (Folkman, 1995), and insufficient angiogenesis is a feature of ischemic heart and limb disease, stroke and gastrointestinal ulcers (Carmeliet and Jain, 2000).

The process of angiogenesis plays a crucial role in cancer metastasis – the major cause of mortality in cancer patients. In tumor diseases, angiogenesis is stimulated by the secretion of signaling molecules, e.g. VEGFA, by either the tumor cells themselves or tumor-infiltrating macrophages. In most cancers, tumor angiogenesis is crucial for disease progression, as it supplies the tumor cells with nutrients and oxygen, enabling them to survive and spread (Folkman, 2002). Notably, tumor-supporting vessels tend to be disorganized and leaky; thus vessel function is suboptimal and angiogenesis is further stimulated by hypoxia-driven expression of VEGFA in the tumor tissue. These findings have stimulated great interest in targeting tumor vessels as a means of developing novel cancer therapies. Indeed, intensive research efforts toward this end have revealed that, in patients with metastatic colorectal cancer, supplementing chemotherapy with a neutralizing antibody against VEGFA (Avastin/Bevacizumab) results in significantly improved survival (McCarthy, 2003).

Angiogenesis can also be regulated by microRNA (miRNA) (Wang and Olson, 2009). MicroRNA is a class of highly conserved, single stranded, non-coding small RNAs influencing gene expression by inhibiting translation of protein from mRNA or by promoting the degradation of mRNA (Bartel, 2004; Kim, 2005). The direct evidence of miRNA importance in angiogenesis was provided by observation of defective vascular remodeling during developmental angiogenesis in hypomorphic mouse line with EC-specific deletion of Dicer, one of key enzymes involved in miRNA generation (Otsuka et al., 2008; Yang et al., 2005). Endothelial cell primarily express miRNA-221/222, miRNA-21, the Let-7 family, the miR-17-92 cluster, the miRNA-23-24 cluster, and miRNA-126 (Harris et al., 2008; Kuehbacher et al., 2007; Suarez et al., 2007). miRNA-210 which gets activated upon hypoxia is an important regulator of EC survival, migration and differentiation during angiogenesis (Fasanaro et al., 2008). miRNA-210 overexpression under normoxic conditions stimulates angiogenesis and VEGF-induced cell migration whereas its blockade by anti-mRNA inhibits tube formation stimulated by hypoxia (Fasanaro et al., 2008). miRNA-210 may play an important role in pathological angiogenesis since hypoxia is associated with tumor development and organ ischemia. miRNA-21 and miRNA-31 are the other pro-angiogenic miRNAs which are upregulated in various various cancers to stimulate invasion and metastasis in cancer (Tsai et al., 2009).

3. Ligands and receptors in angiogenesis

At the molecular level, the initiation of vascular development is dependent on a number of cell-surface receptors and their respective ligands. Upon binding to a wide range of peptide growth factors, members of the receptor tyrosine kinase (RTK) family of transmembrane proteins transduce proliferative and morphogenic signals, thereby fine-tuning the orchestration of vascular remodeling and angiogenic processes. Although angiogenesis is controlled by a wide range of extracellular signals, the most potent pro-angiogenic signaling is initiated by binding of VEGF (vascular endothelial growth factor) to EC-resident VEGF receptors (VEGFRs) like VEGFR1 [Flt (Fms-like tyrosine kinase)-1], VEGFR2 [Flk-1 (fetal liver kinase 1)/KDR (kinase insert domain receptor)] and VEGFR3 (Flt-4) (Zachary, 2003).

Remodeling from existing vessels during angiogenesis is governed by VEGF-mediated EC proliferation, and their sprouting from points of loose contact between capillaries and the extracellular matrix. The nascent capillary network then matures through the actions of TGF-β and platelet-derived growth factor (PDGF). The arterial and venous ECs within the final primary capillary express Ephrin B2 and its receptor EphB4, respectively, in their cell membranes; this enables correct fusion between arterial and venous vessels.

3.1 The VEGF-VEGFR system coordinates the process of angiogenesis

3.1.1 VEGF

The VEGF family is a branch of the PDGF/VEGF supergene family and its members have a homodimeric structure (Ferrara and Davis-Smyth, 1997). The VEGF family consists of five related growth factors: VEGFA, VEGFB, VEGFC, VEGFD and PlGF (placental growth factor). Although VEGFs are homodimeric polypeptides, naturally occurring heterodimers have also been reported (DiSalvo et al., 1995). VEGFA, which was also isolated as vascular permeability factor (VPF), is alternatively spliced to generate VEGFA121, VEGFA145, VEGFA165 and VEGFA189 (the numbers indicate final residue in each polypeptide in humans). Alternative splicing and processing regulates ligand binding to VEGF receptors, heparan sulfate and neuropilins (NRPs) (Grunewald et al., 2010). VEGFA165 and VEGFA189 bind to both heparan sulfate and NRP1. VEGFA plays an important role in the proliferation and migration of ECs, and also acts on monocytes and macrophages, neurons, cancer cells, and kidney epithelial cells. VEGFA is known to be regulated by hypoxia-inducible factor (HIF) (Germain et al., 2010), an event that leads to increased expression during embryonic development and wound healing, and also in the context of cancer. VEGFA produced by most parenchymal cells, act in paracrine manner on adjacent ECs to regulate signaling by the VEGF receptors. Autocrine VEGFA is essential for EC survival (Lee et al., 2007), and is consistent with their requirement for complete development of the vasculature in mice; both homozygosity and heterozygosity for knockout of the VEGFA gene result in embryonic lethality characterized by incomplete development of the vasculature (Carmeliet et al., 1996; Ferrara et al., 1996). The biological activity of VEGF is manifested after it binds to VEGF receptors, which are of 3 different types in human, and bind VEGF with distinct affinities.

3.2 VEGF receptors

Orthologs of each of the VEGF receptor tyrosine kinases (VEGFRs) – namely VEGFR1, VEGFR2 and VEGFR3 – have been identified in humans, mice and other mammals. Structurally, the VEGFRs have a common organization consisting of: an extracellular, ligand-binding domain that features 7 immunoglobulin (Ig)-like loops, a transmembrane domain; a juxtamembrane domain; a split kinase domain and a C-terminal tail (**Figure 3**). Structurally, the VEGFRs are distantly related to the PDGFRs, which have five extracellular Ig-like domains (Matthews et al., 1991; Terman et al., 1991). All three VEGFRs undergo alternative splicing to generate more than one receptor form. The truncated form of VEGFR1, known as soluble VEGFR1 (sVEGR1, sFlt-1) (Kendall and Thomas, 1993), is implicated as causative agent in preeclampsia, a major disorder that can occur during pregnancy (Levine et al., 2004). A naturally occurring soluble form of VEGFR2 has also been described; it could potentially arise as a result of alternative splicing or through proteolytic processing (Ebos et al., 2004). In humans, alternative splicing of VEGFR3 generates two isoforms with distinct C-terminal tails (Hughes, 2001).

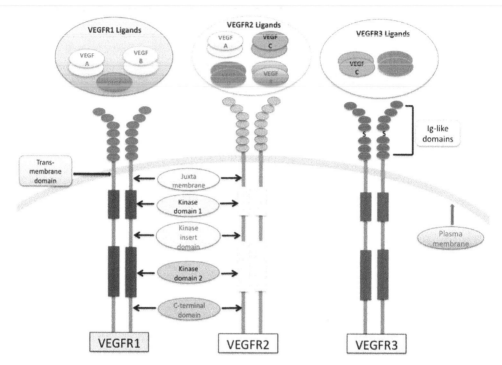

Fig. 3. VEGF receptors and their ligands. Schematic presentation of VEGF receptors (VEGFR1, VEGFR2 and VEGFR3). The signaling domain of all three receptors is present within cytosol. The Ig-like domains of VEGFRs are involved in VEGF binding, shown in elliptical structures that are present extracellularly. More than one kind of VEGF can bind to one receptor with different affinities.

3.2.1 VEGFR1

VEGFR1 (also known as Flt1 in mouse) is a glycoprotein of 150-184 kDa (de Vries et al., 1992; Shibuya et al., 1990) that gets activated upon binding of VEGFA, VEGFB and PLGF. VEGFR1 is expressed in vascular ECs at relatively high levels, throughout development and in the adult (Peters et al., 1993). It is also expressed in various other cell types such as monocytes, macrophages, human trophoblasts, renal mesangial cells, vascular smooth muscle cells, dendritic cells and a variety of human tumor-cell types (Barleon et al., 1996; Dikov et al., 2005; Sawano et al., 2001).

Alternative splicing of VEGFR1 generates soluble VEGFR1 (sVEGFR1), which is abundantly expressed in the placenta. Although the affinity of VEGFR1 for VEGFA is greater than that of VEGFR2, VEGFR1 transduces only weak signals for EC and pericyte growth and survival, as well as for macrophage migration (Barleon et al., 1996; Nomura et al., 1995). In response to ligand binding, VEGFR1 undergoes autophosphorylation at various tyrosines within the intracellular domain (TYRs1169, 1213, 1242, 1327, 1333) (Ito et al., 1998; Sawano et al., 1997). Phosphorylation of TYR1169 allows binding and activation of phospholipase C (PLC)γ1, which regulates EC proliferation via the mitogen-activated protein kinase (MAPK) pathway (Sawano et al., 1997). Tyr1213 binds a variety of SH2-containing proteins, including PLCγ, growth-factor-receptor bound protein (GRB) 2, non-catalytic region of tyrosine kinase adaptor protein (Nck) and SH2-domain-containing protein tyrosine phosphatase 2 (SHP-2) (Igarashi et al., 1998; Ito et al., 1998). Tyr1309 is however phosphorylated in response to PLGF but not VEGF (Autiero et al., 2003) (**Figure 4**). Although the exact role of VEGFR1

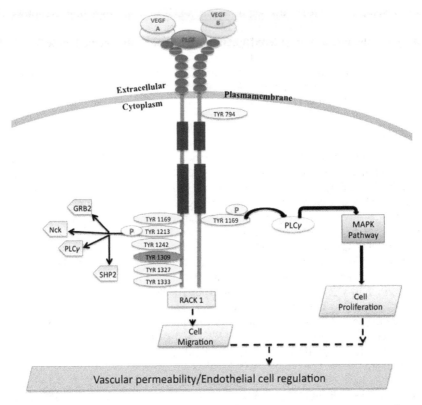

Fig. 4. VEGFR1 tyrosine phosphorylation and signaling. Schematic presentation of intracellular dimerized VEGFR1. VEGFA/VEGFB binding induces tyrosine phosphorylation of VEGFR1 at different tyrosine (TYR) positions shown in yellow ellipses. PLGF binding stimulates phosphorylation at TYR1309 shown in orange ellipse. Signaling molecules (shown within boxes) binds to certain phosphorylated tyrosine residues (circled P) and activates downstream signaling events leading to specific physiological outcome (shown in purple boxes) required for vascular permeability and endothelial cell regulation. PLCγ, phospholipase C-γ; MAPK, mitogen-activated protein; RACK1, receptor for activated C-kinase 1; SHP2, SH2-domain-containing protein tyrosine phosphatase 2.

remains a subject of debate, studies using VEGFR1-neutralizing antibodies have implicated this receptor in actin reorganization within, and the migration of ECs (Kanno et al., 2000), and suggested that receptor for activated C-kinase 1 (RACK1) is its downstream effector in this context (Wang et al., 2011). VEGFR1-dependent activation of PI3K/Akt may play a role in EC differentiation and organization (Huang et al., 2001) (Figure 4). Under *in vitro* conditions, VEGFR1 and VEGFR2 are known to form heterodimers on cells co-expressing these receptors (Huang et al., 2001), so it is believed that VEGFR1 can regulate EC functions via cross-talk with VEGFR2, through dimerization as a result of VEGFA binding to both. Binding of PLGF can also lead to crosstalk between VEGFR2 and VEGFR1 through transphosphorylation, leading to sensitization of VEGFR2 subsequent to activation by VEGFA (Autiero et al., 2003). Soluble VEGFR1 (sVEGFR1, sFlt1) can negatively influence vascular development, either by sequestering VEGFA from signaling receptors or by forming non-functional heterodimers with VEGFR2 (Kendall et al., 1994). Although, VEGFR1 and sVEGFR1 are considered VEGF decoys that control signaling by VEGFR1 and the formation of angiogenic sprouts (Kappas et al., 2008), the importance of VEGFR1 in angiogenesis is demonstrated by the fact that the VEGR1 null (*vegfr1-/-*) mouse dies at embryonic day 9, due to increased proliferation of ECs, disorganization and dysfunction of the vascular system (Fong et al., 1995).

3.2.2 VEGFR2

VEGFR2 (also known as KDR or Flk-1) is generally accepted to be the main receptor tyrosine kinase responsible for transducing the angiogenic activities of VEGFA, a factor that stimulates vascular-cell survival/growth and promotes angiogenesis. VEGFR2 knockout results in embryonic lethality due to deficiencies in vasculogenesis and hematopoiesis (Shalaby et al., 1995). VEGFR2 is highly expressed in vascular endothelial progenitors during early embryogenesis and generates a variety of angiogenic signals, not only for the proliferation of ECs but also their migration and morphogenesis, and as such has an important role in vascular tube formation. VEGFR2 expression is upregulated under conditions that trigger pathological angiogenesis, such as in tumors (reviewed in (Matsumoto and Claesson-Welsh, 2001). The binding of VEGF to VEGFR2 leads to receptor dimerization and promotes EC differentiation, proliferation, migration and vascular-tube formation. Both homo- and heterodimerization occurs following the trans-phosphorylation of tyrosine in the receptor intracellular domain. The major phosphorylation sites on VEGFR2 are TYR951 (in the kinase-insert domain), TYR1054 and TYR1059 (within the kinase domain), and TYR1175 and TYR1214 (in the C-terminal domain) (Matsumoto et al., 2005; (Takahashi et al., 2001). Additional phosphorylation sites on VEGFR2 have been identified at postions 1223, 1305, 1309 and 1319, but their function remains to be established (Matsumoto et al., 2005). Although TYR801 within the juxtamembrane can be phosphorylated when the intracellular portion of VEGFR2 is tested in isolation (Solowiej et al., 2009), its phosphorylation in the context of the intact protein has not yet been demonstrated. Phosphorylation at TYR951, within the kinase-insert domain, leads to binding and tyrosine phosphorylation of the SH2-domain–containing signaling molecule T-cell specific adapter (TSAd)(Matsumoto et al., 2005). TSAd, which is equipped with Src Homology 2 (SH2) and protein tyrosine binding (PTB) domains, in turn associates with the cytoplasmic tyrosine kinase Src, thereby regulating actin stress fiber organization and the migratory responses of ECs to VEGFA (**Figure 5**). Phosphorylation at TYR1054 and TYR1059, both of which are located within the kinase domain activation loop (Kendall et al., 1999), is preceded by autophosphorylation at TYR801 (Solowiej et al., 2009). Phosphorylation at TYR1059 induces Src binding, which in turn phosphorylates TYR1175 of VEGFR2, as well as residues within downstream signal transducers, such as the actin binding protein IQ-motif-contaning GTPase-activating protein 1 (IQGAP1), which is implicated in the regulation of cell-cell contacts, proliferation and migration (Meyer et al., 2008; Yamaoka-Tojo et al., 2006).

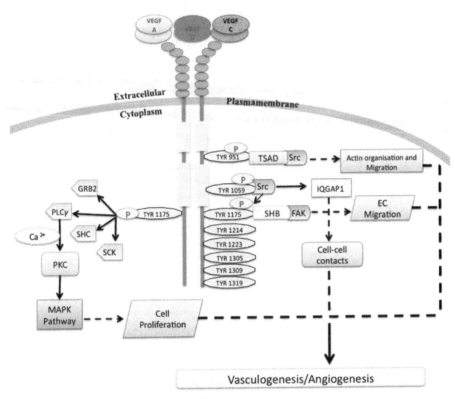

Fig. 5. VEGFR2 tyrosine phosphorylation and signaling. Schematic presentation of dimerized VEGFR2. VEGFA/VEGFB/VEGFC binding induces tyrosine phosphorylation of VEGFR2 at different tyrosine (TYR) positions shown in ellipses. Signaling molecules (shown within boxes) binds to certain phosphorylated TYR residues (circled P) and activates network of downstream signaling events required for variety of physiological outcomes (shown in purple boxes) essential during vasculogenesis and angiogenesis.

Phosphorylation at TYR1175 is required for the binding of PLCγ, which mediates activation of the mitogen-activated protein kinase (MAPK)/extracellular-signal-regulated kinase-1/2 (ERK1/2) cascade and the proliferation of ECs (Takahashi et al., 2001). Binding of PLCγ stimulates the protein kinase C (PKC) pathway, leading to inositol triphosphate generation and calcium mobilization. In addition to interacting with PLCγ, phosphorylated TYR1175 binds to the SH2-domain–containing adaptor protein B (SHB) and Src homology and collagen homology (Sck/SHC) (Holmqvist et al., 2004; Warner et al., 2000). SHB binds to Tyrosine-phosphorylated focal adhesion kinase (FAK) in VEGF-treated cells (Abu-Ghazaleh et al., 2001) and thereby contributes to EC attachment and migration (Holmqvist et al., 2003). The binding of SHC to TYR1175-phosphorylated VEGFR2 is believed to control Ras activation and mitogenicity in response to VEGF (Meadows et al., 2001).

3.2.3 VEGFR3

VEGFR3, also denoted Flt4, is a protein with a molecular weight of around 195 kDa, and becomes activated when bound to VEGFC or VEGFD. VEGFR3 is an essential protein; its inactivation results in embryonic death at E9.5, due to abnormal remodeling of the primary vascular plexus (Dumont et al., 1998). Although VEGFR3 plays a role in vascular development in the early embryo, its expression is later largely confined to ECs of the lymphatic system (Kaipainen et al., 1995). The exception is when its expression is induced in vascular ECs during active phases of angiogenesis, for example in the tumor vasculature or the endothelial tip cells of angiogenic sprouts in the retina (Tammela et al., 2008). VEGFR3 has five tyrosine phosphorylation sites – at positions 1230, 1231, 1265, 1337 and 1363 in the C-terminal tail (Dixelius et al., 2003) – that are activated and phosphorylated upon binding of VEGFC or VEGFD. TYR1337 when phosphorylated is known to bind to Shc and Grb2 to initiate signaling by the MAPK pathway. Both TYR1063 and TYR1068, which are located within the kinase activation domain, are crucial for kinase activity. Phosphorylation of TYR1230 and TYR1231 creates a docking site for SHC–GBR2, which promotes signaling by the ERK1/2 and PI3K/Akt pathways **(Figure 6)**. Phosphorylated TYR1063 has been shown to interact with adaptor protein C10 regulator of kinase (CRK I/II), which activates the c-Jun N-terminal kinase (JNK) pathway to promote cell survival (Salameh et al., 2005).

3.2.4 Neuropilins (NRP)

The cell-surface glycoprotein neuropilin is a transmembrane protein with a small cytoplasmic tail that lacks intrinsic catalytic function (Fujisawa et al., 1997). The neuropilin homolog NRP1 is expressed in arteries, whereas NRP2, is expressed in the venous and lymphatic vessels (Yuan et al., 2002). NRP1 was originally identified as a receptor for the collapsin/semaphorin family of neuronal guidance molecule (Chen et al., 1997). Later it was reported to also be expressed in ECs, where it acts as a coreceptor for VEGFA164 and VEGFA165 in mice and humans, respectively (Miao et al., 1999; Soker et al., 1998). NRP1 modulates VEGFR signaling, leading to enhanced survival and migration of ECs *in vitro* (Favier et al., 2006). NRP1 has also been implicated in VEGFR2-mediated vascular permeability (Becker et al., 2005) and VEGFA-induced vessel sprouting and branching (Kawamura et al., 2008). Although the exact influence of NRP1 on VEGFA mediated VEGFR2 signaling remains to be deciphered, the importance of NRP1 in angiogenesis was established by the fact that overexpression or deletion of NRP1 in mice leads to embryonic lethality and vascular abnormalities (Kawasaki et al., 1999). Neuropilin is also expressed in tumors and is believed to enhance tumor angiogenesis (Miao et al., 2000); it probably does so by stabilizing VEGF/VEGFR signaling on adjacent cell in trans.

3.3 Role of the extracellular matrix (ECM) in endothelial-cell interactions during angiogenesis

The angiogenic process is influenced not only by ligand/receptor systems, but also overall composition of extracellular matrix (ECM) surrounding the vasculature. Indeed, the ECM

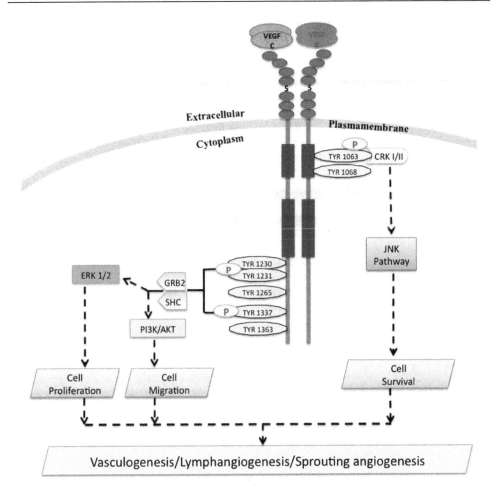

Fig. 6. VEGFR3 tyrosine phosphorylation and signaling. Schematic presentation of intracellular dimerized VEGFR3. VEGFC/VEGFD binding induces tyrosine phosphorylation of VEGFR3 at different tyrosine (TYR) positions shown in green ellipses. Signaling molecules (shown within boxes) binds to certain phosphorylated tyrosine residues (circled P) and activates network of downstream signaling events required for variety of physiological outcomes (shown in purple boxes) essential during vasculogenesis and angiogenesis

provides an essential connection between ECs and the surrounding tissues and affect angiogenesis either positively or negatively (Nyberg et al., 2005). ECs are attached to a basement membrane (BM), which forms a continuous coat around the vessels. The main components of the vascular BM are type IV collagen, laminins, fibronectin, heparan-sulphate proteoglycans and nidogens. The BM provides structural support to the ECs (Kalluri, 2003), and interaction of ECs with components in the BM is important for maintaining integrity of the vessel wall (Hallmann et al., 2005). When ECs are exposed to angiogenic growth factors such as VEGFA, several kind of matrix-degrading enzymes, such as matrix metalloproteinases, dissolve the BM. Matrix-degrading enzymes are produced by ECs and stromal cells, as well as by tumor and inflammatory cells (Egeblad and Werb, 2002). Endothelial sprouting is activated not only by growth factors, but also signals from the matrix proteins. Degradation of the BM reveals so-called cryptic sites that can activate the angiogenic properties of ECs. As the BM is degraded and vascular permeability increases, the blood-clotting protein fibrinogen leaks out of the vessels and polymerizes into a fibrin gel (Iivanainen et al., 2003). Constituents of the degraded BM, fibrin, and EC-produced extracellular matrix (ECM) components then form a provisional matrix that ECs invade with guidance from both growth factors and matrix proteins. Once through the provisional matrix, the endothelial sprout further invades the interstitial matrix, which is composed of many proteins including fibrillar collagens (such as collagen I) and fibronectin. These proteins may also promote angiogenesis, collagen I for example, has pro-angoigenic effects (Davis and Senger, 2005; Senger et al., 2002). The signals from the ECM are transmitted by cell-surface expressed adhesion receptors called integrins, which bind to different ECM proteins in a specific manner (Stupack and Cheresh, 2004). In conjunction with the fusion of newly formed vessel sprouts to allow perfusion, the BM reassembles and pericytes are recruited to the vessel. ECs recruit pericytes by secreting PDGF, which binds to the PDGFβ-receptor expressed on pericytes; this process is crucial for vessel stabilization, and lack of pericyte engagement causes remodelling defects and leaky vessels (Uemura et al., 2002)

3.4 Role of Integrin in endothelial-cell dynamics during angiogenesis

Integrins are heterodimeric transmembrane glycoproteins consisting of non-covalently associated α and β subunits, and they promote cell-matrix adhesion and migration on the surrounding ECM. Integrins have no intrinsic enzymatic or kinase activity, but activate signaling pathways by co-clustering with kinases and adaptor proteins in a focal adhesion complex comprising: protein kinases such as FAK and Src; adaptor proteins such as Shc; signaling intermediates such as GTPases of the Rho family; and actin-binding cytoskeletal proteins such as talin, α-actinin, paxillin, tensin and vinculin (Mitra et al., 2005; Mitra and Schlaepfer, 2006). Integrin signaling promotes cell migration, proliferation and survival (Avraamides et al., 2008). Eighteen α and eight β subunits can associate to form 24 unique integrin heterodimers. EC integrins that regulate cell growth, survival and migration during angiogenesis include heterodimers $\alpha1\beta1$, $\alpha2\beta1$, $\alpha4\beta1$, $\alpha5\beta1$, $\alpha6\beta1$, $\alpha6\beta4$, $\alpha9\beta1$, $\alpha v\beta3$ and $\alpha v\beta5$ (Avraamides et al., 2008). Integrin $\alpha v\beta3$ (a receptor for RGD-containing ECM proteins such as vitronectin, fibronectin, fibrinogen and osteopontin) was the first αv integrin shown to regulate EC survival and migration during angiogenesis. The expresssion of $\alpha v\beta3$ integrin on resting ECs is negligible, but is upregulated by the presence of angiogenic growth factors such as bFGF, TNFα and IL8 (Brooks et al., 1994). Integrin $\alpha v\beta3$ also regulate pathological angiogenesis during processes such as wound healing. The VEGFR2–$\alpha v\beta3$-integrin association is important for full VEGFR2 signaling activity, for activation of p38MAPK and FAK, and for the recruitment of actin-binding vinculin as needed to initiate EC migration (Mahabeleshwar et al., 2008). The ligation of endothelial $\alpha v\beta3$ integrin has also been shown to activate FAK, Src, and other kinases, resulting in cell proliferation, differentiation and migration (Eliceiri et al., 2002). Whereas $\alpha v\beta3$ dimers initiate angiogenesis in response to bFGF and TNFα, the related integrin $\alpha v\beta5$ is required for TNFα- and VEGF-mediated angiogenesis (Friedlander et al., 1995). $\beta1$

integrin, which pairs with variety of α integrin subunits, plays an important role in angiogenesis. Mice with EC-specific deletion of β1 integrin die during embryonic stages due to severe vascular defects (Tanjore et al., 2008). Matrix-bound VEGF induces the formation of a complex between VEGFR2 and β1 integrin, which leads to prolonged phosphorylation of VEGFR2 at TYR 1214 and association of β1 integrin with focal adhesions (Chen et al., 2010).

Fibronectin secreted by ECs is a key ECM component. It is deposited by ECs during normal and tumor angiogenesis (Clark et al., 1982; Kim et al., 2000). Fibronectin interacts with integrins such as α5β1, αvβ5 and αvβ3 (Plow et al., 2000). During embryonic vascular development, as well as during tumor angiogenesis, the ECM protein fibronectin serves as an adhesive support and signals through α5β1 integrin to regulate the spreading, migration and contractility of ECs (Francis et al., 2002). Although the expression of α5β1 in quiescent endothelium is low, it is upregulated by exposure to a subset of angiogenic stimuli including bFGF, IL8 and the ECM protein (Kim et al., 2000). Integrin α5β1 promotes EC migration and survival in *in vivo* and *in vitro* models of angiogenesis by suppressing the activity of protein kinase A (PKA) (Kim et al., 2000b(Kim et al., 2002). Further, our recent study has demonstrated that integrin α5β1 recycling is essential for EC adhesion and migration on fibronectin (Tiwari et al., 2011), a process required during angiogenesis. Integrin α5β1 promotes the formation of focal adhesions and signaling through FAK (Schlaepfer and Hunter, 1998), which is required for EC migration (Mitra et al., 2005). The reduction in EC surface associated adhesion through integrin α5β1 in the context of impaired recycling leads to further reduction in total and activated FAK (Tiwari et al., 2011). During embryogenesis, integrin α5 is required for the development of early blood vessels and other tissues, as revealed by the fact that α5 integrin-deficient mice exhibit a mesodermal defect and are embryonic lethal (Yang et al., 1993). Integrin α4β1, another fibronectin receptor, affects the adhesion and extravasation of lymphocytes by binding to VCAM1, a member of the immunoglobulin superfamily, that is expressed on inflamed ECs. Deletion of integrin α4 in a mouse model leads to defects in plancentation, heart development and coronary artery development, and thus to embryonic lethality (Yang et al., 1995). Integrin α4β1 promotes adhesion of the endothelium to VCAM1-expressing vascular smooth muscle cells during blood vessel formation (Garmy-Susini et al., 2005). Integrin α4β1–VCAM1 facilitates cell-cell attachment between ECs expressing the pericyte chemoattractant PDGF and pericytes expressing VEGF, in response to growth and survival signals that emanate from each cell type during angiogenesis (Garmy-Susini et al., 2005). Integrin α9β1 is another fibronectin-binding integrin known to have role in angiogenesis (Vlahakis et al., 2007). Although structurally similar to integrin α4β1, integrin α9β1 can bind to a number of ECM proteins and cell-surface receptors including tenascin C, thrombospondin, osteopontin, fibronectin, VCAM1 and other ligands (Liao et al., 2002; Marcinkiewicz et al., 2000; Staniszewska et al., 2007). α4β1 binds only to VEGF, and promotes VEGFA-induced angiogenesis. β1 integrin, which pairs with variety of alpha integrin subunits, plays a key role in angiogenesis. Mice with an EC-specific deletion of β1 integrin die at embryonic stages due to a severe vascular defect (Tanjore et al., 2008). Matrix-bound VEGF induces the formation of complex between VEGFR2 and β1 integrin, which leads to prolonged phosphorylation of VEGFR2 at TYR 1214 and to an association of β1 integrin with focal adhesions (Chen et al., 2010).

4. Membrane trafficking

Membrane trafficking is an active process that relocates proteins from one region of a cell to another, and contributes to the regulation of cell migration (Ulrich and Heisenberg, 2009). Signaling by the membrane-resident proteins/receptors is regulated by their availability at the cell surface or correct locations that are controlled by membrane trafficking events. The trafficking of membrane receptors and their signaling are intertwined: trafficking itself affects signal transduction, and signaling by RTKs regulates the trafficking machinery (Sorkin and von Zastrow, 2009). The secretory and endocytic pathways, which are made up of a network of membrane-bound compartments, modify newly synthesized proteins, deliver them to their appropriate locations, and regulate the uptake and turnover of those that are targeted to the cell surface. Trafficking accomplishes the specific and regulated transfer of molecules between distinct membrane-enclosed organelles. The transport process involves the budding of vesicular or tubular carriers from donor membranes, followed by their delivery to specific acceptor membranes. Budding requires the formation of cargo-laden vesicles or tubules at a donor compartment, and also the involvement of (i) specific coat proteins like COPI or COPII; (ii) adaptor proteins such as clathrin, AP-1, 2, 3; and (iii) membrane-deforming proteins like Bar-family proteins (Doherty and McMahon, 2009). The cargo-containing donor vesicle then docks to the acceptor compartment with the help of rab GTPases and a tether. Finally, fusion of the donor and acceptor membranes for the delivery of the cargo is accomplished with the help of N-ethylmaleimide-sensitive factor (NSF)-attachment protein receptor (SNARE) protein complexes (Jahn and Scheller, 2006; Sudhof and Rothman, 2009).

4.1 Biosynthetic/secretory pathway

After being synthesized in the cytoplasm, new proteins are translocated to the endoplasmic reticulum (ER) (Lee et al., 2004) and then move to Golgi via membranous vesicles. After moving through the cis and medial cisternae of the Golgi, the ER-derived cargoes move to trans-Golgi cisternae, where the proteins destined for secretion or presentation on the PM are packed into secretory vesicle that subsequently fuse with the PM (Emr et al., 2009). The Golgi apparatus is the major sorting compartment of the cell; its cargo is sorted not only to the PM for presentation or secretion, but also to endosomes and lysosomes, or back to the ER (Emr et al., 2009).

4.2 Endocytic and exocytic pathways

The endocytic pathway regulates internalization and recycling of proteins internalized from the PM, through a variety of mechanisms, to early and/or late endosomes. Depending on the receptor type and the particular requirements of a particular cell, protein from the endosomes are either sorted to the lysosome, a major degradation site for both internalized and cellular proteins, or recycled back to the PM (Doherty and McMahon, 2009).

Efficient protein trafficking within endomembrane system is further regulated by cross-talk between the two pathways. Endosomal and lysosomal proteins that maintain their integrity and functionality shuttle from the ER, via the Golgi, to endosomes and lysosomes (Ghosh et al., 2003). In polarized cells, movement of the proteins from one side of the cell to the other, via the transcytotic pathway, involves both the biosynthetic/secretory and the endo/exocytic routes (Tuma and Hubbard, 2003). Thus, the membrane trafficking events control the cell communication network connected with signaling events, determining not only the intensity and duration, but also the final biological outcome.

The membrane trafficking process is also important for the signaling activities required for cell survival and migration during the normal physiological response, as well as for those that take place during angiogenesis. In ECs, modulation of receptor tyrosine activity through endocytosis and vesicle trafficking affects downstream targets such as endothelial nitric oxide synthase (eNOS) and VE-cadherin. Further, activation of RTKs results in the dissolution of EC–specific adhesion through endocytosis of VE-cadherin, thereby promoting cell migration and vascular permeability (Mukherjee et al., 2006). Directional cell migration requires the trafficking of adhesion and growth factor receptors including VEGFR2, which is involved with angiogenesis (Lanahan et al., 2010). The angiogenic signals generated in response to VEGFR2 receptor activation are highly regulated by sorting pathways during intracellular trafficking (Manickam et al., 2011). VEGFR2 signaling is regulated by a broad range of angiogenic regulators that in turn regulates receptor trafficking through the endosomal system (Manickam et al., 2011; Scott and Mellor, 2009). Rab GTPases regulate key events in VEGFR2 trafficking between the PM, early endosomes and late endosomes (Bruns et al., 2009). In addition, the Golgi (which is the central hub for membrane trafficking across the mammalian cell) coordinates the cell-surface expression of VEGFR2 by regulating the secretory transport of newly synthesized VEGFR2 (Manickam et al., 2011).

4.3 Endocytic trafficking of VEGFR2

Resting ECs have two pools of VEGFR2: a stable cell-surface pool that can form a complex with VE-cadherin at cell-cell junctions and does not undergo rapid internalization (Lampugnani et al., 2006), and a pool that continuously cycles between the surface and sorting endosomes and is independent of VEGF binding (Gampel et al., 2006). The VEGFR2 is associated with the caveolin-containing and cholesterol-enriched membrane microdomain (Labrecque et al., 2003). Binding of VEGF to extracellular domain of VEGFR2 triggers internalization of receptor subsequent to its dimerization and phosphorylation at TYR1054 and TYR1059. Upon activation, VEGFR2 dissociates from caveolin and transported to endosomes (Salikhova et al., 2008). Multiple modes of VEGFR2 internalization exist, since VEGF-stimulated endocytosis of VEGFR2 is clathrin-dependent (Lampugnani et al., 2006), and VEGFR2 is known to be translocated to perinuclear caveosomes through caveolar endocytosis (Bauer et al., 2005; Labrecque et al., 2003). Thus, the intracellular distribution of VEGFR2 depends on VEGF stimulation. Endosomal trafficking and the signaling of VEGFR2 is dependent on the Rab5a protein, a Ras-related small GTPase associated with early endosomes (Jopling et al., 2009). Depletion of Rab5a enhances VEGFR2 tyrosine phosphorylation and MAPK signaling, whereas overexpression of a Rab5a GTPase-deficient (constitutively active mutant, Q79L) causes VEGFR2 accumulation within endosomes (Jopling et al., 2009). Rab7a GTPase regulates VEGFR2 trafficking from early to late endosomes. Rab7a depletion is inhibitory whereas Rab5a depletion is stimulatory for EC migration (Jopling et al., 2009). VEGF stimulation also can increase the rate of VEGFR2 recycling from sorting endosomes. The vesicles containing VEGFR2 /Src complex traffic to a late endosomal compartment after a longer duration (30 mins) of VEGF stimulation (Gampel et al., 2006). Since Src is an important downstream target of VEGFR2 in an angiogenesis and vascular permeability pathway (Zachary, 2003), it is believed that recycling of VEGFR2/Src to the PM would sensitize pro-angiogenic signals. VEGF stimulation direct VEGFR2 from sorting endosomes to late endosomes finally directs it toward lysosomes for degradation (Gampel et al., 2006).

Regulation of VEGFR2 degradation is important for angiogenesis since VEGFR2 down-regulation controls the sensitivity of ECs to VEGF stimulation. Reports of VEGFR2 degradation upon VEGF stimulation are varied. One study suggests that VEGFR2 degradation is complete upon VEGF A stimulation (Ewan et al., 2006), whereas another study revealed degradation of only 30-40% of the total receptor population (Gampel et al., 2006). Degradation of activated VEGFR2 is promoted by its ubiquitination by c-Cbl, a protein that forms a complex with phospholipase Cγ1 (PLCγ1), a mediator of VEGFR2 signaling (Singh et al., 2007). VEGFR2 trafficking can also be regulated by the co-receptors such as VEGFR1 and NRP1, which can interact with VEGFR2. VEGFR1 is ubiquitylated upon VEGF stimulation and recruits Cbl (Kobayashi et al., 2004). As discussed above, VEGFR1 forms a heterodimer with VEGFR2 upon VEGF binding, so that the decision for sorting of VEGFR2 along a degradative pathway could be influenced by VEGFR1. NRP1, one of the other VEGFR2 co-receptors, which forms a complex with VEGFR2 upon VEGF binding, could stabilize VEGFR2 on the EC surface since loss of NRP1 increases the degradation of VEGFR2 upon VEGF stimulation (Holmes and Zachary, 2008).

4.4 Secretory transport of VEGFR2

Although the endocytic transport of VEGFR2 has been characterized in detail, the reports on secretory transport, i.e transport of newly synthesized VEGFR2, are scant. The Golgi apparatus regulates the trafficking of newly synthesized VEGFR2, since the Golgi receives newly synthesized proteins and lipids from the endoplasmic reticulum (ER), the central organelle in which trafficking-route decisions are made. Recently, studies from our group demonstrated that a significant amount of VEGFR2 is present in the Golgi apparatus, and that VEGF mobilizes this pool from the Golgi compartment (Manickam et al., 2011). The post-Golgi trafficking of cargo occurs in vesicular fashion, where the cargo-loaded vesicles bud from Golgi, delivering the cargoes to their target destinations by membrane fusion events. Membrane fusion steps in eukaryotic cells require SNAREs (Chen and Scheller, 2001; Hong, 2005). The SNAREs are classified into 2 major groups based on the presence of a glutamine (Q SNAREs or t-SNAREs) or an arginine (R SNAREs or v-SNAREs) in the center of the SNARE motif. The trans-Golgi network- and endosome-localized t-SNARE syntaxin 6 (STX6), but not syntaxin 10 and syntaxin 16, regulates secretory transport of VEGFR2 as well as VEGF-induced angiogenic processes (Manickam et al., 2011). Earlier studies demonstrated that STX6 participates in post-Golgi transport of components of membrane microdomains to the PM (Choudhury et al., 2006). Inhibition of STX6 either by loss-of-function approaches, applying an siRNAs against STX6 or by expressing the inhibitory, cytosolic domains of STX6 interferes with trafficking of Golgi-resident pool of VEGFR2 and targets it to lysosomes for degradation in human ECs, as described in model **(Figure 7)**. Further, inhibition of STX6 in cell culture reduced VEGF-induced cell proliferation, cell migration, and vascular tube formation (Manickam et al., 2011). Thus, the t-SNARE STX6 plays a crucial role in maintaining cellular VEGFR2 levels and, subsequently, in physiological processes associated with VEGF-mediated angiogenesis.

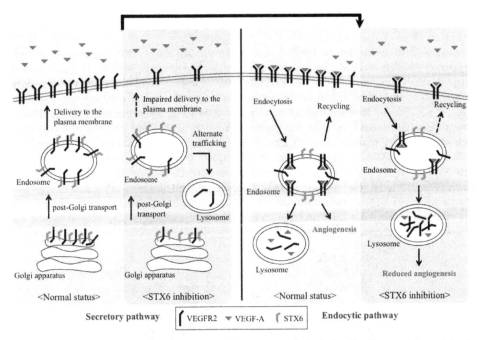

Fig. 7. Schematic summary of VEGFR2 trafficking. In endothelial cells, VEGFR2 is enriched in the plasma membrane, endosomes and Golgi apparatus. These VEGFR2 pools are maintained by endocytic and secretory transport pathways. The subcellular localization of VEGFR2 is essential for VEGF mediated signaling and angiogenesis, and is regulated by syntaxin 6, which colocalizes with VEGFR2 at the Golgi apparatus and endosomes. When syntaxin 6 function is inhibited, the cellular pool of VEGFR2 is depleted as a consequence of enhanced degradation in lysosomes. Syntaxin 6 contributes to trafficking of VEGFR2 from the Golgi and/or endosomes and the maintenance of proper levels of this receptor in different subcellular compartments required for efficient receptor signaling and angiogenesis. (Modified from Manickam et al., 2011. Blood *117*, 1425-1435. © the American Society of Hematology.)

4.5 VEGFR2 trafficking and angiogenesis

The process of angiogenesis is regulated by the response of VEGFR2 to VEGF binding. The availability of VEGFR2 at the PM may directly control the signaling response of ECs to VEGF for the onset of pro-angiogenic events. Thus, the trafficking mechanisms, such as secretory transport, recycling or degradation that affects the surface level VEGFR2, would determine the response of ECs to VEGF during angiogenesis. The EC-surface proteins that stabilize VEGFR2 at the plasma membrane contribute to the VEGF-driven cellular response during angiogenesis. A reduction in the engagement of VE-cadherin with ECs present in the stable vasculature leads to a reduction in surface levels of VEGFR2, thus reducing the sensitivity of ECs to VEGF (Lampugnani et al., 2006). The trafficking of VEGF receptors becomes more important under pathological conditions such as wound healing or ischemic heart disease, which may require rapid recycling and/or secretory transport of VEGF receptors to the surface, ensuring continuous activation of the VEGF/VEGFR pathway to guide angiogenic events.

As discussed above, a study by our group (Manickam et al., 2011) demonstrated that enhanced VEGFR2 degradation due to reduced secretory transport of VEGFR2 from the Golgi to PM (due to lack of functional STX6) leads to reductions in VEGF-induced proliferation, migration, and tube formation. Such *in vitro* effects may be responsible for reduced VEGFA-induced angiogenesis in the context of interference with STX6 function via adenoviral gene transfer of cytosolic domain of STX6 (STX6-cyto, inhibitory form) in ear angiogenesis assay in nude mice **(Figure 8)**. This ear angiogenesis model demonstrated that trafficking of VEGFR2 is essential for angiogenesis. Also, in our most recent study, we demonstrated that STX6 is essential for maintenance of EC surface-localized integrin α5β1, which plays a crucial role in angiogenesis (Tiwari et al., 2011). The finding that expressing a cytosolic form of STX6 significantly blocks VEGF-induced angiogenesis raises the prospect that pharmacologic manipulation of STX6 function in the setting of vascular disorders may be an effective therapeutic tool.

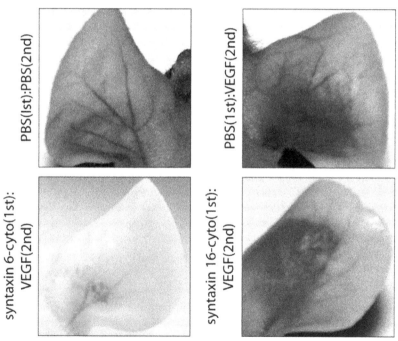

Fig. 8. Mice Ear Angiogenesis Assay: Representative images showing gross appearance of angiogenesis in mock, syntaxin 6-cyto- or syntaxin 16-cyto–injected mouse ears, 5 days before adenovirus expressing VEGF164 (Ad-VEGF164) administration. Nude mice (Nu/Nu strain) were given 2 injections under anesthesia. The first set of injections (1st) was PBS, syntaxin 6-cyto, or syntaxin 16-cyto. The second (2nd) was PBS or Ad-VEGF164, and given 2 days later at the site of first injection. At 7 days after the first set of injections, animals were euthanized and the ears were photographed. (from Manickam et al., 2011. Blood *117*, 1425-1435. © the American Society of Hematology).

5. Conclusions

Angiogenesis is regulated by VEGF-stimulated sensitization of the VEGF receptor and subsequent signaling events that are required during this process. Intracellular trafficking of VEGFR2 controls the VEGF signals that govern angiogenesis. Deciphering the mechanism underlying this trafficking and the roles of mediators in the transport of other VEGF receptors, as well as identifying other angiogenic components that play a role in the formation of new vessels, may provide better insight into angiogenesis. Syntaxin 6-regulated membrane trafficking events control outside-in signaling via the haptotactic and chemotactic mechanisms that regulate integrin α5β1-mediated EC movement on fibronectin and VEGF-mediated VEGFR2 signaling– important components of the angiogenic process (Manickam et al., 2011; Tiwari et al., 2011). A great deal has been deciphered about angiogenesis-related signaling pathways, but a detailed investigation of the intracellular and membrane trafficking of molecules associated directly or indirectly with angiogenesis would add to our knowledge of the angiogenic process, as well as help us to design therapeutic strategies for pathological angiogenesis therapeutic strategies for pathological angiogenesis.

6. Acknowledgement

Supported by grant from National Institutes of Health, National Heart, Lung, and Blood Institute (HL089599 to AC).

7. References

Abu-Ghazaleh, R., Kabir, J., Jia, H., Lobo, M., and Zachary, I. (2001). Src mediates stimulation by vascular endothelial growth factor of the phosphorylation of focal adhesion kinase at tyrosine 861, and migration and anti-apoptosis in endothelial cells. Biochem J 360, 255-264.

Autiero, M., Waltenberger, J., Communi, D., Kranz, A., Moons, L., Lambrechts, D., Kroll, J., Plaisance, S., De Mol, M., Bono, F., et al. (2003). Role of PlGF in the intra- and intermolecular cross talk between the VEGF receptors Flt1 and Flk1. Nat Med 9, 936-943.

Avraamides, C.J., Garmy-Susini, B., and Varner, J.A. (2008). Integrins in angiogenesis and lymphangiogenesis. Nat Rev Cancer 8, 604-617.

Barleon, B., Sozzani, S., Zhou, D., Weich, H.A., Mantovani, A., and Marme, D. (1996). Migration of human monocytes in response to vascular endothelial growth factor (VEGF) is mediated via the VEGF receptor flt-1. Blood 87, 3336-3343.

Baron, M. (2001). Induction of embryonic hematopoietic and endothelial stem/progenitor cells by hedgehog-mediated signals. Differentiation 68, 175-185.

Bartel, D.P. (2004). MicroRNAs: genomics, biogenesis, mechanism, and function. Cell 116, 281-297.

Bauer, P.M., Yu, J., Chen, Y., Hickey, R., Bernatchez, P.N., Looft-Wilson, R., Huang, Y., Giordano, F., Stan, R.V., and Sessa, W.C. (2005). Endothelial-specific expression of caveolin-1 impairs microvascular permeability and angiogenesis. Proc Natl Acad Sci U S A 102, 204-209.

Becker, P.M., Waltenberger, J., Yachechko, R., Mirzapoiazova, T., Sham, J.S., Lee, C.G., Elias, J.A., and Verin, A.D. (2005). Neuropilin-1 regulates vascular endothelial growth factor-mediated endothelial permeability. Circ Res 96, 1257-1265.

Bruns, A.F., Bao, L., Walker, J.H., and Ponnambalam, S. (2009). VEGF-A-stimulated signalling in endothelial cells via a dual receptor tyrosine kinase system is dependent on co-ordinated trafficking and proteolysis. Biochem Soc Trans 37, 1193-1197.

Caplice, N.M., and Doyle, B. (2005). Vascular progenitor cells: origin and mechanisms of mobilization, differentiation, integration, and vasculogenesis. Stem Cells Dev 14, 122-139.

Carmeliet, P., Ferreira, V., Breier, G., Pollefeyt, S., Kieckens, L., Gertsenstein, M., Fahrig, M., Vandenhoeck, A., Harpal, K., Eberhardt, C., et al. (1996). Abnormal blood vessel development and lethality in embryos lacking a single VEGF allele. Nature 380, 435-439.

Carmeliet, P., and Jain, R.K. (2000). Angiogenesis in cancer and other diseases. Nature 407, 249-257.

Chen, H., Chedotal, A., He, Z., Goodman, C.S., and Tessier-Lavigne, M. (1997). Neuropilin-2, a novel member of the neuropilin family, is a high affinity receptor for the semaphorins Sema E and Sema IV but not Sema III. Neuron 19, 547-559.

Chen, Y.A., and Scheller, R.H. (2001). SNARE-mediated membrane fusion. Nat Rev Mol Cell Biol 2, 98-106.

Choi, K. (2002). The hemangioblast: a common progenitor of hematopoietic and endothelial cells. J Hematother Stem Cell Res 11, 91-101.

Choudhury, A., Marks, D.L., Proctor, K.M., Gould, G.W., and Pagano, R.E. (2006). Regulation of caveolar endocytosis by syntaxin 6-dependent delivery of membrane components to the cell surface. Nat Cell Biol 8, 317-328.

Clark, R.A., DellaPelle, P., Manseau, E., Lanigan, J.M., Dvorak, H.F., and Colvin, R.B. (1982). Blood vessel fibronectin increases in conjunction with endothelial cell proliferation and capillary ingrowth during wound healing. J Invest Dermatol 79, 269-276.

Davis, G.E., and Senger, D.R. (2005). Endothelial extracellular matrix: biosynthesis, remodeling, and functions during vascular morphogenesis and neovessel stabilization. Circ Res 97, 1093-1107.

de Vries, C., Escobedo, J.A., Ueno, H., Houck, K., Ferrara, N., and Williams, L.T. (1992). The fms-like tyrosine kinase, a receptor for vascular endothelial growth factor. Science 255, 989-991.

Dikov, M.M., Ohm, J.E., Ray, N., Tchekneva, E.E., Burlison, J., Moghanaki, D., Nadaf, S., and Carbone, D.P. (2005). Differential roles of vascular endothelial growth factor receptors 1 and 2 in dendritic cell differentiation. J Immunol 174, 215-222.

DiSalvo, J., Bayne, M.L., Conn, G., Kwok, P.W., Trivedi, P.G., Soderman, D.D., Palisi, T.M., Sullivan, K.A., and Thomas, K.A. (1995). Purification and characterization of a naturally occurring vascular endothelial growth factor.placenta growth factor heterodimer. J Biol Chem 270, 7717-7723.

Dixelius, J., Makinen, T., Wirzenius, M., Karkkainen, M.J., Wernstedt, C., Alitalo, K., and Claesson-Welsh, L. (2003). Ligand-induced vascular endothelial growth factor receptor-3 (VEGFR-3) heterodimerization with VEGFR-2 in primary lymphatic endothelial cells regulates tyrosine phosphorylation sites. J Biol Chem *278*, 40973-40979.

Doherty, G.J., and McMahon, H.T. (2009). Mechanisms of endocytosis. Annu Rev Biochem *78*, 857-902.

Dumont, D.J., Jussila, L., Taipale, J., Lymboussaki, A., Mustonen, T., Pajusola, K., Breitman, M., and Alitalo, K. (1998). Cardiovascular failure in mouse embryos deficient in VEGF receptor-3. Science *282*, 946-949.

Ebos, J.M., Bocci, G., Man, S., Thorpe, P.E., Hicklin, D.J., Zhou, D., Jia, X., and Kerbel, R.S. (2004). A naturally occurring soluble form of vascular endothelial growth factor receptor 2 detected in mouse and human plasma. Mol Cancer Res *2*, 315-326.

Egeblad, M., and Werb, Z. (2002). New functions for the matrix metalloproteinases in cancer progression. Nat Rev Cancer *2*, 161-174.

Eliceiri, B.P., Puente, X.S., Hood, J.D., Stupack, D.G., Schlaepfer, D.D., Huang, X.Z., Sheppard, D., and Cheresh, D.A. (2002). Src-mediated coupling of focal adhesion kinase to integrin alpha(v)beta5 in vascular endothelial growth factor signaling. J Cell Biol *157*, 149-160.

Emr, S., Glick, B.S., Linstedt, A.D., Lippincott-Schwartz, J., Luini, A., Malhotra, V., Marsh, B.J., Nakano, A., Pfeffer, S.R., Rabouille, C., *et al.* (2009). Journeys through the Golgi--taking stock in a new era. J Cell Biol *187*, 449-453.

Ewan, L.C., Jopling, H.M., Jia, H., Mittar, S., Bagherzadeh, A., Howell, G.J., Walker, J.H., Zachary, I.C., and Ponnambalam, S. (2006). Intrinsic tyrosine kinase activity is required for vascular endothelial growth factor receptor 2 ubiquitination, sorting and degradation in endothelial cells. Traffic *7*, 1270-1282.

Fasanaro, P., D'Alessandra, Y., Di Stefano, V., Melchionna, R., Romani, S., Pompilio, G., Capogrossi, M.C., and Martelli, F. (2008). MicroRNA-210 modulates endothelial cell response to hypoxia and inhibits the receptor tyrosine kinase ligand Ephrin-A3. J Biol Chem *283*, 15878-15883.

Favier, B., Alam, A., Barron, P., Bonnin, J., Laboudie, P., Fons, P., Mandron, M., Herault, J.P., Neufeld, G., Savi, P., *et al.* (2006). Neuropilin-2 interacts with VEGFR-2 and VEGFR-3 and promotes human endothelial cell survival and migration. Blood *108*, 1243-1250.

Ferrara, N., Carver-Moore, K., Chen, H., Dowd, M., Lu, L., O'Shea, K.S., Powell-Braxton, L., Hillan, K.J., and Moore, M.W. (1996). Heterozygous embryonic lethality induced by targeted inactivation of the VEGF gene. Nature *380*, 439-442.

Ferrara, N., and Davis-Smyth, T. (1997). The biology of vascular endothelial growth factor. Endocr Rev *18*, 4-25.

Folkman, J. (1995). Angiogenesis in cancer, vascular, rheumatoid and other disease. Nat Med *1*, 27-31.

Folkman, J. (2002). Role of angiogenesis in tumor growth and metastasis. Semin Oncol *29*, 15-18.

Fong, G.H., Rossant, J., Gertsenstein, M., and Breitman, M.L. (1995). Role of the Flt-1 receptor tyrosine kinase in regulating the assembly of vascular endothelium. Nature *376*, 66-70.

Francis, S.E., Goh, K.L., Hodivala-Dilke, K., Bader, B.L., Stark, M., Davidson, D., and Hynes, R.O. (2002). Central roles of alpha5beta1 integrin and fibronectin in vascular development in mouse embryos and embryoid bodies. Arterioscler Thromb Vasc Biol *22*, 927-933.

Friedlander, M., Brooks, P.C., Shaffer, R.W., Kincaid, C.M., Varner, J.A., and Cheresh, D.A. (1995). Definition of two angiogenic pathways by distinct alpha v integrins. Science *270*, 1500-1502.

Fujisawa, H., Kitsukawa, T., Kawakami, A., Takagi, S., Shimizu, M., and Hirata, T. (1997). Roles of a neuronal cell-surface molecule, neuropilin, in nerve fiber fasciculation and guidance. Cell Tissue Res *290*, 465-470.

Gampel, A., Moss, L., Jones, M.C., Brunton, V., Norman, J.C., and Mellor, H. (2006). VEGF regulates the mobilization of VEGFR2/KDR from an intracellular endothelial storage compartment. Blood *108*, 2624-2631.

Garmy-Susini, B., Jin, H., Zhu, Y., Sung, R.J., Hwang, R., and Varner, J. (2005). Integrin alpha4beta1-VCAM-1-mediated adhesion between endothelial and mural cells is required for blood vessel maturation. J Clin Invest *115*, 1542-1551.

Gerhardt, H., and Betsholtz, C. (2003). Endothelial-pericyte interactions in angiogenesis. Cell Tissue Res *314*, 15-23.

Gerhardt, H., Golding, M., Fruttiger, M., Ruhrberg, C., Lundkvist, A., Abramsson, A., Jeltsch, M., Mitchell, C., Alitalo, K., Shima, D., *et al.* (2003). VEGF guides angiogenic sprouting utilizing endothelial tip cell filopodia. J Cell Biol *161*, 1163-1177.

Germain, S., Monnot, C., Muller, L., and Eichmann, A. (2010). Hypoxia-driven angiogenesis: role of tip cells and extracellular matrix scaffolding. Curr Opin Hematol *17*, 245-251.

Ghosh, P., Dahms, N.M., and Kornfeld, S. (2003). Mannose 6-phosphate receptors: new twists in the tale. Nat Rev Mol Cell Biol *4*, 202-212.

Grunewald, F.S., Prota, A.E., Giese, A., and Ballmer-Hofer, K. (2010). Structure-function analysis of VEGF receptor activation and the role of coreceptors in angiogenic signaling. Biochim Biophys Acta *1804*, 567-580.

Hallmann, R., Horn, N., Selg, M., Wendler, O., Pausch, F., and Sorokin, L.M. (2005). Expression and function of laminins in the embryonic and mature vasculature. Physiol Rev *85*, 979-1000.

Harris, T.A., Yamakuchi, M., Ferlito, M., Mendell, J.T., and Lowenstein, C.J. (2008). MicroRNA-126 regulates endothelial expression of vascular cell adhesion molecule 1. Proc Natl Acad Sci U S A *105*, 1516-1521.

Hiratsuka, S. (2011). Vasculogenensis, angiogenesis and special features of tumor blood vessels. Front Biosci *16*, 1413-1427.

Holmes, D.I., and Zachary, I.C. (2008). Vascular endothelial growth factor regulates stanniocalcin-1 expression via neuropilin-1-dependent regulation of KDR and synergism with fibroblast growth factor-2. Cell Signal *20*, 569-579.

Holmqvist, K., Cross, M., Riley, D., and Welsh, M. (2003). The Shb adaptor protein causes Src-dependent cell spreading and activation of focal adhesion kinase in murine brain endothelial cells. Cell Signal *15*, 171-179.

Holmqvist, K., Cross, M.J., Rolny, C., Hagerkvist, R., Rahimi, N., Matsumoto, T., Claesson-Welsh, L., and Welsh, M. (2004). The adaptor protein shb binds to tyrosine 1175 in vascular endothelial growth factor (VEGF) receptor-2 and regulates VEGF-dependent cellular migration. J Biol Chem *279*, 22267-22275.

Hong, W. (2005). SNAREs and traffic. Biochim Biophys Acta *1744*, 493-517.

Huang, K., Andersson, C., Roomans, G.M., Ito, N., and Claesson-Welsh, L. (2001). Signaling properties of VEGF receptor-1 and -2 homo- and heterodimers. Int J Biochem Cell Biol 33, 315-324.

Hughes, D.C. (2001). Alternative splicing of the human VEGFGR-3/FLT4 gene as a consequence of an integrated human endogenous retrovirus. J Mol Evol 53, 77-79.

Igarashi, K., Isohara, T., Kato, T., Shigeta, K., Yamano, T., and Uno, I. (1998). Tyrosine 1213 of Flt-1 is a major binding site of Nck and SHP-2. Biochem Biophys Res Commun 246, 95-99.

Iivanainen, E., Kahari, V.M., Heino, J., and Elenius, K. (2003). Endothelial cell-matrix interactions. Microsc Res Tech 60, 13-22.

Ito, N., Wernstedt, C., Engstrom, U., and Claesson-Welsh, L. (1998). Identification of vascular endothelial growth factor receptor-1 tyrosine phosphorylation sites and binding of SH2 domain-containing molecules. J Biol Chem 273, 23410-23418.

Jahn, R., and Scheller, R.H. (2006). SNAREs--engines for membrane fusion. Nat Rev Mol Cell Biol 7, 631-643.

Jopling, H.M., Odell, A.F., Hooper, N.M., Zachary, I.C., Walker, J.H., and Ponnambalam, S. (2009). Rab GTPase regulation of VEGFR2 trafficking and signaling in endothelial cells. Arterioscler Thromb Vasc Biol 29, 1119-1124.

Kaipainen, A., Korhonen, J., Mustonen, T., van Hinsbergh, V.W., Fang, G.H., Dumont, D., Breitman, M., and Alitalo, K. (1995). Expression of the fms-like tyrosine kinase 4 gene becomes restricted to lymphatic endothelium during development. Proc Natl Acad Sci U S A 92, 3566-3570.

Kalluri, R. (2003). Basement membranes: structure, assembly and role in tumour angiogenesis. Nat Rev Cancer 3, 422-433.

Kanno, S., Oda, N., Abe, M., Terai, Y., Ito, M., Shitara, K., Tabayashi, K., Shibuya, M., and Sato, Y. (2000). Roles of two VEGF receptors, Flt-1 and KDR, in the signal transduction of VEGF effects in human vascular endothelial cells. Oncogene 19, 2138-2146.

Kappas, N.C., Zeng, G., Chappell, J.C., Kearney, J.B., Hazarika, S., Kallianos, K.G., Patterson, C., Annex, B.H., and Bautch, V.L. (2008). The VEGF receptor Flt-1 spatially modulates Flk-1 signaling and blood vessel branching. J Cell Biol 181, 847-858.

Kawamura, H., Li, X., Goishi, K., van Meeteren, L.A., Jakobsson, L., Cebe-Suarez, S., Shimizu, A., Edholm, D., Ballmer-Hofer, K., Kjellen, L., et al. (2008). Neuropilin-1 in regulation of VEGF-induced activation of p38MAPK and endothelial cell organization. Blood 112, 3638-3649.

Kawasaki, T., Kitsukawa, T., Bekku, Y., Matsuda, Y., Sanbo, M., Yagi, T., and Fujisawa, H. (1999). A requirement for neuropilin-1 in embryonic vessel formation. Development 126, 4895-4902.

Kendall, R.L., Rutledge, R.Z., Mao, X., Tebben, A.J., Hungate, R.W., and Thomas, K.A. (1999). Vascular endothelial growth factor receptor KDR tyrosine kinase activity is increased by autophosphorylation of two activation loop tyrosine residues. J Biol Chem 274, 6453-6460.

Kendall, R.L., and Thomas, K.A. (1993). Inhibition of vascular endothelial cell growth factor activity by an endogenously encoded soluble receptor. Proc Natl Acad Sci U S A 90, 10705-10709.

Kendall, R.L., Wang, G., DiSalvo, J., and Thomas, K.A. (1994). Specificity of vascular endothelial cell growth factor receptor ligand binding domains. Biochem Biophys Res Commun 201, 326-330.

Kim, S., Bakre, M., Yin, H., and Varner, J.A. (2002). Inhibition of endothelial cell survival and angiogenesis by protein kinase A. J Clin Invest 110, 933-941.

Kim, S., Bell, K., Mousa, S.A., and Varner, J.A. (2000). Regulation of angiogenesis in vivo by ligation of integrin alpha5beta1 with the central cell-binding domain of fibronectin. Am J Pathol 156, 1345-1362.

Kim, V.N. (2005). MicroRNA biogenesis: coordinated cropping and dicing. Nat Rev Mol Cell Biol 6, 376-385.

Kobayashi, S., Sawano, A., Nojima, Y., Shibuya, M., and Maru, Y. (2004). The c-Cbl/CD2AP complex regulates VEGF-induced endocytosis and degradation of Flt-1 (VEGFR-1). FASEB J 18, 929-931.

Kuehbacher, A., Urbich, C., Zeiher, A.M., and Dimmeler, S. (2007). Role of Dicer and Drosha for endothelial microRNA expression and angiogenesis. Circ Res 101, 59-68.

Labrecque, L., Royal, I., Surprenant, D.S., Patterson, C., Gingras, D., and Beliveau, R. (2003). Regulation of vascular endothelial growth factor receptor-2 activity by caveolin-1 and plasma membrane cholesterol. Mol Biol Cell 14, 334-347.

Lampugnani, M.G., Orsenigo, F., Gagliani, M.C., Tacchetti, C., and Dejana, E. (2006). Vascular endothelial cadherin controls VEGFR-2 internalization and signaling from intracellular compartments. J Cell Biol 174, 593-604.

Lanahan, A.A., Hermans, K., Claes, F., Kerley-Hamilton, J.S., Zhuang, Z.W., Giordano, F.J., Carmeliet, P., and Simons, M. (2010). VEGF receptor 2 endocytic trafficking regulates arterial morphogenesis. Dev Cell 18, 713-724.

Lee, M.C., Miller, E.A., Goldberg, J., Orci, L., and Schekman, R. (2004). Bi-directional protein transport between the ER and Golgi. Annu Rev Cell Dev Biol 20, 87-123.

Lee, S., Chen, T.T., Barber, C.L., Jordan, M.C., Murdock, J., Desai, S., Ferrara, N., Nagy, A., Roos, K.P., and Iruela-Arispe, M.L. (2007). Autocrine VEGF signaling is required for vascular homeostasis. Cell 130, 691-703.

Levine, R.J., Maynard, S.E., Qian, C., Lim, K.H., England, L.J., Yu, K.F., Schisterman, E.F., Thadhani, R., Sachs, B.P., Epstein, F.H., et al. (2004). Circulating angiogenic factors and the risk of preeclampsia. N Engl J Med 350, 672-683.

Liao, Y.F., Gotwals, P.J., Koteliansky, V.E., Sheppard, D., and Van De Water, L. (2002). The EIIIA segment of fibronectin is a ligand for integrins alpha 9beta 1 and alpha 4beta 1 providing a novel mechanism for regulating cell adhesion by alternative splicing. J Biol Chem 277, 14467-14474.

Mahabeleshwar, G.H., Chen, J., Feng, W., Somanath, P.R., Razorenova, O.V., and Byzova, T.V. (2008). Integrin affinity modulation in angiogenesis. Cell Cycle 7, 335-347.

Manickam, V., Tiwari, A., Jung, J.J., Bhattacharya, R., Goel, A., Mukhopadhyay, D., and Choudhury, A. (2011). Regulation of vascular endothelial growth factor receptor 2 trafficking and angiogenesis by Golgi localized t-SNARE syntaxin 6. Blood 117, 1425-1435.

Marcinkiewicz, C., Taooka, Y., Yokosaki, Y., Calvete, J.J., Marcinkiewicz, M.M., Lobb, R.R., Niewiarowski, S., and Sheppard, D. (2000). Inhibitory effects of MLDG-containing heterodimeric disintegrins reveal distinct structural requirements for interaction of the integrin alpha 9beta 1 with VCAM-1, tenascin-C, and osteopontin. J Biol Chem *275*, 31930-31937.

Matsumoto, T., Bohman, S., Dixelius, J., Berge, T., Dimberg, A., Magnusson, P., Wang, L., Wikner, C., Qi, J.H., Wernstedt, C., *et al.* (2005). VEGF receptor-2 Y951 signaling and a role for the adapter molecule TSAd in tumor angiogenesis. EMBO J *24*, 2342-2353.

Matsumoto, T., and Claesson-Welsh, L. (2001). VEGF receptor signal transduction. Sci STKE *2001*, re21.

Matthews, W., Jordan, C.T., Gavin, M., Jenkins, N.A., Copeland, N.G., and Lemischka, I.R. (1991). A receptor tyrosine kinase cDNA isolated from a population of enriched primitive hematopoietic cells and exhibiting close genetic linkage to c-kit. Proc Natl Acad Sci U S A *88*, 9026-9030.

McCarthy, M. (2003). Antiangiogenesis drug promising for metastatic colorectal cancer. Lancet *361*, 1959.

Meadows, K.N., Bryant, P., and Pumiglia, K. (2001). Vascular endothelial growth factor induction of the angiogenic phenotype requires Ras activation. J Biol Chem *276*, 49289-49298.

Meyer, R.D., Sacks, D.B., and Rahimi, N. (2008). IQGAP1-dependent signaling pathway regulates endothelial cell proliferation and angiogenesis. PLoS One *3*, e3848.

Miao, H.Q., Lee, P., Lin, H., Soker, S., and Klagsbrun, M. (2000). Neuropilin-1 expression by tumor cells promotes tumor angiogenesis and progression. FASEB J *14*, 2532-2539.

Miao, H.Q., Soker, S., Feiner, L., Alonso, J.L., Raper, J.A., and Klagsbrun, M. (1999). Neuropilin-1 mediates collapsin-1/semaphorin III inhibition of endothelial cell motility: functional competition of collapsin-1 and vascular endothelial growth factor-165. J Cell Biol *146*, 233-242.

Mitra, S.K., Hanson, D.A., and Schlaepfer, D.D. (2005). Focal adhesion kinase: in command and control of cell motility. Nat Rev Mol Cell Biol *6*, 56-68.

Mitra, S.K., and Schlaepfer, D.D. (2006). Integrin-regulated FAK-Src signaling in normal and cancer cells. Curr Opin Cell Biol *18*, 516-523.

Mukherjee, S., Tessema, M., and Wandinger-Ness, A. (2006). Vesicular trafficking of tyrosine kinase receptors and associated proteins in the regulation of signaling and vascular function. Circ Res *98*, 743-756.

Nomura, M., Yamagishi, S., Harada, S., Hayashi, Y., Yamashima, T., Yamashita, J., and Yamamoto, H. (1995). Possible participation of autocrine and paracrine vascular endothelial growth factors in hypoxia-induced proliferation of endothelial cells and pericytes. J Biol Chem *270*, 28316-28324.

Nyberg, P., Xie, L., and Kalluri, R. (2005). Endogenous inhibitors of angiogenesis. Cancer Res *65*, 3967-3979.

Otsuka, M., Zheng, M., Hayashi, M., Lee, J.D., Yoshino, O., Lin, S., and Han, J. (2008). Impaired microRNA processing causes corpus luteum insufficiency and infertility in mice. J Clin Invest *118*, 1944-1954.

Peters, K.G., De Vries, C., and Williams, L.T. (1993). Vascular endothelial growth factor receptor expression during embryogenesis and tissue repair suggests a role in endothelial differentiation and blood vessel growth. Proc Natl Acad Sci U S A *90*, 8915-8919.

Risau, W. (1997). Mechanisms of angiogenesis. Nature *386*, 671-674.

Salameh, A., Galvagni, F., Bardelli, M., Bussolino, F., and Oliviero, S. (2005). Direct recruitment of CRK and GRB2 to VEGFR-3 induces proliferation, migration, and survival of endothelial cells through the activation of ERK, AKT, and JNK pathways. Blood *106*, 3423-3431.

Salikhova, A., Wang, L., Lanahan, A.A., Liu, M., Simons, M., Leenders, W.P., Mukhopadhyay, D., and Horowitz, A. (2008). Vascular endothelial growth factor and semaphorin induce neuropilin-1 endocytosis via separate pathways. Circ Res *103*, e71-79.

Sawano, A., Iwai, S., Sakurai, Y., Ito, M., Shitara, K., Nakahata, T., and Shibuya, M. (2001). Flt-1, vascular endothelial growth factor receptor 1, is a novel cell surface marker for the lineage of monocyte-macrophages in humans. Blood *97*, 785-791.

Sawano, A., Takahashi, T., Yamaguchi, S., and Shibuya, M. (1997). The phosphorylated 1169-tyrosine containing region of flt-1 kinase (VEGFR-1) is a major binding site for PLCgamma. Biochem Biophys Res Commun *238*, 487-491.

Scappaticci, F.A. (2002). Mechanisms and future directions for angiogenesis-based cancer therapies. J Clin Oncol *20*, 3906-3927.

Schlaepfer, D.D., and Hunter, T. (1998). Integrin signalling and tyrosine phosphorylation: just the FAKs? Trends Cell Biol *8*, 151-157.

Scott, A., and Mellor, H. (2009). VEGF receptor trafficking in angiogenesis. Biochem Soc Trans *37*, 1184-1188.

Senger, D.R., Perruzzi, C.A., Streit, M., Koteliansky, V.E., de Fougerolles, A.R., and Detmar, M. (2002). The alpha(1)beta(1) and alpha(2)beta(1) integrins provide critical support for vascular endothelial growth factor signaling, endothelial cell migration, and tumor angiogenesis. Am J Pathol *160*, 195-204.

Shalaby, F., Rossant, J., Yamaguchi, T.P., Gertsenstein, M., Wu, X.F., Breitman, M.L., and Schuh, A.C. (1995). Failure of blood-island formation and vasculogenesis in Flk-1-deficient mice. Nature *376*, 62-66.

Shibuya, M., Yamaguchi, S., Yamane, A., Ikeda, T., Tojo, A., Matsushime, H., and Sato, M. (1990). Nucleotide sequence and expression of a novel human receptor-type tyrosine kinase gene (flt) closely related to the fms family. Oncogene *5*, 519-524.

Singh, A.J., Meyer, R.D., Navruzbekov, G., Shelke, R., Duan, L., Band, H., Leeman, S.E., and Rahimi, N. (2007). A critical role for the E3-ligase activity of c-Cbl in VEGFR-2-mediated PLCgamma1 activation and angiogenesis. Proc Natl Acad Sci U S A *104*, 5413-5418.

Soker, S., Takashima, S., Miao, H.Q., Neufeld, G., and Klagsbrun, M. (1998). Neuropilin-1 is expressed by endothelial and tumor cells as an isoform-specific receptor for vascular endothelial growth factor. Cell *92*, 735-745.

Solowiej, J., Bergqvist, S., McTigue, M.A., Marrone, T., Quenzer, T., Cobbs, M., Ryan, K., Kania, R.S., Diehl, W., and Murray, B.W. (2009). Characterizing the effects of the juxtamembrane domain on vascular endothelial growth factor receptor-2 enzymatic activity, autophosphorylation, and inhibition by axitinib. Biochemistry *48*, 7019-7031.

Sorkin, A., and von Zastrow, M. (2009). Endocytosis and signalling: intertwining molecular networks. Nat Rev Mol Cell Biol *10*, 609-622.

Staniszewska, I., Zaveri, S., Del Valle, L., Oliva, I., Rothman, V.L., Croul, S.E., Roberts, D.D., Mosher, D.F., Tuszynski, G.P., and Marcinkiewicz, C. (2007). Interaction of alpha9beta1 integrin with thrombospondin-1 promotes angiogenesis. Circ Res *100*, 1308-1316.

Stupack, D.G., and Cheresh, D.A. (2004). Integrins and angiogenesis. Curr Top Dev Biol *64*, 207-238.

Suarez, Y., Fernandez-Hernando, C., Pober, J.S., and Sessa, W.C. (2007). Dicer dependent microRNAs regulate gene expression and functions in human endothelial cells. Circ Res *100*, 1164-1173.

Sudhof, T.C., and Rothman, J.E. (2009). Membrane fusion: grappling with SNARE and SM proteins. Science *323*, 474-477.

Takahashi, T., Yamaguchi, S., Chida, K., and Shibuya, M. (2001). A single autophosphorylation site on KDR/Flk-1 is essential for VEGF-A-dependent activation of PLC-gamma and DNA synthesis in vascular endothelial cells. EMBO J *20*, 2768-2778.

Tammela, T., Zarkada, G., Wallgard, E., Murtomaki, A., Suchting, S., Wirzenius, M., Waltari, M., Hellstrom, M., Schomber, T., Peltonen, R., *et al.* (2008). Blocking VEGFR-3 suppresses angiogenic sprouting and vascular network formation. Nature *454*, 656-660.

Tanjore, H., Zeisberg, E.M., Gerami-Naini, B., and Kalluri, R. (2008). Beta1 integrin expression on endothelial cells is required for angiogenesis but not for vasculogenesis. Dev Dyn *237*, 75-82.

Terman, B.I., Carrion, M.E., Kovacs, E., Rasmussen, B.A., Eddy, R.L., and Shows, T.B. (1991). Identification of a new endothelial cell growth factor receptor tyrosine kinase. Oncogene *6*, 1677-1683.

Tiwari, A., Jung, J.J., Inamdar, S.M., Brown, C.O., Goel, A., and Choudhury, A. (2011). Endothelial cell migration on fibronectin is regulated by syntaxin 6-mediated {alpha}5{beta}1 integrin recycling. J Biol Chem.

Tuma, P.L., and Hubbard, A.L. (2003). Transcytosis: crossing cellular barriers. Physiol Rev *83*, 871-932.

Uemura, A., Ogawa, M., Hirashima, M., Fujiwara, T., Koyama, S., Takagi, H., Honda, Y., Wiegand, S.J., Yancopoulos, G.D., and Nishikawa, S. (2002). Recombinant angiopoietin-1 restores higher-order architecture of growing blood vessels in mice in the absence of mural cells. J Clin Invest *110*, 1619-1628.

Vlahakis, N.E., Young, B.A., Atakilit, A., Hawkridge, A.E., Issaka, R.B., Boudreau, N., and Sheppard, D. (2007). Integrin alpha9beta1 directly binds to vascular endothelial growth factor (VEGF)-A and contributes to VEGF-A-induced angiogenesis. J Biol Chem *282*, 15187-15196.

Wang, F., Yamauchi, M., Muramatsu, M., Osawa, T., Tsuchida, R., and Shibuya, M. (2011). RACK1 regulates VEGF/Flt1-mediated cell migration via activation of a PI3K/Akt pathway. J Biol Chem *286*, 9097-9106.

Wang, S., and Olson, E.N. (2009). AngiomiRs--key regulators of angiogenesis. Curr Opin Genet Dev *19*, 205-211.

Warner, A.J., Lopez-Dee, J., Knight, E.L., Feramisco, J.R., and Prigent, S.A. (2000). The Shc-related adaptor protein, Sck, forms a complex with the vascular-endothelial-growth-factor receptor KDR in transfected cells. Biochem J *347*, 501-509.

Yamaoka-Tojo, M., Tojo, T., Kim, H.W., Hilenski, L., Patrushev, N.A., Zhang, L., Fukai, T., and Ushio-Fukai, M. (2006). IQGAP1 mediates VE-cadherin-based cell-cell contacts and VEGF signaling at adherence junctions linked to angiogenesis. Arterioscler Thromb Vasc Biol *26*, 1991-1997.

Yang, J.T., Rayburn, H., and Hynes, R.O. (1993). Embryonic mesodermal defects in alpha 5 integrin-deficient mice. Development *119*, 1093-1105.

Yang, J.T., Rayburn, H., and Hynes, R.O. (1995). Cell adhesion events mediated by alpha 4 integrins are essential in placental and cardiac development. Development *121*, 549-560.

Yang, W.J., Yang, D.D., Na, S., Sandusky, G.E., Zhang, Q., and Zhao, G. (2005). Dicer is required for embryonic angiogenesis during mouse development. J Biol Chem *280*, 9330-9335.

Yuan, L., Moyon, D., Pardanaud, L., Breant, C., Karkkainen, M.J., Alitalo, K., and Eichmann, A. (2002). Abnormal lymphatic vessel development in neuropilin 2 mutant mice. Development *129*, 4797-4806.

Zachary, I. (2003). VEGF signalling: integration and multi-tasking in endothelial cell biology. Biochem Soc Trans *31*, 1171-1177.

Permissions

The contributors of this book come from diverse backgrounds, making this book a truly international effort. This book will bring forth new frontiers with its revolutionizing research information and detailed analysis of the nascent developments around the world.

We would like to thank Charles H. Lawrie, for lending his expertise to make the book truly unique. He has played a crucial role in the development of this book. Without his invaluable contribution this book wouldn't have been possible. He has made vital efforts to compile up to date information on the varied aspects of this subject to make this book a valuable addition to the collection of many professionals and students.

This book was conceptualized with the vision of imparting up-to-date information and advanced data in this field. To ensure the same, a matchless editorial board was set up. Every individual on the board went through rigorous rounds of assessment to prove their worth. After which they invested a large part of their time researching and compiling the most relevant data for our readers. Conferences and sessions were held from time to time between the editorial board and the contributing authors to present the data in the most comprehensible form. The editorial team has worked tirelessly to provide valuable and valid information to help people across the globe.

Every chapter published in this book has been scrutinized by our experts. Their significance has been extensively debated. The topics covered herein carry significant findings which will fuel the growth of the discipline. They may even be implemented as practical applications or may be referred to as a beginning point for another development. Chapters in this book were first published by InTech; hereby published with permission under the Creative Commons Attribution License or equivalent.

The editorial board has been involved in producing this book since its inception. They have spent rigorous hours researching and exploring the diverse topics which have resulted in the successful publishing of this book. They have passed on their knowledge of decades through this book. To expedite this challenging task, the publisher supported the team at every step. A small team of assistant editors was also appointed to further simplify the editing procedure and attain best results for the readers.

Our editorial team has been hand-picked from every corner of the world. Their multi-ethnicity adds dynamic inputs to the discussions which result in innovative outcomes. These outcomes are then further discussed with the researchers and contributors who give their valuable feedback and opinion regarding the same. The feedback is then collaborated with the researches and they are edited in a comprehensive manner to aid the understanding of the subject.

Apart from the editorial board, the designing team has also invested a significant amount of their time in understanding the subject and creating the most relevant covers. They scrutinized every image to scout for the most suitable representation of the subject and create an appropriate cover for the book.

The publishing team has been involved in this book since its early stages. They were actively engaged in every process, be it collecting the data, connecting with the contributors or procuring relevant information. The team has been an ardent support to the editorial, designing and production team. Their endless efforts to recruit the best for this project, has resulted in the accomplishment of this book. They are a veteran in the field of academics and their pool of knowledge is as vast as their experience in printing. Their expertise and guidance has proved useful at every step. Their uncompromising quality standards have made this book an exceptional effort. Their encouragement from time to time has been an inspiration for everyone.

The publisher and the editorial board hope that this book will prove to be a valuable piece of knowledge for researchers, students, practitioners and scholars across the globe.

List of Contributors

Katja Fiedler and Cornelia Brunner
University Ulm, Germany

Goossens Steven and Haigh J. Jody
VIB and Ghent University, Belgium

Laura Velazquez
UMR U978 Inserm/Université Paris 13, UFR SMBH, Bobigny, France

Vladan P. Čokić and Gordana Jovčić
Laboratory of Experimental Hematology, Institute for Medical Research, Belgrade, Serbia

Bojana B. Beleslin-Čokić
Clinic of Endocrinology, Diabetes and Diseases of Metabolism, School of Medicine, University Clinical Center, Belgrade, Serbia

Raj K. Puri
Division of Cellular and Gene Therapies, Center for Biologics Evaluation and Research, Food and Drug Administration, Bethesda, USA

Alan N. Schechter
Molecular Medicine Branch, National Institute of Diabetes and Digestive and Kidney Diseases, National Institutes of Health, Bethesda, USA

Daniel Jimenez-Teja, Nadia Martin-Blanco and Matilde Canelles
Instituto de Parasitología y Biomedicina, CSIC, P. T. Ciencias de la Salud, Granada, Spain

Amanda Chen and W. Beau Mitchell
Laboratory of Platelet Biology, New York Blood Center, USA

Haiqiang Yu and Haiteng Deng
Proteomics Resources Center, The Rockefeller University, USA

Doris Cerecedo
Laboratorio de Hematobiología, Escuela Nacional de Medicina y Homeopatía, Instituto Politécnico Nacional (IPN), México DF, México

Sara Massena and Mia Phillipson
Department of Medical Cell Biology, Integrative Physiology, Uppsala University, Sweden

Kamalvishnu P. Gottimukkala, Mithila Burute and Sanjeev Galande
Indian Institute of Science Education and Research, Sai Trinity, Garware Circle, Pashan, Pune, India

Ajit Tiwari, Jae-Joon Jung, Shivangi M. Inamdar and Amit Choudhury
Department of Anatomy and Cell Biology, University of Iowa, Iowa City, USA